6·5·00
$63.-

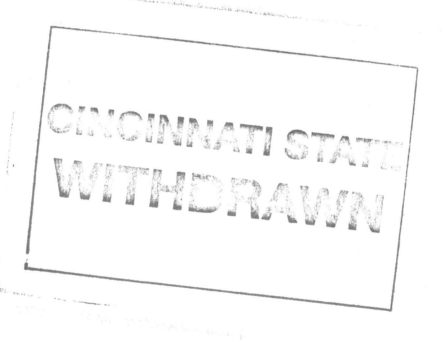

Back and Neck
DISORDERS
SOURCEBOOK

Health Reference Series

Volume Twenty-four

Back and Neck
DISORDERS
SOURCEBOOK

*Basic Information about
Disorders and Injuries of the
Spinal Cord and Vertebrae,
Including Facts on Chiropractic
Treatment, Surgical Interventions,
Paralysis, and Rehabilitation,
Along with Advice for Preventing
Back Trouble*

Edited by
Karen Bellenir

Omnigraphics, Inc.

Penobscot Building / Detroit, MI 48226

BIBLIOGRAPHIC NOTE

Since this page cannot legibly accommodate all the copyright notices, the Preface constitutes an extension of the copyright notice.

Edited by Karen Bellenir

Peter D. Dresser, Managing Editor, *Health Reference Series*

Omnigraphics, Inc.

Matthew P. Barbour, *Production Manager*
Laurie Lanzen Harris, *Vice President, Editorial*
Peter E. Ruffner, *Vice President, Administration*
James A. Sellgren, *Vice President, Operations and Finance*
Jane J. Steele, *Marketing Consultant*

Frederick G. Ruffner, Jr., *Publisher*

Copyright © 1997, Omnigraphics, Inc.

Library of Congress Cataloging-in-Publication Data

Back and neck disorders sourcebook ; basic information about
    disorders and injuries of the spinal cord and vertebrae,
    including facts on chiropractic treatment, surgical
    interventions, paralysis, and rehabilitation, along with advice
    for preventing back trouble / edited by Karen Bellenir.
        p. cm. -- (Health reference series ; v. 24)
    Includes bibliographical references and index.
    ISBN 0-7808-0202-0
    1. Spine--Diseases--Popular works. 2. Spinal cord--Wounds
and injuries--Popular works. 3. Spine--Abnormalities--Popular
works. 4. Neck--Diseases--Popular works. I. Bellenir, Karen.
II. Series.
RD766.B28 1997   97-1006
616.7'3--dc21   CIP

∞

This book is printed on acid-free paper meeting the ANSI Z39.48 Standard. The infinity symbol that appears above indicates that the paper in this book meets that standard.

Printed in the United States

Contents

Preface ix

Part I: General Information about the Spinal Column

Chapter 1—Anatomy of a Backache 3
Chapter 2—Straighten Up and Stay Healthy: A Perfect
              Posture Guide for Everyone 11
Chapter 3—Physical Fitness and Healthy Low Back
              Function 19
Chapter 4—Glossary of Back and Neck Terms 29

Part II: Disorders of the Back and Neck

Chapter 5—Back Talk: Advice for Suffering Spines 45
Chapter 6—Acute and Chronic Low Back Pain 55
Chapter 7—Sciatica 73
Chapter 8—Spina Bifida 85
Chapter 9—Scoliosis 89
Chapter 10—Degenerative Problems of the Back 95
Chapter 11—Spinal Stenosis 99
Chapter 12—Osteoporosis 103
Chapter 13—Syringomyelia 125
Chapter 14—Spondylitis 133
Chapter 15—Spinal Cord Tumors 155

Chapter 16—Neck Pain and Disorders of the Cervical
  Spine 181
Chapter 17—Spasmodic Torticollis 185
Chapter 18—Stiff Neck: An Occupational Hazard 189

Part III: Treatment and Rehabilitation

Chapter 19—Treatment for Acute Low Back Problems
  in Adults 195
Chapter 20—Motion and Progress in Low-Back Pain 219
Chapter 21—General Information about Physical
  Therapy 231
Chapter 22—Herniated Disk: New Laser Therapy Is
  More Efficient and Rapid than Standard
  Technique 239
Chapter 23—Back Surgery 243
Chapter 24—Pedicle Screws 253
Chapter 25—Electrical Bone-Growth Stimulation and
  Spinal Fusion 267
Chapter 26—What to Do About a Pain in the Neck 275

Part IV: Chiropractic Care

Chapter 27—Basic Facts about Chiropractic 283
Chapter 28—What Is Manipulation? 287
Chapter 29—Advice from the International Chiropractors
  Association on Whiplash and Arm and
  Shoulder Pain 291
Chapter 30—Chiropractic Offers Long-Term Headache
  Relief 297
Chapter 31—Studies Regarding the Effectiveness of
  Chiropractic Care 299
Chapter 32—Glossary of Chiropractic Terms 305

Part V: Information for Spinal Cord Injury Patients

Chapter 33—Spinal Cord Injuries: Causes and Statistics 311
Chapter 34—General Spinal Cord Injury Anatomy and
  Physiology 323

Chapter 35—Psychosocial Adjustment to a Spinal
　　　　　　　Cord Injury 341
Chapter 36—Sexuality and Spinal Cord Injuries 371
Chapter 37—Chronic Pain Management for People
　　　　　　　with Spinal Cord Injuries 389
Chapter 38—Spinal Cord Injuries: Science Meets
　　　　　　　Challenge 403
Chapter 39—Milestones in Spinal Cord Injury
　　　　　　　Research 413
Chapter 40—What's New in Spinal Cord Injury Cure
　　　　　　　and Treatment Research 421
Chapter 41—Disability and Social Security 437
Chapter 42—Information for the Air Traveler with a
　　　　　　　Spinal Cord Injury 451
Chapter 43—Assistive Technology for People with
　　　　　　　Spinal Cord Injuries 473
Chapter 44—The National Spinal Cord Injury Hotline
　　　　　　　and Other Resources for People with Spinal
　　　　　　　Cord Injuries 487

Appendix: Other Sources for Further Help and Information

Chapter 45—Public Education Books and Videos on
　　　　　　　Low Back Pain 511
Chapter 46—Directory of National Information Sources
　　　　　　　and Related Services for Back Patients 513

Index **525**

Preface

About This Book

The spinal column is one of the most vital parts of the human body. When its function is impaired, the consequences can be painful and even disabling. According to estimates, about 80 percent of Americans will experience low back pain at least once in their lives. Some will develop chronic or degenerative spinal disorders. In addition, trauma-related spinal cord injuries leave another 8,000 Americans paralyzed every year.

This book presents basic information for the back and neck patient, his or her family members, and other interested laypeople. Topics include the function of the spinal column, specific back and neck disorders, treatment options, rehabilitation, research, and sources of additional information.

Bibliographic Note

This volume contains publications issued by the following government agencies: Agency for Health Care Policy and Research (AHCPR); Food and Drug Administration (FDA); National Information Center for Children and Youth with Disabilities; National Institute of Arthritis and Musculoskeletal and Skin Disease (NIAMS); National Institute on Disability and Rehabilitation Research (NIDRR); National Institute of Neurological Disorders and Stroke (NINDS); President's

Council on Physical Fitness and Sports; Social Security Administration; and the U.S. Department of Transportation.

This volume also contains copyrighted documents from the following organizations: Abledata, American Chiropractic Association, American Paralysis Association, American Physical Therapy Association, International Chiropractors Association, The Johns Hopkins Medical Institutions, KRA Corporation, National Board of Chiropractic Examiners, National Osteoporosis Foundation, National Rehabilitation Information Center, National Spinal Cord Injury Association, National Spinal Cord Injury Statistical Center, Paralyzed Veterans of America, The Research and Training Center on Independent Living, and the Spondylitis Association of America.

Copyrighted articles from the following journals are also included: *Arthritis Today*, *Chiropractic Online Today*, *Consumer Reports Health Letter*, *The Johns Hopkins Medical Letter*, *Mayo Clinic Health Letter*, *Modern Medicine*, *Patient Care*, *The Physician and Sportsmedicine*, and the *Washington Post*.

All copyrighted material is reprinted with permission. Document numbers where applicable and specific source citations are provided on the first page of each chapter. Every effort has been made to secure all necessary rights to reprint the copyrighted material. If any omissions have been made, contact Omnigraphics to make corrections for future editions.

How to Use this Book

This book is divided into parts and chapters. Parts focus on broad areas of interest. Chapters are devoted to single topics within a part.

Part I: General Information about the Spinal Column provides important anatomical information, advice on posture, and tips for exercising to maintain spinal health. The glossary of neck and back terms in this section will help readers understand the terms used throughout this book.

Part II: Disorders of the Back and Neck describes common, specific and non-specific spinal ailments such as low back pain, sciatica, spinal stenosis, spondylitis, and spasmodic torticollis.

Part III: Treatment and Rehabilitation provides explanations of many of the different kinds of treatment options available to back and neck patients.

Part IV: Chiropractic Care offers answers to many questions about the common, and sometimes controversial, practice of chiropractic care.

Part V: Information for Spinal Cord Injury Patients describes different types of spinal cord injuries, their possible outcomes, coping strategies for patients facing long-term disabilities, and resources for additional assistance. The section also includes reports on current research initiatives and information about assistive technologies.

The *Appendix* provides lists of resources and organizations able to offer further help and information.

Acknowledgements

Several people and organizations contributed the materials that make up the information in this book. The editor gratefully acknowledges the assistance and cooperation of Abledata, American Chiropractic Association, American Paralysis Association, American Physical Therapy Association, International Chiropractors Association, The Johns Hopkins Medical Institutions, KRA Corporation, National Board of Chiropractic Examiners, National Osteoporosis Foundation, National Rehabilitation Information Center, National Spinal Cord Injury Association, National Spinal Cord Injury Statistical Center, Paralyzed Veterans of America, The Research and Training Center on Independent Living, and the Spondylitis Association of America. In addition, thanks go to Margaret Mary Missar for obtaining many of the documents reproduced in this volume, to Matthew Barbour for his Internet expertise, and to Bruce the Scanman for all his production assistance and guidance.

Note from the Editor

This book is part of Omnigraphics' *Health Reference Series*. The series provides basic information about a broad range of medical concerns. It is not intended to serve as a tool for diagnosing illness, in prescribing treatments, or as a substitute for the physician/patient relationship. All persons concerned about medical symptoms or the possibility of disease are encouraged to seek professional care from an appropriate health care provider.

Part One

General Information about the Spinal Column

Chapter 1

Anatomy of a Backache

The Spine and Its Parts

Knowing a little about the spine and its parts makes it easier to understand why things can go wrong with the back. Though humans are born with 33 separate vertebrae (the bones that form the spine), by adulthood most have only 24. The nine vertebrae at the base of the spine grow together. Five form a triangular bone called the sacrum—those two dimples in most everyone's back are where the sacrum joins the hipbones (the sacroiliac joint). The lowest four form the tailbone, or coccyx, often united with the sacrum above.

Physicians use a code to identify the vertebrae. The seven in the neck, the cervical vertebrae that support and provide movement for the head, are called C1 to C7. The thoracic vertebrae, numbered T1 to T12, join with and are supported by the ribs, which protect the heart and lungs. Because they're fairly rigid, thoracic vertebrae don't permit much movement, and, consequently, aren't injured as often as the other vertebrae. The lumbar vertebrae, below the thoracic vertebrae and above the sacrum, are most frequently involved in back pain, because they carry most of the body's stress. They are known as L1 to L5.

Text for this chapter is taken from *FDA Consumer*, April 1989, and *Low Back Pain*, a Johns Hopkins White Paper, ©1996 Medletter Associates, Inc.; reprinted with permission. Illustrations are taken from *FDA Consumer*, April 1989, NIH 81-160, NIH 93-504, and AHCPR Pub. No. 95-0644.

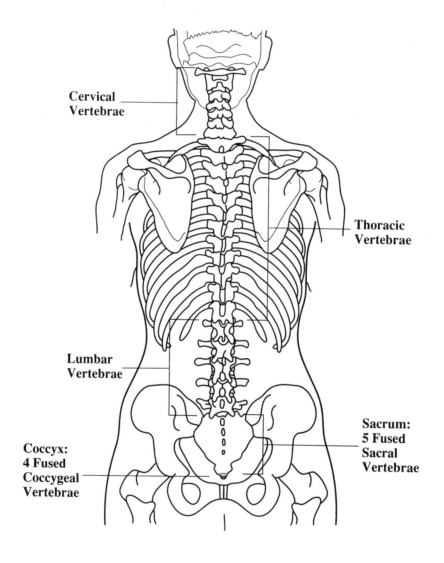

Cervical
Vertebrae

Thoracic
Vertebrae

Lumbar
Vertebrae

Sacrum:
5 Fused
Sacral
Vertebrae

Coccyx:
4 Fused
Coccygeal
Vertebrae

Figure 1.1. *Parts of the spine.*

Spinal Architecture

The architecture of the spine provides both strength and flexibility. Each vertebra meets its neighbor at a slight angle, resulting in an S-shaped curvature that helps to absorb the shock of movement, but still provides stable support. Between each vertebra is a flexible pad (intervertebral disk) that supplies further cushioning against shock and contributes to the spine's great range of motion.

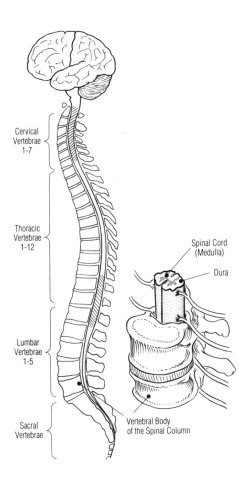

Cervical Vertebrae 1-7

Thoracic Vertebrae 1-12

Spinal Cord (Medulla)

Dura

Lumbar Vertebrae 1-5

Sacral Vertebrae

Vertebral Body of the Spinal Column

Figure 1.2. *The cervical vertebrae are numbered C1 to C7. The thoracic vertebrae are numbered T1 to T12. The lumbar vertebrae are numbered L1 to L5.*

The vertebrae grow progressively larger and stronger from top to bottom. The smallest—the cervical vertebrae—have the greatest flexibility, allowing easy movement of the neck in all directions. The thoracic vertebrae are slightly larger to support the weight of the arms and trunk. Performing the majority of the back's weight-bearing task are the lumbar vertebrae—the thickest and sturdiest in the spine. Because the lumbar region endures the highest stress, it is the most

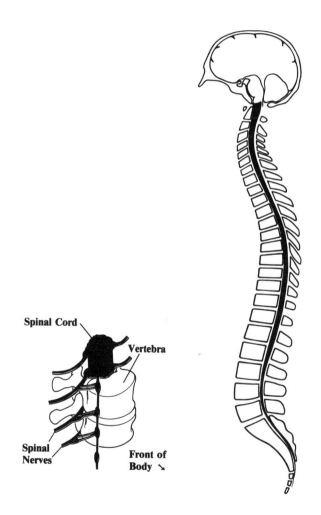

Figure 1.3. *The spinal cord extends from the brain to the lower back. The detail shows the snug fit of the cord inside the spinal column. Both incoming and outgoing nerve signals are carried in the spinal nerves which exit from the sides of the cord through the spaces between the vertebrae.*

common site for back pain. At the base, the sacrum and coccyx affix to the pelvic bones in the hip to form a solid pedestal for the entire structure.

The vertebrae are held together by the ligaments running down the length of the spine, as well as those that attach at the facet joints — the points where the bony processes jutting from the rear of each vertebra connect to one another. This intricate, interlocking design creates a rigid, stable shell to protect the delicate spinal cord, while allowing the spinal nerves to emerge through small openings between each vertebra.

The spinal cord, an extension of the brain, extends as far as L1, where it ends in a sheaf of nerves (cauda equina) resembling a horse's tail. Throughout the length of the spine, 31 pairs of nerves branch off from the spinal cord and serve all parts of the body, transmitting sensory messages to the brain (the pot is hot), and messages from the brain to the muscles (withdraw your hand). Where the nerves exit from the spinal cord through spaces (foramina) between adjacent vertebrae they are called nerve roots. Few people are aware that when the neck is bent forward as far as it will go, the whole spinal cord moves upwards in the spinal canal. Anything that prevents the cord and nerves from moving freely, such as abnormal bone growth within the spinal canal, will cause tingling or pain.

Spinal Disks

Sandwiched between each pair of adjacent vertebrae is a spinal disc, 23 discs in all. Discs are flat, round structures — about one-quarter to three-quarters of an inch thick — of tough outer rings of tissue that contain a soft, white jelly-like center. Each disc is connected to the vertebrae above and below it by flat, circular plates of cartilage. The discs not only keep the vertebra apart, but act as shock absorbers. They compress when weight is put on them, and spring back when the weight is removed.

While we need the strong, solid parts of the lumbar vertebrae (vertebral bodies) to bear the body's weight, only joints will allow us to bend backward and forward, twist and turn. These joints are found in a ring-like structure of bone, known as the arch, at the rear of each vertebra. The arch has a hollow center and little bones that go off in several directions, serving as anchors for muscles and ligaments. A pair of vertical bones projecting upward and another pair projecting downward — the facet joints — glide on similar smooth-surfaced bones in the vertebrae above and below them, creating an interlocking column of bones. The hollow areas of the arches form a channel (spinal canal) that encloses and protects the spinal cord. The only parts of the spine that we can feel with our fingers are projections from the bony rings called spinous (thorn-like) processes. Each spinous process bends down slightly over the one below to form an extra shield for the spinal cord.

Disks and Muscles: How the Spine Moves

The remarkable flexibility of the spine—which can bend forward, backward, and sideways, as well as rotate—is largely made possible by the intricate construction of the intervertebral disks. The outer ring, or annulus fibrosus, of each disk is made up of many overlapping layers of collagen fibers which expand and contract as the body moves. Each layer of fibers extends at an angle from one vertebra to the next, and criss-crosses with the next layer of fibers, which lies in the opposite direction. This alternating structure permits movement in any direction.

Inside the annulus is a gel-like center, called the nucleus pulposus. Its high water content not only exerts outward pressure against the annulus—keeping the fibers taut enough to support the spine—but also allows the nucleus to change shape as the disk bends. While each individual disk can only bend to a limited degree, their combined flexibility permits a great range of motion.

Despite the elasticity of the disks, however, it would be impossible for the back to bend without the assistance of the ligaments running down the front and rear of the spine and the enveloping layers of back and abdominal muscles. The tough, fibrous ligaments hold the disks and vertebrae in place even as they bend and twist, and the muscles supply stability and strength to absorb much of the stress of movement. The innermost layer of back muscles and disks stretch to reinforce the spine as it bends.

Major Causes of Back Pain

Thirty-three vertebrae, 23 discs, 31 pairs of spinal nerves, 140 muscles that hook on to the vertebrae, plus ligaments, tendons, cartilage—all very complicated and all potential sources of back trouble.

The four most frequent causes of back pain in older adults are degenerative changes of the spine, spinal stenosis, vertebral compression fracture, and herniated disk. Although they may cause similar symptoms, each of these conditions affects the vertebrae and disks differently.

Degenerative Changes

Degenerative changes result from years of wear and tear on the disks and facet joints. Disks begin to lose moisture and shrink, decreasing the cushion between the vertebrae and pushing the facet joints out of alignment. This added stress leads to the development of bony outgrowths known as osteophytes or bone spurs. In addition, the cartilage lining the facet joints may wear away, causing a roughening of the bone.

Spinal Stenosis

Spinal stenosis is most commonly caused by an osteophyte that grows large enough to narrow the spinal canal (central stenosis) or

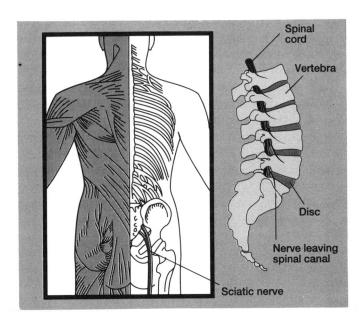

Figure 1.4. The lower part of the back holds most of the body's weight. Even a minor problem with the bones, muscles, ligaments or tendons in this area can cause pain when a person stands, bends, or moves around. Less often, a problem with a disc can pinch or irritate a nerve from the spinal cord, causing pain that runs down the leg, below the knee called sciatica.

one of the smaller exit canals through which spinal nerves branch away (lateral stenosis). In central stenosis, the outgrowth of bone impinges on the spinal cord or cauda equina, causing localized back pain that may radiate down one or both legs; lateral stenosis entraps a spinal nerve, resulting in pain along the path of the affected nerve.

Vertebral Compression Fracture

Aging may lead to osteoporosis—a loss of bone density that greatly weakens bones throughout the body. One serious complication of this disorder is a vertebral compression fracture, in which minor trauma, such as a sneeze, causes a fragile vertebra to collapse forward into a wedge shape. This may cause no symptoms, but can result in sudden, intense pain in the region of the fracture or elsewhere in the body if pain is referred along a compressed nerve.

Herniated Disk

Minor trauma may also cause a herniated disk in a spine weakened by degenerative changes. Commonly known as a "slipped disk," herniation occurs when the inner core (nucleus pulposus) of the disk bulges out through the thinned outer shell (annulus fibrosus), causing local back pain. If the protruding disk presses on a spinal nerve, pain may spread to the area of the body served by that nerve.

Between each vertebra in the spine, a pair of spinal nerves branches off from the spinal cord to a specific part of the body. Any portion of the skin that experiences hot or cold, pain, or touch refers that sensation to the brain via one of these nerves. In turn, pressure on a spinal nerve—resulting, for example, from a herniated disk—causes pain in the portion of the body served by that nerve. By determining the precise areas of pain and testing for loss of sensation in the legs and buttocks, doctors can pinpoint the spinal nerve that is entrapped.

Chapter 2

Straighten Up and Stay Healthy: A Perfect Posture Guide for Everyone

Good Posture Is Good Health

We're a health conscious society today and good posture is a part of it. Because good posture means your bones are properly aligned and your muscles, joints and ligaments can work as nature intended. It means your vital organs are in the right position and can function at peak efficiency. Good posture helps contribute to the normal functioning of the nervous system.

Without good posture, your overall health and total efficiency may be compromised. Because the long-term effects of poor posture can affect bodily systems (such as digestion, elimination, breathing, muscles, joints and ligaments), a person who has poor posture may often be tired or unable to work efficiently or move properly.

Even for younger people, how you carry yourself when working, relaxing, or playing can have big effects. Did you know that just fifteen minutes reading or typing when using the wrong positions exhausts the muscles of your neck, shoulders and upper back?

Poor Posture—How Does It Happen?

Often, poor posture develops because of accidents or falls. But bad posture can also develop from environmental factors or bad habits. This means that you have control.

International Chiropractors Association, nd; reprinted with permission.

Today, posture-related problems are increasing—

- as we become a society that watches more television than any previous generation;

- as we become a more electronic society, with more and more people working at sedentary, desk jobs or sitting in front of computer terminals;

- as more and more cars are crowding our roads, resulting in accidents and injuries;

- and as we drive in cars with poorly designed seats.

In most cases, poor posture results from a combination of several factors, which can include:

1. Accidents, injuries and falls.
2. Poor sleep support (mattress).
3. Excessive weight.
4. Visual or emotional difficulties.
5. Foot problems or improper shoes.
6. Weak muscles, muscle imbalance.
7. Careless sitting, standing, sleeping habits.
8. Negative self image.
9. Occupational stress.
10. Poorly designed work space.

Poor Posture and Pain

A lifetime of poor posture can start a progression of symptoms in the average adult. It can start with ...

- **Fatigue**—your muscles have to work hard just to hold you up if you have poor posture. You waste energy just moving, leaving you without the extra energy you need to feel good.

- **Tight, achy muscles in the neck, back, arms and legs**—by this stage, there may be a change in your muscles and ligaments and you may have a stiff, tight painful feeling. More than 80% of the neck and back problems are the result of tight, achy muscles brought on by years of bad posture.

12

- **Joint stiffness and pain**—at risk for "wear-and-tear" arthritis, or what is termed degenerative osteoarthritis. Poor posture and limited mobility increase the likelihood of this condition in later years.

Self-Test for Posture Problems

The Wall Test

Stand with the back of your head touching the wall and your heels six inches from the baseboard. With your buttocks touching the wall, check the distance with your hand between your lower back and the wall, and your neck and the wall. If you can get within an inch or two at the low back and two inches at the neck, you are close to having excellent posture. It not, your posture may need professional attention to restore the normal curves of your spine.

The Mirror Test

Front view. Stand facing a full length mirror and check to see if: 1. your shoulders are level, 2. your head is straight, 3. the spaces between your arms and sides seem equal, 4. your hips are level, your kneecaps face straight ahead, and 5. your ankles are straight.

Side view. This is much easier to do with the help of another, or by taking a photo. Check for the following: 1. head is erect, not slumping forward or backwards, 2. chin is parallel to the floor, not tilting up or down, 3. shoulders are in line with ears, not drooping forward or pulled back, 4. stomach is flat, 5. knees are straight, 6. lower back has a slightly forward curve (not too flat or not curved too much forward, creating a hollow back).

The 'Jump' Test. Feel the muscles of your neck and shoulders. Do you find areas that are tender and sensitive? Are the buttock muscles sore when you apply pressure? What about the chest muscles?

Lifestyle Tips for Lifelong Good Posture

- **Keep your weight down**—Excess weight, especially around the middle, pulls on the back, weakening stomach muscles.

- **Develop a regular program of exercise**—Regular exercise keeps you flexible and helps tone your muscles to support proper posture.

- **Buy good bedding**—A firm mattress will support the spine and help maintain the same shape as a person with good upright posture.

- **Pay attention to injuries from bumps, falls and jars**—injuries in youth may cause growth abnormalities or postural adaptations to the injury or pain that can show up later in life.

- **Have your eyes examined**—a vision problem can affect the way you carry yourself as well as cause eye strain.

- **Be conscious of where you work**—is your chair high enough to fit your desk? Do you need a footrest to keep pressure off your legs?

What Does Perfect Posture Look Like?

Normal Posture

Perfect standing posture is when the following are properly aligned—the points between your eyes, chin, collarbone, breastbone, pubic area and midpoint between your ankles.

- from the side, you can easily see the three natural curves in your back

- from the front, your shoulders, hips and knees are of equal height

- your head is held straight, not tilted or turned to one side

- from the back, the little bumps of your spine should be in a straight line down the center of your back.

Obviously, no one spends all day in this position. But, if you naturally assume a relaxed standing posture, you will carry yourself in a more balanced position and with less stress in your other activities.

14

Poor Posture

When you have poor posture, the body's proper vertical position is out of alignment and the back's natural curves become distorted.

Head Forward or Slouched Posture:

- rounded shoulders
- head forward, rounded upper back
- arched lower back
- protruding buttocks
- chest flattens
- abdominal organs sag, crowding and making more work for heart and lungs
- seen often in women who have osteoporosis in later years

Military Posture:

- head pulled back
- shoulder blades tightly pulled back
- arched lower back
- knees locked (straight)
- minimizes the spinal column's ability to be a shock absorber for the body

Slumped Sitting Posture:

- upper back humped or too rounded
- head forward
- rounded lower back
- often starts in teenage years

Kids, Parents and Posture

Standing up straight is important for everyone, but at no time is it more crucial to develop the habits of good posture than in childhood. Many adults with chronic back pain can trace the problem to years of bad posture habits or injuries in childhood.

Because they are growing and more active, children may be at even more risk for injury to the back and spine. According to studies, there is a significantly high risk associated with football, trampolining and gymnastics. More than 1/3 of all high school football players sustain some type of injury. As a parent, seek professional help for children in the event of even a minor sports injury. Parents should also be aware that babies who are not strapped into an auto safety seat run the risk of injury and even death in the event of a quick stop or an accident.

Good Posture and Aging

Poor posture extracts a high price as you age because it can:

- **Limit your range of motion**—muscles can be permanently shortened or stretched when a slumped over position becomes your normal position. Muscles and ligaments that have been shortened or stretched no longer function as they should.

- **Increase discomfort and pain**—it can often cause headaches and pain in the shoulders, arms, hands and around the eyes resulting from a forward-head position. Rounded shoulders can trigger the headaches at the base of your skull where the shoulder muscles attach.

- **Create pain in the jaw**—a forward-head position can lead to jaw pain. This kind of pain (known as TMJ, temporomandibular joint disease) was once considered only a dental problem. Today we know that TMJ pain also may be caused or aggravated by faulty posture.

- **Decrease lung capacity**—reducing the amount of oxygen in your body can decrease the space in your chest cavity, restricting efficient functioning of your lungs.

- **Cause low back pain**—one of the most common consequences of bad posture. For people over 35, low back pain is often interpreted as a sure sign of age, although it may have been developing since childhood.

- **Cause nerve interference**—Your spine is the basis of your posture. If your posture is bad, your spine can be misaligned. Spinal misalignments may cause interference in nerve function.

- **Affect proper bowel function**—even this important bodily task may be affected by faulty posture. If you have a rounded shoulder, head-forward posture, it may affect your bowels. If your spine arches and sways forward, your intestines may sag and cause constipation.

- **Make you look older than you are**—when you are slumped over, or hunched over, not standing straight, you can add years to your appearance. For women, the more rounded the shoulders, the more breasts may sag. Any woman, no matter what her age, can help reduce the sag in her breasts by nearly 50% by simply standing tall.

Improving Your Posture

- **When standing**—hold your head high, chin firmly forward, shoulders back, chest out, and stomach tucked in to increase your balance. If you stand all day in a job like a cashier or clerk, rest one foot on a stool or take breaks to get off your feet for a while.

- **When sitting**—use a chair with firm low-back support. Keep desk or table top elbow high, adjust the chair or use a footrest to keep pressure off the back of the legs, and keep your knees a little higher than your hips. Get up and stretch frequently— every hour if you sit for long periods of time. Do not sit on a fat wallet; it can cause hip imbalance!

- **When working on a computer**—take a one or two minute task break every 20 minutes when you work at a computer screen. Keep the screen 15 degrees below eye level. Place reference materials on a copy stand even with and close to the terminal.

- **When sitting in the car**—adjust the seat forward so your knees are higher than your hips. Put a small pillow or cushion in the small of your back.

- **When sleeping**—sleep on your side with your knees bent and head supported by a pillow, to make your head level with your spine. Or, sleep on your back, avoiding thick pillows under your

17

head. Use a small pillow under your neck instead. Don't sleep on your stomach.

- **When lifting**—let your legs do the work in order to prevent injury to your low back. Stand close to the object, then where possible squat down and straddle it. Grasp the object, and slowly lift the load by straightening your legs as you stand up. Carry the object close to your body.

- **When bending**—never twist from the waist and bend forward at the same time. To lift or reach something on the floor, bend the knees while keeping the back straight.

If you follow these practices, but still feel discomfort and pain related to specific activities, visit your doctor of chiropractic periodically for spinal checkups and for a postural evaluation for yourself and for your children.

Good Posture...Just How Important Is It?

Posture ranks right up at the top of the list when you are talking about good health. It is as important as eating right, exercising, getting a good night's sleep and avoiding potentially harmful substances like alcohol, drugs and tobacco. Good posture is a way of doing things with more energy, less stress and fatigue. Without good posture, you can't really be physically fit.

Surprised? Well, you're not alone. The importance of good posture in an overall fitness program is often overlooked by fitness advisers and fitness seekers alike. In fact, the benefits of good posture may be among the best kept secrets of the current fitness movement.

The good news is that most everyone can avoid the problems caused by bad posture...and you can make improvements at any age!

Chapter 3

Physical Fitness and Healthy Low Back Function

The following key points are discussed in detail in this chapter:

- At some time in their lives, 60-80% of all individuals experience low back pain. The condition is disabling to 1-5% of this population.

- To have a healthy, well-functioning back, flexible lumbar muscles, hamstrings, and hip flexors and strong fatigue-resistant abdominal and back extensor muscles are necessary.

- The Healthy People 2000 goals aim to decrease disability from chronic disabling disease and to increase the proportion of the population who regularly perform activities to enhance muscular strength, endurance, and flexibility. In terms of low back health, the latter goal may be one way of achieving the former goal.

- Exercises to maintain or increase muscular function in the low back region are presented in Figure 3.1.

- The anatomical logic (presented in Figure 3.2) linking low back health and physical activity is stronger than the research evidence at this time.

by Sharon Ann Plowman, Northern Illinois University, *Physical Activity and Fitness Research Digest*, produced by the President's Council on Physical Fitness and Sports, August 1993.

Studies support the fact that individuals who have suffered low back pain (LBP) have weaker, more fatigable, and less flexible muscles in the trunk region even after the acute pain episode has subsided than do those who are pain free. Continued weakness, low endurance and restricted range of movement appear to be contributing factors to recurrent LBP. The ability to predict first-time LBP from muscular strength, endurance or flexibility values has not been established. Likewise, a direct relationship between LBP and cardiovascular or body composition fitness has not been established. On the other hand, with one exception which is noted in the following text, the studies reviewed have not shown that high levels of any of these fitness components are in any way linked as causal factors to LBP. Therefore, it appears prudent at this point to continue recommending a specific program of truncal muscular fitness as a part of a comprehensive physical fitness activity program. This recommendation is in accordance with the Healthy People 2000 goal, which states the aim of increasing to at least 40 percent the proportion of the population 6 years old and above who regularly perform physical activities that enhance and maintain muscular strength, muscular endurance, and flexibility (Public Health Service, 1990). A comprehensive program would, of course, utilize the entire body and, along with the trunk region, stress upper arm and shoulder girdle areas. While baseline data suggests that the goal is close to being met for high school students, for the total population the 1991 estimate is that only 16% are involved in such programs.

For the trunk and low back region, it is imperative that the neuromuscular program go beyond traditional sit-ups for abdominal strength (actually, partial curls should be substituted for sit-ups) and modified hurdler's stretches for hamstring flexibility. The exercise program should be designed to include all five major anatomical areas and abilities listed in Figure 3.1 without overemphasizing lumbar flexibility. Ignoring any element in the whole may lead to imbalances. Figure 3.1 presents suggested flexibility and muscular strength/endurance exercises for the five identified areas with a progression from relatively easy to reasonably hard. Individual selections can be made from this chart for each area. Even if these components have not been shown irrevocably to be protective against the development of LBP, truncal muscular strength, endurance and flexibility are important aspects of a healthy, fully functioning, fit body.

Neuromuscular Fitness Components	Low	Moderate	High
a. Lumbar mobility*	Knee To Chest — In supine lying position bring one or both knees to the chest, grasping the leg, under the thigh(s), raise and lower head slowly.	"Mad Cat" — Kneeling on all fours alternate head up with sway back and head tucked with rounded back.	Crossed Leg Flexion — Sitting position with knees flexed and ankles crossed. Slowly bend forward until head approaches floor.
b. Hamstring flexibility*	Modified Hurdler's Stretch — Sit with one leg straight, the other flexed. Move the flexed knee to the side and bend forward.	PNF Supine Position — Place jump rope around foot or ankle with leg raised as straight as possible. Contract against rope, relax and pull leg straighter. Repeat.	Standing Stretch — Stand with one leg placed on a support at about 90° hip flexion. Keeping back straight with shoulders back, flex forward.
c. Hip flexor flexibility*	Hip Extension — Stand with pelvis in neutral position. Extend leg backward at hip.	Lying Stretch — Lie on table with knees over the edge and back flat. Pulling one leg to the chest (hands on thigh) stretches the opposite hip.	Standing Stretch — Stand in forward backward stride position. Bend front knee and thrust back hip forward. Keep front knee over ankle.
d. Abdominal strength/ endurance**	Pelvic Tilt — In supine lying or standing position – press pelvis to floor or wall.	Partial Curl (crunch) — Hook lying position, feet not held, tilt pelvis, curl up, sliding hands at side 3-4 1/2 inches.	Oblique Curl — Lying on side – twist trunk and curl up reaching for top leg with opposite arm.
e. Back extensor strength/endurance**	Hyperextension – 1 — Lying in prone position with hands at thighs. Keep neck and chin in neutral position and raise shoulders off floor.	Hyperextension – 2 — Lying in prone position with arms and hands extended forward. Keep neck and chin in neutral position and raise shoulders off floor.	Hyperextension – 3 — Lying in prone position on a table or bench with body supported and stabilized from top of pelvis down. Flex waist to 90° and extend to several inches above level.

* Move into stretch positions slowly and hold for 10-60 seconds.
** Repeat controlled movements 5-25 times.

Table 3.1. Suggested exercises for various fitness levels.

The Problem

The incidence of low back pain has been and continues to be consistently high. At some time in their lives, 60-80% of all individuals experience back pain. Both sexes are affected equally. Most cases occur between the ages of 25 and 60 years, but no age is completely immune. Approximately 12-26% of children and adolescents are LBP sufferers. Fortunately, most LBP is acute and, with or without treatment of any kind, resolves itself within three days to six weeks. After six weeks to a year, the condition is considered to be chronic. For the 1-5% so afflicted, the condition is disabling. This statistic speaks directly to the Healthy People 2000 priority of reducing disability from chronic disease, for while LBP is not the most prevalent disabling disease in the U.S., it is one of the many (Public Health Service, 1990). The psychological, social and physical costs to individuals cannot begin to be calculated. The medical, insurance and business/industry costs have been estimated into the billions of dollars per year (Cailliet, 1988; Plowman, 1992).

Most cases of acute LBP arise spontaneously from no known cause. Without knowing the exact cause, or causes of, LBP, it is difficult to determine risk factors which might predispose an individual to LBP. Among the possible risk factors most commonly linked with LBP is a lack of physical fitness. Indeed, LBP has often been labeled as a hypokinetic disease, that is, as a disease caused by and/or associated with a lack of exercise (Kraus and Raab, 1961).

The Theoretical Link Between Physical Activity, Physical Fitness and LBP

The theoretical link between physical activity, physical fitness and LBP is largely based on functional anatomy. Anatomically, back pain is primarily located in the lumbosacral region of the back which normally forms a lordotic curve. Twenty-four vertebrae comprise the entire spine. Effective functioning of the back requires coordination of all of the vertebra, the pelvis, the hip and thigh joints, and the muscles, fascia and ligaments which originate and insert on these bones. Such coordination is task-specific, but to be normal it should be completed with minimal and equalized stresses within the spine (Cailliet, 1988; Gracovetsky, 1990).

Figure 3.2 presents the theoretical relationships between all of the components of health-related physical fitness and healthy and unhealthy functioning of the low back. It can be seen that there is a strong anatomical rationale for all components of fitness. The actual research-based support is not as strong as the anatomical relationships.

The Research Link Between Physical Activity, Physical Fitness and Low Back Pain

Studies which have attempted to determine the relationship between physical activity and/or fitness and low back function or pain/injury are of two primary types. The first are retrospective studies. In a retrospective study, the relationship between the activity or fitness component and LBP is examined, or an attempt is made to distinguish between those who do and do not have low back pain based on the activity or fitness score. Retrospective studies must be interpreted cautiously since there are at least three possible confounding problems. First, activity or fitness measures in individuals already suffering from LBP may represent less than maximal effort due to real or feared pain. Second, physical activity is generally spontaneously decreased in individuals suffering from LBP, with the result that scores may reflect detraining as much as LBP per se. Third, these studies statistically establish just relationships (some of which may be statistically significant but not practically meaningful) and not cause and effect.

The second type of study is prospective. Prospective studies are longitudinal studies which test either normal individuals with no history of LBP, individuals with a history of LBP, or both, and then wait a specified time to see who develops LBP. The initial activity or fitness variables are then statistically analyzed to determine which, if any, had the most predictive value for the development of LBP. Perspective studies are obviously more valuable but they are also harder to conduct.

Throughout this section it has been emphasized that either physical activity or physical fitness can be used to determine the linkage with low back health or pain. In point of fact, very few studies have even attempted to relate physical activity per se in non-athletic populations with LBP. Those which have examined activity are weak in design and contradictory in outcome, precluding any meaningful comments or conclusions. The biggest difficulty is the inconsistent classification of physical activity and a primary reliance on frequency of participation to the exclusion of duration and intensity (Plowman, 1992). Even the most direct study by Porter, Adams, and Hutton (1989), which found a significant positive relation between spinal

23

Physical Fitness Component	Normal Anatomical Function in Low Back-Healthy	Dysfunction	Results of Dysfunction-Unhealthy
Cardiovascular-Respiratory Endurance	Discs obtain nutrients and dispose of wastes by absorption from adjacent blood supply.	Poor circulation, low CVR endurance	May speed up disc degeneration.
Body Composition	High musculature allows for proper functioning as outlined below and provides mechanical loading on the vertebrae for maintenance of bone mass.	High % body fat content	Increases the weight the spine must support; may lead to increased pressure on discs or other vertebral structures.
Neuromuscular a. Lumbar flexibility	Allows the lumbar curve to almost be reversed in forward flexion.	Inflexible	Disrupts forward and lateral movement; places excessive stretch on hamstrings leading to low back and hamstring pain.
b. Hamstring flexibility	Allows anterior rotation (tilt) of the pelvis in forward flexion and posterior rotation in sitting position.	Inflexible	Restricts anterior pelvic rotation and exaggerates posterior tilt; both cause increased disc compression; excessive stretching causes strain and pain.
c. Hip flexor flexibility	Allows achievement of neutral pelvic position.	Inflexible	Exaggerates anterior pelvic tilt if not counteracted by strong abdominal muscles, thereby increasing disc compression.
d. Abdominal strength/endurance	Maintains pelvic position; reinforces back extensor fascia and pulls it laterally on forward flexion providing support.	Weak, easily fatigued	Allows abnormal pelvic tilt; increases strain on back extensor muscles.
e. Back extensor strength/endurance	Provides stability for spine; maintains erect posture; controls forward flexion.	Weak, easily fatigued	Increases loading on spine; causes increased disc compression.

Table 3.2. *Theoretical relationship between physical fitness components and healthy/unhealthy low back/spinal function.*

motion segment compressive strength and physical activity in young men killed in motorcycle accidents, relied only on a sports history obtained from the next of kin. Thus, no exercise prescription guidelines specific for low back health can be documented from the literature. This is a fertile area for research.

The rest of this report will concentrate on the linkage between physical fitness and low back health or pain. Some specific studies will be mentioned for illustrative purposes, but the primary emphasis will be on general consensus. For a more in-depth presentation of the research literature, the reader is referred to Plowman (1992). Complete references are also provided there.

Cardiovascular Fitness and LBP

As stated in Figure 3.2, a properly functioning cardiovascular system is necessary for disc nourishment and to slow disc degeneration. The exact relationship with total body cardiovascular fitness has received little attention. Only two retrospective studies have measured cardiovascular fitness, and neither established a definitive linkage with low back function (Plowman, 1992).

Likewise, only two prospective studies have designs specific enough to draw conclusions from, but unfortunately the conclusions that must be drawn are in opposition to each other. The first study was completed on fire fighters by Cady, Thomas, and Karwasky (1985). Cardiovascular condition was assessed by physical working capacity (PWC). The 20 fire fighters with the lowest PWC incurred much higher low back injury costs than the 20 with the highest PWC, showing a beneficial effect. The second study is the study with the stronger design. It was conducted by Battié et al. (1989). Maximal oxygen consumption (VO_2max) was predicted from a submaximal treadmill test on over 2400 Boeing airplane employees. VO_2max was not found to be predictive of the 228 back problems which occurred in these employees over the subsequent 4 years.

There is no evidence that a highly fit cardiovascular system is detrimental in any way, but the evidence of benefit is minimal. This is another area which requires further research.

Body Composition and LBP

The skeletal system in general and the spine in particular are the primary supporting structures of the body. As pointed out in Figure

3.2, if the weight the spine supports is largely muscular and the muscles are both strong and flexible, healthy functioning should result. However, if a large portion of the body mass is fat, this adds excess weight and pressure on the discs without any positive assistance. The few studies which have utilized body mass index (WT/HT^2) as an indication of body composition have shown split results. No studies have been done on LBP in which body composition has been directly assessed by a laboratory criterion measure such as underwater weighing (Plowman, 1992).

Neuromuscular Fitness and LBP

The most important components of fitness in relation to healthy functioning of the low back are muscular strength, muscular endurance and flexibility. It is necessary that each separate muscle group possess both strength/endurance and flexibility, and that anatomically opposing muscle groups are balanced in strength/endurance and flexibility. The goal in relation to the low back region is that the vertebra will be kept in proper alignment without excessive disc pressure throughout the full range of possible motions. In addition, the pelvis must freely rotate both posteriorly and anteriorly without strain on the muscles or fascia. Figure 3.2 presents the specific actions of the back, hip, abdominal and hamstring muscles and what can theoretically happen if these muscles are allowed to become weak, easily fatigued and/or inflexible.

The research evidence shows that regardless of the testing mode (that is, whether the test is one of static or dynamic function), individuals with low back pain exhibit lower strength values of both the abdominals and back extensor groups than do individuals without LBP. Only two studies looked at trunk extensor endurance specifically, but both of these found that individuals with LBP severe enough to limit function had scores lower than those without such limitations (Plowman, 1992).

Perhaps the most interesting studies in this area are those utilizing electromyographic (EMG) analysis of back extensor fatigue. In each of the three studies (DeVries, 1968; Roy, DeLuca, and Casavant, 1989; Roy et al., 1990), 80-100% of those with LBP showed increased electrical activity during sustained static muscle contraction. While these were not intended to be prospective studies, in one case an individual who showed high EMG activity but no history of LBP developed LBP the following year. Retrospective studies of low back pain and hamstring flexibility have shown the same trend. That is, that there is a significant relationship between tightness in those muscle groups and LBP (Plowman, 1992).

Prospective studies of neuromuscular fitness are neither as numerous nor as definitive as the retrospective ones. Only one strength/endurance study found any variable predictive of first-time low back pain, and this showed the predictive variable to be limited (low) back extensor endurance (Biering-Sorensen, 1984a). Unfortunately, this was the only study using this variable, but since it is consistent with the results of the retrospective studies it would seem that back extensor endurance needs to be given more attention. Recurrent back pain has been successfully predicted in about half of the studies of trunk and back extensor strength/endurance with, as expected, low scores preceding the reoccurrence of back pain (Plowman, 1992).

One prospective study found lumbar flexibility to be predictive of first time LBP (Biering-Sorensen, 1984b). In it, increased (not decreased as might be expected) lumbar mobility was found to be predictive of first-time back pain in males but not females. It is anatomically possible that extreme lumbosacral flexion stresses the discs at that site (Sharpe, Liehmon, and Snodgrass, 1988). Recurrent back pain has been found to be predictable from both low lumbar extension range of motion and low hamstring flexibility.

No specific level of strength, endurance and/or flexibility has emerged as critical in any of these studies. Hopefully, further research to clarify these issues will be forthcoming.

References

Battié, M.C., Bigos, S.J., Fisher, L.D., Hansson, T.H., Nachemson, A.L., Spengler, D.M., Wortley, M.D., & Zeh J. (1989). A prospective study of the role of cardiovascular risk factors and fitness in industrial back pain complaints. *Spine*, 12:141-147.

Biering-Sorensen, F. (1984a). A one-year prospective study of low back trouble in a general population. *Danish Medical Bulletin*, 31:362-375.

Biering-Sorensen, F. (1984b). Physical measurements as risk indicators for low-back trouble over a one-year period. *Spine*, 9:106-119.

Cady, L.D., Thomas P.C., & Karwasky, R.J. (1985). Program for increasing health and physical fitness for fire fighters. *Journal of Occupational Medicine*, 27:110-114.

Cailliet, R. (1988). *Low Back Pain Syndrome*, 4th edition. Philadelphia, PA: F.A. Davis.

DeVries, H.A. (1968). EMG fatigue curves in postural muscles. A possible etiology for idiopathic low back pain. *American Journal of Physical Medicine*, 47:175-181.

Gracovetsky, S., Kary, M., Levy, S., Ben Said, R., Pitchen, I., & Helie, J. (1990). Analysis of spinal and muscular activity during flexion/extension and free lifts. *Spine*, 15:1333-1339.

Kraus, H., & Raab, W. (1961). *Hypokinetic Disease*. Springfield, IL: Charles C. Thomas.

Plowman, S.A. (1992). Physical activity, physical fitness, and low back pain. In: Holloszy, J.O. (ed.), *Exercise and Sport Sciences Review*, 20:221-242.

Porter, R.W., Adams, M.A., & Hutton, W.C. (1989). Physical activity and the strength of the lumbar spine. *Spine*, 14:201-203.

Public Health Service. (1990). *Healthy People 2000*. Washington, D.C.: U.S. Government Printing Office.

Roy, S.H., DeLuca, C.J., Casavant, D.A. (1989). Lumbar muscle fatigue and chronic lower back pain. *Spine*, 14:992-1001.

Roy, S.H., DeLuca, C.J., Snyder-Mackler, L., Emley, M.S., Crenshaw, R.L., & Lyons, J.P. (1990). Fatigue, recovery, and low back pain in varsity rowers. *Medicine and Science in Sports and Exercise*, 22:463-469.

Sharpe, G.L., Liehman, W.P., & Snodgrass, L.B. (1988). Exercise prescription and the low back—kinesiological factors. *Journal of Health, Physical Education, Recreation and Dance*, 59(8):74-78.

Chapter 4

Glossary of Back and Neck Terms

A

Acromiohumeral region. Pertaining to the area of the scapula (shoulder blade) and humerus (upper arm bone).

Acute stage. The time right after your injury when you are in the hospital and may have many kinds of medical problems.

Adaptive equipment. Equipment that is used to help adapt your environment to your personal needs. Examples include ramps, splints to hold pens or forks, and hand controls to drive vehicles.

ADL (activities of daily living). Self-care activities such as bathing, dressing, toileting, eating, grooming, etc.

Advocate. Someone who goes to bat for you and represents your best interests in a given situation.

Airway management. Helping you get the air you need from the outside into your lungs.

Definitions in this chapter were compiled from publications of the National Institute of Arthritis and Musculoskeletal and Skin Diseases (1992), the *Washington Post* (©1995), and the Paralyzed Veterans of America (©1989); copyrighted definitions reprinted with permission.

Anemia. A lack of red blood cells to carry oxygen to the tissues of the body.

Appliance. A device used to perform or help you perform a certain activity.

Atherosclerosis. Thickening of artery walls, hardening of the arteries.

Atrophy. A condition in which muscles diminish in size due to lack of stimulation from nerves.

Attendant. An individual (family, friend, stranger, etc.) hired to assist with household tasks or personal care on a routine basis.

Automobile adaptive equipment. Items/devices necessary to permit the safe operation of, or the ability to get in and out of, an automobile or other types of vehicle.

B

Bedridden. When you are confined to bed for medical treatment.

Braces. Splints used to support, align, or hold parts of your body in correct position.

C

Carbohydrates. Sugars and starches.

Caregiver. General term used to describe any person who gives you physical, emotional, psychological, or social care.

Cath. Slang for Catheterization (see Intermittent Catheterization Program).

Catheterization (Cath or Intermittent Catheterization Program). Inserting a small special tube into your bladder to empty urine.

Cauda equina syndrome. Compression, usually due to the pressure of a massive herniated disc, on a sheaf of nerve roots from the lower spinal cord that spread out like the tail of a horse, hence cauda equina. Symptoms include weakness of the legs, loss of sensation in the skin over the perineum (called saddle anesthesia) and urine retention or incontinence from loss of function in the sphincter muscle. Usually requires prompt surgery.

Cervical. Refers to conditions or things associated with the levels of your spine at the neck.

Chemonucleolysis. Injection of a disc-dissolving enzyme, such as chymopapain, into the jelly-like center of a herniated disc.

Cholesterol. A waxy-like, non-fat substance found in blood that is made by your liver or taken in from food sources of animal origin.

Chronic pain. Pain that has usually been present longer than six months and is out of proportion to physical and laboratory test results, for which pain medication does not work and that becomes central to the lifestyle of the sufferer.

Chux. Absorbent pads used to protect a mattress, also known as "blue pads."

Cirrhosis of the liver. A disease aggravated by excessive alcohol consumption.

Clothing allowance. An annual sum of money, specified by Congress, to be paid to each veteran who, because of his or her service-connected disability, wears or uses a prosthetic or orthotic appliance (including a wheelchair), which tends to wear out or tear the clothing of the veteran.

Contracture. Permanent limitation of joint movement usually due to not doing range-of-motion exercises, poor positioning, and/or severe spasms.

Contraindicated. Something that is bad for your health.

Credé. A method of emptying the bladder by firm pressure on the abdomen with the hands to push the urine out.

CT-myelography. Multi-view X-ray enhanced through computers after a contrasting dye has been injected into membranes covering the spinal cord.

CT scan (computerized tomography scanning). A diagnostic technique in which the combined use of a computer and x-rays passed through the body at difference angles produces clear cross-sectional images of the tissue being examined. CT scanning is more sensitive than x-rays, which, alone, do not permit cross-sectional views.

D

Decompression. Relief of pressure, such as that exerted on the spinal cord or nerve roots by a disc or part of the bone of the spine.

Decubitus ulcer. Bed sore, pressure sore, pressure ulcer—a reddened area or an open sore usually found on the skin over bony areas like your hip bone or tail bone. It is usually caused by too much pressure on those areas.

Diskectomy (discectomy). Surgical removal of part of a disc compressing a nerve root. Called microdiskectomy when microscopic or visually aided surgical techniques are used.

Discography (diskography). A diagnostic technique in which a dye visible on x-ray films is injected into an intervertebral disc to assess damage and locate the source of pain.

Distended. Bloated and stretched due to overfilling.

Dosage. The amount of medication you should take and when to take it.

Drugs. This is a confusing word. It may mean medicines you take to get better, or it may mean substances that are abused.

DVB. Department of Veterans Benefits

E

Edema (swelling). Generally caused by fluid collecting in the given area that is swollen.

Eligibility. The determination of whether you qualify for certain entitlement programs. VA benefit payments are based on certain facts, among them being your period of service, whether you had an honorable or other discharge from the service, income guidelines, and/or a documented physical disability.

Embolus. A thrombus, or blood clot, that has broken loose and is passing freely through the bloodstream.

EMG (electromyogram). A test to find out how your nerves and muscles are working, using electronic equipment.

Evaluation. The careful study of something to determine its significance or value.

Extension. Unbending of a joint, an example of which is straightening your arm.

Extremity. A medical term referring to your arm or leg.

- *Upper extremity*: includes your arm, forearm, and hand.
- *Lower extremity*: includes your thigh, lower leg, and foot.

F

Fabricate. To construct, assemble, or manufacture.

Flaccid. Lack of muscle tone.

Flexion. Bending of a joint, as in when you bend your leg at the knee.

Foley. Short for a Foley catheter. Used to continuously drain urine from your bladder.

Fusion. Surgical fusing of two vertebrae together by inserting fragments of the patient's own bone (graft) usually taken from the pelvic bone. Space between the two vertebrae may be bridged with bone or held together with metal, such as rods or screws.

G

Gait. Description of your individual style of walking.

H

Halo. A metal ring worn around your head used to treat broken necks. When used with a plastic vest, this keeps your neck and body straight.

HBHC (Hospital Based Home Care). The service offered by the hospital that tends to the care of people in their own homes.

Health promotion. Those activities and attitudes that help you live a healthy life.

Health risks. Those things, such as living conditions, heredity, attitudes or activities, which increase your chances for poor health.

Herniated or ruptured disc. Extrusion of the central, jelly-like material of a spinal disc through its fibrous outer covering.

Hubbard tank. A tank of water used for exercise or treatment of pressure sores.

Hygiene. Condition or practices leading to health.

I

ICP *see* Intermittent Catheterization Program.

Impaction. Something that gets lodged in and clogs a space, such as an impaction of the bowel.

Incentive spirometer. A device used to build up lung volume and control.

Incontinence. A bowel or bladder accident.

Independent living unit (ILU). A full apartment on the SCI unit where patients can test new skills and be evaluated on what they have learned in therapy sessions.

Intermittent catheterization program (ICP or Cath). A routine program by which the bladder is emptied at regular intervals by catheterization to prevent urinary accidents and infections.

Intervertebral foramena. A normal opening between vertebrae that permits passage of a spinal nerve and blood vessels.

L

Laminectomy. Surgical removal of part or all of one or more of the bony arches of the vertebrae that surround the spinal cord to relieve pressure on the cord or nerve roots.

Laminaplasty. Removal of bony arches of vertebrae, which are thinned and then replaced, resulting in a wider canal.

LPN (licensed practical nurse). This person is trained and licensed to provide routine nursing care.

Lumbar. Refers to a condition or thing in the area of the mid to lower back.

Lung capacity. The volume of air you can breathe and your lungs can hold.

M

MD (doctor of medicine). Someone who has passed four years of medical school. May be an intern, resident, or staff doctor.

Medical history. The important information about your past and present health.

Medication (medicine). A therapeutic substance you take that is prescribed by your doctor or purchased "over the counter."

Medullar vessels. Blood vessels that run along the spinal cord.

MRI (magnetic resonance imaging). Diagnostic technique that provides high quality cross-sectional images without x-rays or other radiation. The patient lies inside a massive, hollow, cylindrical magnet and is exposed to short bursts of powerful magnetic fields and radio waves. The bursts stimulate hydrogen atoms in the tissues to emit signals which are detected and analyzed by computer to create an image of a slice of the tissue.

Myelography (myelogram). Injection of an opaque substance into the spinal column which shows up on x-ray, permitting visualization of pathology. Being replaced by the newer CT scan and MRI techniques.

Myelopathy. Nervous system problems caused by pressure on the spinal cord.

N

NA. Nursing assistant.

Neurogenic. Refers to a condition or thing that is controlled by nerves.

Nutrition. The food you eat and how your body uses it to live, grow, keep healthy, and get the energy you need for work and recreation.

O

Occupational therapy (therapist). The profession or professional that focuses on the range of motion; strength; and coordination of fine, or small, movement of muscles and joints, with or without adaptive devices. The end result is to perform ADL tasks or various vocational skills.

Oral. Pertaining to your mouth.

Orthosis. A device applied to the exterior of the body to support, aid, and align the body and limbs or to influence motion by assisting, resisting, blocking, or unloading part of the body weight. These devices may include, but are not limited to, braces, binders, corsets, belts, and trusses.

Osseous protrusion. A bony projection.

Osteophyte. A bony outgrowth.

OT *see* occupational therapy (therapist).

P

Para (paraplegic). The condition of being completely paralyzed in such a way as to include the legs.

Paralysis. The inability to control movement of a part of your body.

Paralyzed Veterans of America (PVA). An organization that provides free assistance to veterans and other individuals with spinal cord dysfunction. PVA assists all veterans with a disability through a broad range of programs designed to promote fuller access to the community. A local representative of this organization is assigned to each VA Medical Center and will be available to meet with veterans and their families.

Paraparesis. Incomplete paralysis or weakness of the legs only.

Personality. Thoughts, feelings, and behaviors that are specific to an individual, often representing a particular pattern or style of life.

Physiotherapy (physical therapy—therapist). The profession or professional that deals with the strength, coordination, and range of motion of gross movements of your muscles and joints.

Pressure reliefs. Changing positions in wheelchair or bed to let your skin rest and increase circulation of blood flow in the buttocks or areas of pressure.

Primary care. The medical care of routine illness like colds, flu, etc.

Prone. Lying flat on your stomach.

Prosthesis. An artificial substitute for a missing body part.

Prosthetic appliances. All aids, appliances, parts, or accessories that are required to replace, support, or substitute for a deformed, weakened, or missing anatomical portion of the body. Artificial limbs, terminal devices, stump socks, braces, hearing aids and batteries, cosmetic facial or body restorations, eyeglasses, mechanical or motorized wheelchairs, orthopedic shoes, and similar items are included under this broad term.

Psychological. Related to mental and emotional factors that influence behavior (e.g., motivation, awareness, personality, etc.).

PT (physical therapy, physical therapist) *see* Physiotherapy.

Pulmonary. Having to do with your lungs and breathing.

Q

Quad (quadriplegic or tetraplegic). The condition of being completely paralyzed in a way that includes legs and part or all of the arm muscles.

Quadriparesis. Weakness or incomplete paralysis involving the arms and legs.

R

Radiculopathy. Pressure on a nerve root as it branches off the spinal cord, causing symptoms in the area stimulated by the nerve root.

Range of motion (ROM). An arc of movement of a joint of your body.

Rehab (rehabilitation). The process of doing away with, adapting to, or compensating for disabilities.

Residual. In the case of bladder voiding, it is the urine left remaining in the bladder after voiding has taken place.

Respiratory. Having to do with your breathing.

RN (registered nurse). A professional who plans and provides nursing care. Your primary care planner is usually an RN.

RT (respiratory therapy, therapist). The profession or professional that centers on therapy of the lungs and breathing.

S

Sacral. Refers to a condition or thing in the area at the lowest part of your spine around your tailbone.

SCI (spinal cord injury). An injury to the back or neck causing damage to the spinal cord, leading to paralysis.

Sciatica. Pain radiating down the leg below the knee along the distribution of the sciatic nerve, usually related to mechanical pressure and/or inflammation of nerve roots in the lumbar spine, e.g. a herniated disc.

Sensation. Physical feelings of vibration, touch, pain, hot and cold, or awareness of where a body part is in space.

Side effects. The effects of something, usually medication, that are different from the reason for which it was originally planned.

Smoker's robot. A mechanical device that holds a cigarette safely away from the smoker. The cigarette can then be smoked through a piece of tubing.

Spasm. A sudden, often uncontrolled, contraction of a muscle, a muscle jerk.

Spasticity. Movement in your arms and legs due to muscle spasm that may occur as a result of spinal cord injury. It may be somewhat controllable.

Spine immobilizers. Braces or devices that keep you from moving your back or neck.

Spine stabilization. A brace or device that aids in supporting or stabilizing your back or neck.

Splint. A rigid or flexible appliance used for the fixation (holding in place) or support of a displaced or movable part of the body.

Spondylolisthesis. Overlap of a vertebra on the one below. This often results in back pain and can also cause pinching of the nerves that exit at the site of the slip.

Spondylosis. An osteoarthritic condition of the spine.

Stenosis. A narrowing of the spinal canal or intervertebral foramena. Generally affects patients over age 60. Symptoms include leg pain when walking or standing that is relieved by sitting or flexing the spine and occasionally weakness of the legs.

Stones. Solid, hard masses that can become stuck in the urinary tract and block normal urine drainage from the kidney or bladder.

Subluxation. A partial dislocation of a vertebra.

Suctioning. Removal of mucous from the throat and/or lungs by a small tube attached to suction.

Support system. The people who are important to you because they strengthen your emotional, physical, and social well-being. They usually are your family, friends, co-workers, neighbors, members of your church, landlord, or veterans group.

T

Tenodesis. The action of fingers and thumb pinching together when wrist is bent upwards.

Therapy. The treatment of diseases or disorders.

Thoracic. Refers to a condition or thing in the region of the spine at the chest to mid-back levels.

Thrombus. A blood clot anchored somewhere in the bloodstream.

TRS (therapeutic recreation specialist). The person responsible for your recreational therapy.

U

Urinalysis. A sampling test of urine to evaluate the contents of the urine and check for problems.

Urinary system. The body parts that turn wastes into urine, store it, and get rid of it. Kidneys filter blood to wash it clean and make the urine. Ureters are tubes to bring the urine from the kidneys to the bladder. The bladder is a dynamic storage tank for the urine. The urethra is a tube to bring the urine from the bladder to the outside.

V

VA. Department of Veterans Affairs.

Ventilator. A piece of equipment that helps you to breathe when you cannot do it yourself.

Vocational. Work or job-related activity (avocational = hobbies and recreation).

Voc Rehab (vocational rehabilitation). Developing skills to improve work habits or to increase employment potential.

Void. To empty the bladder.

VRS (vocational rehabilitation specialist). The person who assists you in determining changes or improvements in your job or vocational status.

Part Two

Disorders of the Back and Neck

Chapter 5

Back Talk: Advice for Suffering Spines

"Some days," says Linda, "my back hurts so much that I can't stand to have clothes touching me."

If misery loves company, Linda's got plenty of it. At least once in their lives, about 80 percent of Americans will experience a bout of low back pain that can range from a dull, annoying ache to absolute agony. According to *American Family Physician*, on any given day 6.5 million Americans are under some sort of treatment for low back pain.

After headaches, low back pain is the second most common ailment in the United States and is topped only by colds and flu in time lost from work. Low back pain has been described as a 20th century epidemic, the nemesis of medicine, and an albatross of industry. When all the costs connected with it are added up—job absenteeism, medical and legal fees, social security disability payments, workmen's compensation, long-term disability insurance—the bill to business, industry and the government has been estimated to total at least $16 billion each year. Those most often affected are young adults in their most productive years, from ages 17 to 45.

There's no mystery in why Linda's back hurts. Her spine will never be the same because an automobile accident left her with four fractured vertebrae and a destroyed disc. Though accidents are responsible for a fair share of back pain, most backaches are not caused by anything so dramatic.

FDA Consumer, April 1989.

Sedentary Lifestyles

It is believed that many cases of low back pain are due to stresses on the muscles and ligaments that support the spine. Our sedentary jobs and lifestyle make us vulnerable to this type of damage. Too much time in front of the TV, not enough exercise, poor posture, and poor sleeping habits (including sleeping on the stomach) weaken muscles. Weak muscles, especially abdominal muscles, cannot support the spine properly. Obesity, which afflicts 34 million Americans, is another factor—it increases both the weight on the spine and the pressure on the discs.

When the body is in poor shape, it doesn't take much to overstretch (strain) a muscle or put a small tear in (sprain) a ligament. The medical word for backaches arising from either of these conditions is lumbosacral strain (or sprain). Sometimes, a sudden twist or fall can bring on muscle spasm—sudden, involuntary contractions that can be excruciatingly painful. A spasm immobilizes the muscles over the injured area, possibly acting as a kind of splint to protect muscles or joints from further damage.

Jobs that involve bending and twisting, or lifting heavy objects repeatedly—especially when the loads are beyond a worker's strength—are no better for the back than are sedentary jobs. Certain occupations, such as truck driving or nursing, are particularly hard on the back. The truck driver must contend with sitting for long periods (actually worse for the back than standing), the vibration of the vehicle, and lifting and straining at the end of the day when muscles are fatigued and more susceptible to damage. (Truck driving ranks first in workmen's compensation cases for low back pain.) Football, gymnastics, and other strenuous sports can also damage the lower back.

Slipped Discs

Because many people are familiar with the term "slipped" disc, this problem is mistakenly believed to be the chief cause of most low back pain. But in fact, slipped discs are responsible for only 5 percent to 10 percent of the cases. Actually, the term itself is inaccurate because the disc doesn't slip at all; it bulges out between two vertebrae. In some cases, the tough tissues that contain the disc are weakened by injuries that allow the soft gel-like center to protrude. If the protrusion presses on a nerve root, pinching it against the bone, the result is pain in the area of the body served by that nerve. Doctors can tell which disc in the lower back is causing the problem by the part of the body affected, usually the legs.

The protruded part of the disc does not slip back into place. Scar tissue forms around the protrusion and walls it in. If the outer tissues continue to be stressed, they will weaken further and, in time, the slightest activity—a sneeze or cough—may cause the disc to burst through its capsule, or rupture.

As might be expected, pain from disc disease can rank pretty high on the pain index. To make matters worse, if a nerve root is irritated in any one place, it tends to become irritable along its whole length. A ruptured disc that presses on nerve roots in the low back (lower lumbar or high sacral areas) causes sciatica, a condition in which sharp, shooting pains begin in the buttock and run down the back of the thigh and the inside of the leg to the foot. Tingling, numbness and weakness may follow. If the pressure on the nerve root is not relieved, the leg muscles will eventually waste away, or atrophy.

"When sciatica occurs," explains Todd L. Samuels, M.D., Department of Neurology, Georgetown University Hospital, Washington, D.C., "we can pinpoint the specific nerve root or roots that are compressed in most cases by carefully examining the strength of individual muscles and deep tendon reflexes, and by noting where there's loss of sensation."

Samuels says that conservative treatment such as strict bed rest, anti-inflammatory medication, and muscle relaxants often relieve the acute symptoms. In intractable cases, surgery may be necessary to relieve pressure on the nerve root.

A large protrusion may also press on the nerves that branch off the end of the spinal cord (cauda equina), causing back pain, loss of sensation in the buttocks, thighs or genital organs, and bowel and bladder disturbances. When this, or any other symptoms of nerve root pressure, occurs, help should be sought immediately.

Pain That Comes with Aging

Degenerative conditions that go along with aging can also cause low back pain. The bloom may still be on the cheek, but things are slowly falling apart within. Muscles reach their peak capacity by age 20, then decline without proper exercise. Disc degeneration begins in the early 20s. Though discs in babies are about 90 percent water, by age 70 fluid loss reduces the water content to 70 percent, flattening the discs. (Because discs constitute 25 percent of the spine's length, as the discs become flatter and less elastic, people lose height: Most of us can expect to be about a half inch to two inches shorter in old age.) When discs shrink, they lose their ability to act as shock absorbers, putting greater stress on supporting ligaments, causing back pain.

Back pain can also result from osteoporosis, a disorder that robs bones of calcium and makes them porous, so that vertebrae crush or fracture easily. Though both men and women lose bone density after age 35, the disease appears most often in women past menopause. It is thought that failure to develop adequate bone mass during youth, lack of exercise, and a diet low in calcium and other nutrients may be contributing factors. Smoking and overconsumption of alcohol may also be involved.

Spinal joints are also affected by various types of arthritis. One type that most of us will experience if we live long enough is degenerative joint disease, or osteoarthritis. The cartilage that cushions joints gradually breaks down, resulting in back pain and stiffness, especially in the morning. Osteoarthritis may appear as early as the 20s and 30s, though without symptoms, and nearly everybody has it by age 70.

A particularly distressing type of arthritis is ankylosing spondylitis. The lower back and sacroiliac joints become stiff and swollen. Muscle spasm and back pain may be so severe that bending over is the only way to relieve it. If untreated, in some cases the inflamed spinal joints may fuse, preventing the individual from straightening up. The disease affects more men than women, usually starting between the ages of 20 and 40, though it can begin as early as 10. The cause is unknown, but it is believed that some people may be genetically susceptible to this disorder. Posture-maintaining exercises, hot baths, painkillers, and nonsteroidal anti-inflammatory drugs may help relieve symptoms.

Referred Pain

To add insult to injury, pain can be "referred" to the back from other parts of the body. Prostate problems in men, a retroverted or "tipped" uterus in women, peptic ulcers, colitis, gallbladder disease, heart disease, cancer that has spread to the spine from other organs (most often the breast, lung, prostate and kidney), and many other conditions can all be felt as back pain. People can also be born with abnormalities or develop conditions, such as scoliosis, that predispose them to back pain when they grow older. Infections of the spine, although rare, can also cause back pain. And it is possible to have severe back pain of a psychological, rather than physiological, nature.

The good news is that acute low back pain, especially when caused by lumbosacral strain, often goes away by itself in a few days to a few weeks. Sometimes it's not even necessary to see the doctor. Rest is the basic treatment. A day or two in bed to take the weight off the spine, some aspirin or other pain reliever, an ice bag or a hot water bottle on the back—whichever feels more comfortable—are usually all that's needed. Even disc problems respond to rest; the protruding tissue shrinks, and pressure on the nerve lessens.

But rest can be overdone. Dr. Alf Nachemson, the eminent Swedish orthopedist who designed the Volvo automobile seat for good back support, noted at a National Institutes of Health conference on low back pain in 1988 that recovery is quicker when people are moderately active, even if they feel some pain. He warned that prolonged bed rest is not beneficial because it weakens muscles.

Manipulation by chiropractors or osteopaths appears to afford short-term relief in some cases. (But when the problem is disc herniation or osteoporosis, manipulation may make matters worse.)

It is reassuring to know that with or without treatment some 60 percent of back pain sufferers go back to work within a week, and nearly 90 percent return within six weeks.

When to See a Doctor

But, if there's no relief from pain after a few days in bed, or if pain is severe or recurs, it's time to see the family doctor. There's no time to waste if radiating pain, numbness, tingling or weakness occurs in the arms or legs, or if the bowel or bladder doesn't function properly. It also makes sense to consult the doctor if a child or elderly person has back pain. Fever or vomiting with the pain may indicate infection.

Because so many conditions can contribute to back pain, it's not always easy to pinpoint the cause, even using the best technology available. Nevertheless, if the pain won't let up and the cause can't be determined after the doctor has taken a complete medical history and conducted a comprehensive physical examination, referral to a specialist may be needed.

Specialists—orthopedists, neurologists, neurosurgeons, rheumatologists, internists—have an array of diagnostic tests at their disposal:

X-rays can show bone deformities or fractures of the spine. Although the discs themselves cannot be seen, vertebrae that appear too close together may indicate that the disc has ruptured or degen-erated. Though helpful in diagnosing certain diseases, such as ankylosing spondylitis and osteoporosis, X-rays are more valuable for what they rule out—for example, cancer or tuberculosis—than for what they reveal.

CAT scans (computerized axial tomography) are special X-rays used with a computer to produce images of a "slice" of anatomic tissue. They're good for looking at the spinal cord, spinal bones, frac-tures, osteoarthritis damage, narrowed spinal canal (spinal stenosis), tumors, and spinal cord infections.

Magnetic resonance imaging (MRI) uses a strong magnetic field and a computer to create highly detailed images of soft tissues, such as muscles, cartilage, ligaments, tendons, blood vessels, and, to a lesser extent, bone. MRI can also show disc degeneration, protru-sion and rupture, infection, and other spinal disorders.

A myelogram is another type of X-ray examination. Before tak-ing X-rays, the radiologist injects a contrast medium (dye) into the spinal canal. This dye blocks X-rays and outlines the spinal cord and spinal nerves. Myelograms can show a ruptured disc.

An electromyogram (EMG) is a graphic record of muscle con-traction that can show nerve and muscle damage.

When Surgery Is Called For

Although physicians prefer to treat even severe cases of low back pain conservatively with bed rest and painkillers, surgery is clearly called for if pressure on a nerve root causes severe pain lasting for weeks, or if progressive damage to the nerves results in leg weakness or paralysis. Every year, about 200,000 Americans undergo surgery for persistent back pain.

"There are several operations that we do to relieve back pain.... The most common one is the removal of the slipped disc or herniated disc," says Edward R. Laws Jr., M.D., professor and chairman of neurosurgery at George Washington University, Washington, D.C. "We get at the slipped disc by removing only a very small part of the bone—the arch of the vertebra. [This procedure is called a laminectomy.] Then we remove the part of the disc that's out of place and any other loose fragments that are accessible."

Another condition that requires laminectomy is spinal stenosis, an unusual narrowing of the space inside the spinal canal. A narrow spinal canal may cause pressure on the nerve roots and, in rare cases, on the cord itself. "That's the second most common operation that we do," says Laws. "Some people are born with a narrow spinal canal... [others have] buildup of ligaments and bone spurs that narrow the spinal canal. They occur as a result of wear and tear, of having the spine work against gravity over time.

"In some cases, we do spinal fusion," continues Laws. "The spine is made up of a number of joints, and if a joint is unstable and slips, [causing] nerve root pinching, we can stop the slipping by fusing two vertebrae together." To do this, surgeons insert fragments of the patient's own bone, usually taken from the hip, to bridge the space between two adjacent vertebrae. In time, the bones grow together. Fusion relieves pain but reduces mobility.

A 1987 NIH report to Congress estimated that fewer than 1 in 10 people with low back pain requires surgery. Of these, about one fifth have unsuccessful outcomes—a rather unsettling statistic. "I can see where some analyses would turn out that way, because if you take all comers and look at how the patients do three, four, five years after surgery, only about 75 percent have really great results," comments Laws. "Sometimes, the wrong operation is done, or an operation is done on a patient who could have gotten by without one. There's no doubt that there are a lot of mighty sore backs out there." To avoid unnecessary surgery, it is wise to get a second opinion.

A Drug Instead of the Knife

In a small percentage of cases, sciatic pain caused by a herniated disc that would normally require surgery is treated by some physicians with chymopapain. This drug, approved by FDA in 1982, is an enzyme found in papaya that is used to tenderize meat, make beer, and clear cloudy contact lenses. Injected into the disc's jelly-like center, chymopapain dissolves the disc. thus lessening pressure on the nerve root. The drug has had its champions and detractors ever since it was introduced, but when used in patients in whom conservative treatment has failed and who are candidates for surgery, it can be very successful. Its advantages over surgery are a shorter hospital stay, less expense, less scarring, and less trauma. Since some people are highly allergic to the drug, skin tests must be done first to detect chymopapain sensitivity in candidates for treatment.

51

A relatively new technique called aspiration percutaneous lumbar diskectomy (APLD) may be useful for people allergic to chymopapain and those for whom general anesthesia is risky. Using X-ray pictures as a guide, the neurosurgeon or orthopedist inserts a long, thin needle called a nucleotome probe into the center of the protruding disc. The physician loosens the disc material by moving the probe back and forth. A pump attached to the probe suctions up the material and carries it away.

APLD takes about 40 minutes, requires about 10 days recuperation, and costs a great deal less than laminectomy. However, not everybody is a suitable candidate for this procedure. It cannot be used on those who have severely ruptured discs or spinal stenosis.

To Prevent Recurrences

People who've had one backache are not anxious to have another. There are some things they can do to help prevent recurrences:

- Exercise regularly to strengthen back and abdominal muscles. Walking, swimming, bike riding, and walking in chest-deep water are particularly helpful in building up trunk and thigh muscles.

- Before participating in sports that are recommended by the doctor, warm up by gently stretching for a few minutes to reduce tension and strain.

- Stop smoking. (Some researchers believe that a cigarette smoker's cough may contribute to low back pain by putting pressure on the discs.)

- Lose weight, if necessary, to lessen strain on the back.

- Maintain correct posture. Sit with shoulders back and feet flat on the floor, or on a footstool or chair rung. Stand with head and chest high, neck straight, stomach and buttocks held in, and pelvis forward.

- Use comfortable, supportive seats while driving.

- Use a firm mattress, and sleep on the side with knees drawn up or on the back with a pillow under bent knees.

- Lift by bending at the knees, rather than the waist, using leg muscles to do most of the work.

- Avoid standing or working in any one position for too long. Shift weight from one leg to another.

- Try to reduce emotional stress that causes muscle tension.

—by Evelyn Zamula

Evelyn Zamula is a free-lance writer in Potomac, Md.

Chapter 6

Acute and Chronic Low Back Pain

Some 80% of Americans experience low back pain at some point in their lives, but 90% of them do not seek medical attention.[1]

Of those who suffer low back pain, 80% will improve within 8 weeks, but 80% of them will experience a recurrence. Low back pain rivals the common cold as a leading cause of absenteeism from work.

To understand low back pain, it is useful to envision the spinal elements as a "three-joint complex": a disk and two facet joints at each level. Any changes in one element affect the other two. When a person assumes a normal relaxed, standing position, the vertebral bodies are loosely piled one on the other. When disease affects one of the elements, the intrinsic muscles contract and develop protective splinting to prevent any microinstability that may ensue. They can then become ischemic from prolonged contraction and begin to ache, lose tone, and eventually atrophy.

Lumbar Motion

Man is the only vertebrate that has developed a lumbar lordosis—that is, a forward curvature of the spine. The spine curves in response to the body's attempt to maintain an erect posture; it is not present at birth. Lumbar lordosis is largely due to wedging of the disks, and when it is decreased it usually represents disk degeneration.[1]

Reproduced with permission from *Modern Medicine*, Vol. 60, September 1992. Copyright 1992 by Advanstar Communications, Inc.

Lumbar Hyperlordosis

Hyperlordosis (sway-back) is a well-recognized cause of low back pain. The pain occurs when the anterior longitudinal ligament and facet joints are stretched. Hyperlordosis often develops during pregnancy because of poor abdominal tone. It is aggravated by wearing high-heeled shoes and standing for a prolonged period.[2]

Normally, flexion of the lumbar spine proceeds from L1 sequentially to S1, with each functional unit flexing 8 to 10° totalling 45° of lumbar flexion. Simultaneous pelvic rotation via hip flexion increases the flexion to 135°. When straightening, one derotates the pelvis first.

Rotation of the lumbar spine occurs only at T12-L1 and L4-5. In addition, L4-5 is not protected by the pelvis or the pelvic ligaments, as is L5-S1. Therefore, it is subjected to the greatest load-bearing stress and is most often the first disk involved in acute disk herniation.[3]

Lumbar Muscles

The patient can decrease the strain on the disks by tightening the abdominal muscles to transform the abdominal cavity into a semi-rigid cylinder.[4] If degenerative disease causes intrinsic muscle atrophy, extension is achieved almost exclusively from the gluteii. This puts more traction on the greater trochanter. As a result, there is a higher incidence of bursitis of the greater trochanter in degenerative lumbar spondylosis (a term that includes both degenerative disk and joint disease).

The Disk

The disk is the largest avascular structure in the body. Overall, disk metabolism is very slow and anaerobic. The movement of the nucleus pulposus anteriorly during extension and posteriorly during flexion allows for the flow of nutrients into the disk. This is one of the rationales for prescribing exercise. These movements are progressively lost in degenerative disease.

Disk Hydration

The normal disk is a hydrostatic load-bearing structure. Water makes up about 85% of its center (the nucleus pulposus) and 75% of

its perimeter (the annulus fibrosus). During the day, the water content diminishes to some extent. As a result, an individual can lose up
to three-quarters of an inch in height by evening.

Disk prolapse is less likely to occur during the day because the disk
becomes more elastic as its water content decreases.[5] In the work
place, however, any benefit from the extra elasticity is cancelled by
the fatigue that progressively increases throughout the day.

Shock Absorber

A 150-lb person in a normal erect posture exerts 150 lbs per square
inch of pressure on the disk. A normal disk can withstand pressures
of up to 700 psi before rupturing. However, a vertebral end plate will
fracture before that. This is why young persons usually do not suffer
from herniated disks. Therefore, before a prolapse can occur, the patient must already have preexisting disk disease.

Disk pressure doubles from the supine (1 atmosphere) to the sitting position (2 atmospheres) because the disks sit anteriorly and the
entire body weight is shifted over the disks. When a person is standing, approximately one-third of his body weight is shifted posteriorly
onto the facet joints, thus dropping the pressure to 1.50 atmospheres.[6]
Bending in either a sitting or standing position increases diskal pressure by 50%. Using an armrest to get out of a chair can decrease
intradiskal pressure by up to 30%.

The annulus fibrosus is made up of approximately 20 concentric
bands axially; these fibers criss-cross at 45° sagittally. Flexion and
rotation (rotary torque) predispose to disk damage. The annulus is
weakest at the posterolateral corners, the usual site of disk herniation
and nerve root compromise. The nucleus pulposus, which makes up
one-quarter of the disk's volume, sits more posteriorly.

Aging

The nucleus pulposus changes into fibrocartilage from the second
decade on. The loss of elasticity allows shearing forces to cross the
disk unopposed. In addition, annular fibers can undergo localized
myxomatous degeneration. This can lead to an osmotic gradient with
the formation of a cyst within the annulus.[7-8] This cyst can slowly
enlarge and produce atraumatic disk bulging with consequent clinical signs and symptoms (Figure 6.1).

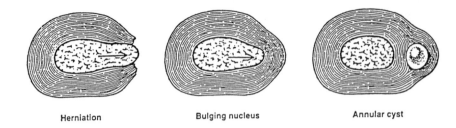

Herniation   Bulging nucleus   Annular cyst

Figure 6.1. *Disk herniation and bulging. The nucleus can herniate or an annular "cyst" can bulge. Usually an annular tear results in a bulging disk.*

Disk Prolapse

Before a prolapse of the nucleus pulposus can occur, the patient must have already experienced circumferential tears that weaken the annulus enough so that the next traumatic episode produces a radial tear. In most of these cases, this results in a bulging disk. The exception occurs when the radial tear extends through Sharpey's fibers. As a result, there is a herniated disk that can separate as a free fragment. In summary, the nucleus can herniate or bulge, or an annular "cyst" can bulge (Figure 6.1).

Clinical Findings

Degenerative disk disease can cause backache, referred pain, or radicular pain. Degenerative joint disease produces the same pain as degenerative disk disease. As a disk degenerates, its height decreases, which causes pressure across the facet joints to increase. Therefore, both disk and joint disease are eventually present together. "Degenerative lumbar spondylosis" refers to both. Therefore, degenerative disk disease can lead to degenerative joint disease and vice versa. When both the disk and the joint become involved, the pain cannot be separated clinically.

Types of Pain

Referred pain produces a sclerotomal distribution of pain (Figure 6.2). This type of pain is similar, although not identical, to the radicular or dermatomal distribution (Figure 6.3). It is not true that referred pain radiates only as far down as the knee and that radicular pain radiates only below the knee. In fact, the only distinguishing feature between the two types of pain is in their quality. Referred pain is an aching or sore type of pain, while radicular pain is a sharp, lancinating, or burning type of pain.

There are four known causes of radicular pain (although the exact mechanism of nerve root compromise is not known):

- direct mechanical compression of the nerve (neuritis)
- compression of the vasa nervorum, which can produce ischemia
- venous obstruction
- chemical irritation of the dural sleeve, which causes inflammation (duritis)

Spinal Osteophytosis

Spinal osteophytosis, a normal function of aging, can be seen on an x-ray. It is produced by traction of the spinal ligaments on the periosteum of the vertebral bodies. It is not related to degenerative lumbar spondylosis.

In spinal osteophytosis, the disk spaces are well preserved. The condition appears to be worse on the right side, probably due to inhibition of spur formation by the pulsating aorta along the left side. Some 90% of men older than 50 have some of these traction osteophytes in the lumbar area.

DISH

When spinal osteophytosis is excessive, it may represent a forme fruste of diffuse idiopathic skeletal hyperostosis (DISH), an ossifying diathesis of ligaments and tendons throughout the patient's body. DISH begins with ossification of the anterior longitudinal ligament of the dorsal spine, and then spreads to the cervical and lumbar spine. It is associated with widespread osteoarthritis as well as spurs where the ligaments and tendons attach to bone (enthesopathy). DISH is typically found in middle-aged men, 80% of whom appear to have adult-onset diabetes. It is also seen as a side effect of isotretinoin (Accutane) and excessive fluorine intake.

Complications

Spinal Stenosis

Degenerative spinal stenosis occurs when facet osteophytes narrow the canal posteriorly and disk bulging narrows the canal anteriorly.[9]

Obstruction of the epidural venous plexus during walking causes varicosities that impinge on the neural foramina and in turn produce neurogenic claudication. The normal buckling of the ligamentum flavum into the spinal canal during standing decreases the volume of an already compromised canal. The obstruction is aggravated by an increased venous return of blood secondary to activity. Neurogenic claudication produces thigh pain spreading distally; vascular

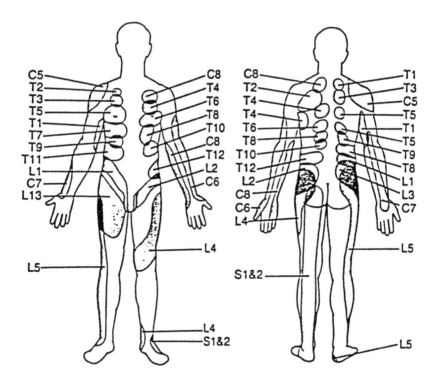

Figure 6.2. Sclerotomal distribution of pain.

claudication produces foot pain spreading proximally. Neurogenic claudication is lessened by climbing stairs, walking uphill, and riding a bicycle because the spine tends to be flexed during these three activities.

Vascular claudication causes aching and cramping. It does not cause the neuropathic pain that is generated by spinal stenosis claudication.

Spondylolisthesis

Degenerative spondylolisthesis is a slippage of the vertebral body without the lysis defect in the pars interarticularis. It is caused by subluxation of degenerated joints (Figure 6.4). Spondylolisthesis almost always occurs at L4-5.

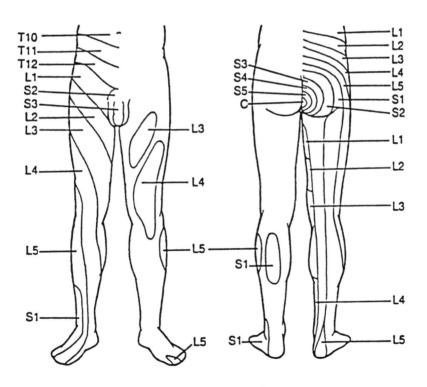

Figure 6.3. *Radicular or dermatomal distribution of pain.*

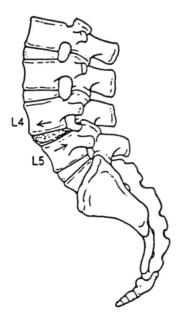

Figure 6.4. Degenerative spondylolisthesis.

Scoliosis

Degenerative scoliosis is a mild scoliosis that is caused by an uneven narrowing on one side of the disk. The scoliosis tends to be primarily rotatory.

Physical Diagnosis

History

The history reveals most of the clues to the correct diagnosis. For example:

- If the pain worsens while the patient is sitting, the probable diagnosis is disk disease.
- If the patient is most uncomfortable while standing, the facet joints are implicated.
- If the pain is aggravated by walking, the cause is most likely spinal stenosis.

- If the pain is worst when the patient is recumbent, you should consider that a space-occupying lesion is the reason.

Physical Exam

During acute pain, muscle spasm will lateralize to the side of the pathology, occasionally producing a pelvic tilt. The maintenance of lordosis at any point between L1 and S1 on flexion indicates a lack of motion and localizes the pathology.

Another cause of low back pain is often unequal leg lengths. This can be measured from the anterior superior iliac spine to the medial malleolus bilaterally.

Tests

A number of tests can assist in making the diagnosis:

- The *straight-leg-raising* (SLR) test for radiculopathy is positive when pain is produced between 30 and 60°. (When a patient's leg is raised less than 30°, no stretch is produced; when it is raised more than 60°, even mechanical pain can produce a positive result.) The SLR is useful for the L4-5 and L5-S1 disks only. Some 98% of herniated disks involve these two levels.

- The *femoral stretch* test for disk disease at L2-4 is performed by flexing the knee while the patient is in the prone position with the hip extended. Older individuals have a higher risk of disk herniation at these upper lumbar levels.[1]

- The *FABER* (for flexion, abduction, and external rotation of the hip) test is useful for localizing the source of pain in the lumbar region if the hip and the S1 joint can be excluded.

Neurologic Exam

Reflexes that have been lost during a previous episode of lumbar radiculopathy rarely return, even when there has been full motor recovery. The same is true for the finding of radiculopathy on electromyelography (EMG); once it is present, it may be permanent. This can lead to an overinterpretation of the EMG on the physical exam during subsequent attacks of low back pain. An experienced neurologist can usually distinguish acute changes from chronic ones on EMG.

Differential Diagnosis

Mechanical Pain

Another cause of mechanical back pain is a compression fracture secondary to trauma or osteopenia. Its acute onset and the severity of the pain should raise your index of suspicion.

Systemic Arthritic Pain

Systemic inflammatory back pain is characterized by morning stiffness for at least 1 hour. The pain is worsened by rest and relieved by activity. The onset of systemic inflammatory back pain is usually insidious. Sometimes there is a family history of this condition. On exam, the straight-leg-raising test will usually be normal. Fever, at least at the onset, adds infection to the differential.

Referred Pain

Referred back pain from a visceral source is usually not worsened by positional changes, as is mechanical low back pain.

Radiology

X-Rays

Plain x-rays are not necessary to diagnose acute low lumbar pain unless the pain is associated with objective radiculopathy.[10] The chance of finding any significant additional information is too small. In my practice, we obtain x-rays only when the pain has lasted beyond a month.

But, again, there are times when x-rays are necessary:

- *Trauma*, of course, requires films to determine if there is any fracture, subluxation, or soft tissue mass.
- *Systemic symptoms*—for example, morning stiffness, weight loss, or fever—also necessitate x-rays.

- X-rays are needed when there is the possibility of a *developmental* or *heritable* condition in a young person.
- When *facet arthritis* is a consideration, oblique films should be included in the survey.

Bone Scans

When back pain remains unexplained, a bone scan should be ordered. In addition, bone scans are indicated when considering inflammatory, neoplastic, metabolic, and traumatic conditions. Early ankylosing spondylitis or osteomyelitis, which cannot be detected on plain radiographs, may very well be detected on a bone scan. Bone scans may also detect osteomalacia and osteoporotic stress fractures that are missed on an x-ray.

CT Scans

CT is an excellent source for detecting bony abnormalities. Degenerative facet joint disease is appreciated best on CT. It is also very good for disk disease.

MRI

Magnetic resonance imaging shows not only the severity of the disk disease, but also its extent. This is because MRI surveys the entire lumbar spine, not just a portion of it, as does CT.

MRI also has an advantage over CT in that it allows for three-dimensional visualization. In addition, MRI is emerging as the technique of choice for diagnosing multilevel spinal stenosis.

Myelography has all but been replaced by MRI, which is less invasive. There are a number of "herniated" disks found on MRI in absolutely asymptomatic persons. Therefore, it is necessary to carefully correlate the MRI findings with the clinical signs and symptoms.

It is important to be familiar with the costs of the various radiographic techniques so that you can order studies more efficiently. In my community, for example, lumbar spine films with obliques cost approximately $300. A bone scan is about $600, a myelogram around $750, and a CT of the lumbar spine about $900. An MRI is almost $1,200 but insurance reimbursement (Blue Cross/Blue Shield and Medicare) averages only 50%. Insurance companies reimburse 80 to 90% for the other procedures.

References

1. Frymoyer JW. Back pain and sciatica. *N Engl J Med* 1988; 318:291-300.
2. Cailliet R. Low back pain. *South Med J* 1969;62:1459-62.
3. Uloka G, Hendrix M. The lumbar disk: Evaluating the causes of pain. *Orthopedics* 1991;14:419-29.
4. King A. Functional anatomy of the lumbar spine. *Orthopedics* 1983; 6:1588-91.
5. Adams M, Dolan P, Hutton WC, Porter RW. Diurnal changes in spinal mechanics and their clinical significance. *J Bone Joint Surg* (Br) 1990;72B:266-70.
6. Nachemson AL. The load on lumbar disks in different positions of the body. *Clin Orthop* 1966;45:107-22.
7. Yasuma T, Essei M, Shiu S, et. al. Histologic development of intervertebral disk herniation. *J Bone Joint Surg* (Am) 1986;68A:1066-72.
8. Yasuma T, Sadao K, Toyoi O, et. el. Histologic changes in aging lumber intervertebral disks. *J Bone Joint Surg* (Am) 1990;72A:220-9.
9. Hall Bartleson J, Onofrio B, et. al. Lumbar spinal stenosis: Clinical features, diagnostic procedures, and results of surgical treatment in 68 patients. *Ann Intern Med* 1985;103:271-5.
10. Gehweiler JA, Daffenr RH. Low back pain: The controversy of radiologic evaluation. *AJR Am J Roentgenol* 1983;140:109-12.

How to Treat, When to Refer

Probably the most important initial therapeutic maneuver that you can offer your patient is instructions on performing and restricting daily activities during exacerbations and intercritical periods of back pain. An inadequate explanation is the greatest source of patient dissatisfaction with their care.[1]

To reduce stress on the disk, standing is preferable to sitting. The patient should avoid bending and twisting. When the patient *is* sitting, he or she can maintain lordosis by using a lumbar roll and keeping the knees above hip level. Using armrests when rising from a sitting to a standing position is also helpful. Women should avoid wearing high-heeled shoes, which can cause hyperlordosis and aggravate pain.

The patient can avoid muscle fatigue and spasm by changing positions frequently. For example, during a long automobile trip, ideally the patient should stop every half hour to stretch. Such hyperextension forces the nucleus pulposus anterior in the disk. At home, sitting in a rocking chair allows for constant, slight changes in position.

Physical Therapy

Heat

Thermal therapy is analgesic. Ice is preferred for acute pain, and heat is preferred for chronic pain. Heat eases muscle spasm, raises the pain threshold, and reduces joint stiffness. Superficial heat in the form of moist packs or electric pads is sufficient.

Deep heat in the form of ultrasound or short-wave diathermy has not been demonstrated to be more effective than superficial heat. Moreover, ultrasound is contraindicated over portions of the spinal cord that have been exposed by a laminectomy.

TENS

Transcutaneous electric nerve stimulation (TENS) operates on the "gate control" theory of analgesia. Nonnoxious electric stimuli travel to the dorsal horn of the spinal cord and stimulate inhibitory neurones that block incoming noxious stimuli. TENS is an effective analgesic for both acute low back pain and radiculopathy. On the other hand, for chronic lumbar pain, it may be no better than placebo.[2]

Supports

The use of lumbosacral supports can decrease pressure on the disks by 30%.[3] They also reinforce the abdominal muscles and relieve any single muscle from bearing the brunt of the force in a particular position. But prolonged use can promote deconditioning. Therefore, lumbosacral supports should be used only for specific activities and/or periods of time, such as late in the day when the patient is apt to become fatigued.

I like supports, especially when degenerative joint disease is the primary cause of symptoms. Supports accomplish the same goal as splints for any peripheral osteoarthritic joint. I do not prescribe braces for uncomplicated degenerative spondylosis because putting them on and taking them off are counterproductive; they tend to excessively restrict normal mobility.

Traction

Traction is supposed to distract opposing vertebral end plates, thus retracting bulging disks. I do not favor using it because with horizontal traction, 50% of a person's body weight is needed to reduce disk herniation and an additional 40 to 60 lbs is needed just to overcome the friction of the bed sheets. Obviously, this is not practical, so the use of inpatient pelvic traction has all but been eliminated.

Inversion therapy, a form of gravity traction, has some proponents. It is potentially hazardous to glaucoma and hypertensive patients. Thus far, inversion therapy has not been studied in controlled trials.

Exercise

In general, exercise increases the endorphin effect, decreases illness behavior, and prevents deconditioning.

Knee-to-chest exercises improve abdominal muscle tone. They stretch the paravertebral muscles, they relieve spastic muscles, and they feel good. The pelvic tilt and the half sit-up with the knees bent are abdominal isometrics. However, McKenzie's philosophy of exercising emphasizes that the extensor muscles are more important in preventing back pain.[4] In an acute situation, McKenzie's exercises "centralize" the pain by hyperextension posturing. Both flexion and extension should be employed.

Once patients can perform these exercises without difficulty, they can replace them with endurance activities, such as swimming, bicycling, and walking. The final step is aerobic conditioning, which improves fitness and prevents further back injury.

In the work place, patients who have chronic or recurrent low back problems should learn to "work to quota, not to tolerance"—that is, they should work until they are just short of developing pain and then rest, rather than working until pain begins and then rewarding themselves by resting.

Manipulation

Manipulation is a high-velocity, thrusting maneuver that is so rapid that reflex muscle contraction is momentarily inhibited. There is a lack of evidence that manipulation provides anything more than temporary relief,[5] but it does appear to shorten the recovery time of acute back pain.[6] Manipulation is relatively contraindicated in the presence of radiculopathy because it can worsen it.[7]

Nevertheless, overall patient satisfaction with chiropractors appears to be much greater than it is with physicians.

Bed Rest

A useful prescription for the patient who has acute lumbar disk pain is bed rest for 2 days, preferably in the semi-Fowler's position (head of the bed raised with the knees and hips flexed).

Minimizing bed rest will prevent muscle atrophy, illness behavior, bone loss, and cardiovascular deconditioning. By the third day, the patient should be able to stand and walk (but not sit). By the end of a week, the patient should be walking 20 minutes for every 3 hours of rest.[1] When the patient is able to sit comfortably, then he or she can begin performing endurance exercises.

Others

Massage, acupuncture, and acupressure may relieve pain by increasing endogenous endorphins.

Drug Therapy

NSAIDs

Nonsteroidal anti-inflammatory drugs are the mainstay of the management of degenerative lumbar spondylosis. Degenerative joint disease in the spine is no different from that in the peripheral joints. Moreover, synovitis is best controlled with NSAIDs. They are also good analgesics for the somatic pain that disk disease causes. You can even find a role for their use in nerve root irritation, which causes a "duritis."

Steroids

Radiculopathy is relieved by administration of epidural steroid injections. Steroid injections are associated with an 85% short-term pain relief, which in turn shortens hospital stays and lessens dependence on narcotic analgesics. They should be tried before you resort to surgery.

Epidural steroids are also very useful for the treatment of chronic radiculopathy. One study has shown that 34% of patients experience relief of pain that lasts more than 6 months.[8] Steroid injections, then, are an important part of the conservative management of spinal stenosis.

Facet-joint steroid injections should work in those individuals who have degenerative joint disease. Unfortunately, they are not helpful clinically because there are always more than one facet joint involved, and each must be injected individually under fluoroscopic control. This also becomes extremely time-consuming and impractical. Trigger-point injections, however, are very easy to administer, and they often afford significant relief of symptoms.

Antidepressants

Radicular pain can also be controlled with low-dose tricyclic antidepressants—for example, amitriptyline HCl (Elavil, Endep, et. al.) at 25 to 100 mg nightly. Tricyclics increase the amount of available serotonin in the spinal column, thus stimulating the release of enkephalin in the dorsal horn of the patient's spinal cord. They are classified as psychoactive analgesics and are not addictive agents.

Muscle Relaxants

The muscle relaxant cyclobenzaprine HCl (Flexeril) is related to amitriptyline and probably exerts its beneficial effect in the same way. The other muscle relaxants probably afford relief by their sedative effect.

Analgesics

When narcotic analgesics are needed for acute pain, they should be used for only a few days at most. Then you should switch to non-narcotic analgesics.

Psychosocial Factors

There are a number of factors that independently contribute to an unfavorable response to therapy.

A patient can use pain as a weapon to manage his life or another's. Other individuals find a form of prestige in being the sick member of the family. Sometimes family members will reinforce pain behavior by providing attention and sympathy.

Another unfavorable factor is drug abuse. Chronic pain, of course, can lead to drug-seeking behavior. The pain then becomes a form of secondary gain to receive narcotics.

The presence of pending legal action is a tip-off to most of us that the patient may be using symptoms to obtain money or to avoid responsibilities. It is almost impossible for this individual to get well during litigation.

Many patients will have unrealistic expectations of getting well. The physician is responsible for preventing unrealistic hopes by explaining to the patient exactly what to expect, not only from the condition itself but from the treatment as well.

Another unfavorable factor is somatization. Patients often internalize their anxiety and stress and develop physical complaints such as low back pain. Finally, there is depression, which is just as often the result of chronic back pain as it is the cause of it.

When the Time Is Right to Refer for Surgery

If, after 6 weeks to 3 months, conservative treatment fails, you should consider referring your patient for surgery. By 6 weeks, most of those patients who respond to medical therapy will have done so. Beyond 3 months, the chance of recovery decreases.

For a herniated lumbar disk, the primary indication for surgery is persistent radiculopathy for a least 1 month. Two exceptions to this guideline are the cauda equina syndrome and progressive neurologic deficit.[9] No more than 10% of patients who have unrelenting sciatica eventually require an operation.

The benefits of surgery last for only 2 years. After that, patients who are operated on do not significantly differ from those who are treated conservatively. After 4 years, back pain will recur in 15% of patients.

Basically, there are three different surgical procedures: laminectomy, disk excision, and fusion—plus combinations thereof. Surgery for chronic degenerative disease is reserved for degenerative spinal stenosis. Laminectomy has been the procedure of choice for patients who have unrelenting pain. However, a recent study of a long follow-up was disappointing.[10]

If the primary care physician provides his patients with a good conservative program and education, they will know what to expect, and 95% of patients will respond to conservative treatment.

References

1. Deyo R, Loser J, Bigos S. Herniated lumbar intervertebral disk. *Ann Intern Med* 1990;112:598-603.
2. Frymoyer JW. Back pain and sciatica. *N Engl J Med* 1988; 318:291-300.
3. Nachemson AL. Mechanical Effectiveness studies of lumbar spin orthoses. *Scand J Rehabil Med Suppl* 1983;9:139-49.
4. McKenzie R. Exercises. In: *The lumbar spine: Mechanical diagnosis and therapy*. Upper Hutt. New Zealand: Spinal Publications. 1981.
5. Laslett M. Use of manipulative therapy for mechanical pain of spinal origin. *Orthop Rev* 1987;16:573-81.
6. Swezey R. The modern thrust of manipulation and traction therapy. *Semin Arthritis Rheum* 1983;12:322-3.
7. Jayson M (ed). The lumbar spine and back pain (Third ed). New York: Churchill Livingston. 1987.
8. Cuckler JM, Bernini P, Wiesel S, et. al. Use of epidural steroids in the treatment of lumbar radicular pain. *J Bone Joint Surg* (Am) 1985;67A:63-6.
9. Kostuik J, Harrington I, Alexander G, et. al. Cauda equina syndrome and lumbar disk herniation. *J Bone Joint Surg* (Am) 1986;68A:386-91.
10. Lipson S. Outcome of decompressive laminectomy for degenerative lumbar stenosis. *J Bone Joint Surg* (Am) 1991;73A: 809-16.

—by Burton Sack, MD

Dr. Sack is on the staff of the Departments of Internal Medicine at Brockton (Mass.) Hospital and Boston University Hospital.

Chapter 7

Sciatica

Contrary to popular belief, sciatica, a symptom of lumbar disk herniation, is relatively uncommon. Characteristics include pain in the posterior thigh, lower leg, or foot that is greater than accompanying low-back pain. Sciatic tension tests confirm the presence of sciatica by reproducing the pain. Many patients who have sciatica recover spontaneously; most others can be treated conservatively with limitation of activity, anti-inflammatory medication, and gradual return to full activity. A variety of surgical options are available for patients who have extruded disks and progressive neurologic deficit or severe, persistent, intolerable pain.

The term *sciatica* has been used since antiquity to refer to pain arising from the hip or thigh (ischiatica). More specifically, sciatica is a symptom that most commonly occurs when a herniated lumbar disk compresses one of the contributing roots of the sciatic nerve. Patients who have sciatica usually have low-back pain in addition to leg pain along the distribution of the sciatic nerve.

Sports and recreational injuries that cause back and leg pain are extraordinarily common. In contrast, true sciatica is relatively uncommon. Yet, because back and leg pain are common among active people and causes may be elusive, physicians often incorrectly label the pain as sciatica. The challenge to physicians is to distinguish radicular pain (caused by an inflamed nerve root) from referred pain (referred from its musculoskeletal origin to other tissues within a sclerotome). Treatment

"Sciatica: Treating a Painful Symptom," *The Physician and Sportsmedicine*, January 1992. Reprinted with permission.

options for patients who have herniated disks or sciatica are controversial; however, correct diagnosis is clearly key to the management decision.

Striking Symptom

The hallmark feature of sciatica is pain in the posterior thigh, lower leg, or foot that is greater than the low-back pain that may accompany it. Typically, patients complain of moderate to severe pain radiating from the buttock down into the leg and foot. Even the most stoic patients may be immobilized by this pain. Patients often give a history of acute low-back pain that began a few days or weeks prior to the leg pain; the leg pain becomes worse than the back pain, which subsides and in some cases nearly disappears. If patients have low-back pain that is greater than that in their legs, the physician should question a diagnosis of herniated disk.

Pain in the buttock, thigh, or lower back alone, with little or no discomfort at or below the knee, is also unusual with a herniated disk. Pain above the knee may instead be caused by irritation of the facets, posterior longitudinal ligament, or the periosteum of the vertebrae. One caveat here, however: Beware the changing character of long-standing sciatica. With time the patient may have a vague aching pain that does not reach the lower leg or foot. The early symptoms over the first few weeks, however, should clearly include pain to or below the knee.

Often no specific trauma, or only a trivial event such as bending over, elicits sciatica. Standing, sitting, lifting, and straining may aggravate it, while lying down—especially with the affected hip extended and the knee flexed—is usually the most comfortable position. Sciatica may have a waxing and waning course with episodic acute aggravation.

Paresthesia, weakness, and diminished bowel or bladder function may accompany sciatica. When present, paresthesia is radicular and roughly follows a dermatomal distribution. The degree of weakness in the affected leg varies from patient to patient. Generally, only patients who have massive paramedian or central herniations have diminished bowel or bladder function.

Identifying True Nerve Compression

Although sciatica may have a variable course and patients may be more or less symptomatic at the time of examination, physicians can still usually use physical signs to identify true nerve compression caused by a large disk herniation.

Posture may be the first physical sign that indicates sciatica. Typically, patients who have sciatica will limp. They have paravertebral muscle spasm, and they have postural lower lumbar scoliosis and flattening of lumbar lordosis induced by listing to relieve pressure on the nerve. For these patients, sitting is more difficult and painful than standing. When they do sit, they slouch to avoid flexing their hips.

A thorough neurologic examination of the lower extremities reveals other physical signs of sciatica. Weakness of the ankle dorsiflexors and of the great toe extensor indicates compression of the L5 nerve root caused by an L4-L5 disk herniation. Weakness of the ankle plantar flexors and toe flexors indicates compression of the first sacral root caused by an L5-S1 herniation. Weakness at several vertebral levels indicates a large midline or far lateral disk herniation.

Sciatic Tension Signs

In addition to these physical signs, physicians can use manipulative maneuvers to reproduce sciatic pain, a key finding in the neurologic examination. The straight leg raise (SLR), or Lasegue's sign,[1] distinguishes sciatica from disease of the hip joint. However, a positive SLR alone is not definitive. Other maneuvers that reproduce pain along the sciatic nerve can be used to confirm the results of the SLR.

Lasegue's sign. Physicians can perform the SLR by slowly lifting the patient's affected leg while keeping his or her knee in extension. The SLR is positive for sciatica when performing it reproduces or aggravates leg or buttock pain on the patient's affected side.[1] Aggravation of low-back pain alone is not positive for sciatica. Tightness in a patient's hamstring, caused by natural tone and tension, will ultimately limit the SLR. To differentiate hamstring stretch pain from sciatic pain, physicians must compare results of the SLR from the affected leg with those of the unaffected leg.

Ankle Dorsiflexion with SLR. While performing the SLR, physicians can lower the patient's leg back down from the height where the test is positive to a height at which the patient feels relief from the pain. With the patient's leg at this height, the physician dorsiflexes the ipsilateral foot. If the patient has sciatica, the sciatic pain is again aggravated.

Bowstring Test Similarly. When a patient's SLR is positive, the physician can relieve the sciatic stretch and the pain by bending the affected leg slightly at the knee. The physician can then press on the point where the sciatic nerve crosses the popliteal space, thereby stretching the nerve again and recreating the sciatic pain.

Contralateral SLR. The contralateral SLR may also elicit pain in a patient's affected leg. Positive results for this test, the most specific for disk herniation, may indicate posterior medial herniation.

Femoral Nerve Stretch Test. This test stretches the femoral nerve and upper lumbar roots. When the patient is prone, holding his or her affected leg flexed 90° at the knee, the physician elevates the patient's thigh. Pain elicited in the anterior thigh is considered a positive result. However, the test may elicit the sciatica (i.e., posterior leg pain) on the affected side, particularly if the disk lesion is at the L4-L5 level.[2]

Diagnostic Studies

Unless symptoms are persistent, severe, or atypical, most patients who have sciatica do not need x-rays or other imaging studies of the intervertebral disks, spinal canal, and neural elements for the first month of their first episode. Imaging is usually done early only if the diagnosis is in question or if the patient is considering surgery. Occasionally, in cases involving professional athletes or compensation for a work-related injury, imaging studies may be done for medicolegal reasons, such as proper documentation and immediate prognosis. But for most patients who have sciatica, further evaluation is not urgent.

Psychosocial evaluation is indicated when patients complain of atypical features or persistent and unusual disability. Laboratory evaluation may be dictated by concurrent medical problems. Also, bladder function symptoms may require urodynamic and urologic studies.

When imaging studies are indicated, magnetic resonance imaging (MRI) is slightly more accurate than computed tomography (CT) myelography for detecting disk herniation (determined by comparing MRI and CT diagnoses with actual surgical findings), and it has no known side effects.[3] However, some patients cannot tolerate the confined space of the MRI scanner, and some patients are too large. For these individuals, a CT myelogram is indicated,[4] CT scanning without contrast is less accurate.

MRI may also be better for detecting the cause of recurrent post-operative sciatica.[5] One study[6] showed Gd-DTPA-enhanced MRI to be very accurate for differentiating between epidural scar (which is not usually amenable to surgery) and recurrent disk herniation (which is). This distinction cannot be made by CT scan.

Note that correlation of radiographic with clinical findings is essential for accurate diagnosis. For example, a study[7] using MRI, CT myelogram, or myelogram alone has demonstrated varying degrees of disk herniation in 20% to 40% of asymptomatic patients. When there is poor correlation among symptoms, signs, and imaging studies, electrophysiologic studies, including conduction velocities and electromyelography, may help to define the area of neural compression.

If Not Herniation, Then What?

The differential diagnosis for back and leg pain includes many uncommon conditions. Most of these conditions cause referred pain without involvement of the sciatic nerve or its roots. A careful history and physical may reveal such conditions: Details of the assessment can differentiate various forms of pain from true sciatica and the diagnosis of lumbar disk herniation.

For example, steady unremitting pain should alert physicians to causes such as tumors or infection. Bilateral radicular pain is very rare with disk herniation and should alert physicians to intrathecal pathology needing urgent investigation.[8]

Mechanical or degenerative lumbar processes, such as spondylolysis or spondylolisthesis, may mimic sciatica. In these conditions pain is *referred* to the hip or thigh without actual nerve root involvement. Referred pain rarely radiates below the knee in these conditions. In addition, the distribution of referred pain is generally not strictly dermatomal, nor is it generally associated with neurologic findings such as weakness.

Differential diagnoses must also include hip and knee conditions such as arthritides or fracture, making careful examination of the patient's hip and knee essential. Other less common conditions to look for include pelvic or psoas abscess, herpes zoster infection, and stress fracture of the ischium or femoral neck. Sensory changes in the lower extremity, including dysesthesia, may indicate multiple sclerosis.

Less frequently, true inflammation of the sciatic nerve itself may be caused by conditions other than disk herniation. Intrapelvic lesions that may cause sciatica include endometriosis, aneurysm and infection.

Other causes of irritation include space-occupying lesions at the sciatic notch, as well as distal nerve entrapment, usually of the common peroneal nerve around the fibular head.

Finally, in patients older than 50, spinal stenosis may cause compression of the cauda equina and exiting roots of the lumbar nerves, resulting in neurogenic claudication and various degrees of radiculopathy. Spinal stenosis is characterized by bilateral symptoms that worsen with activity and spinal extension but improve with sitting and spinal flexion. Physical findings such as weakness are uncommon with spinal stenosis, as are sciatic tension signs.

Choosing Effective Treatment

The progression of sciatica depends on the size of the herniation and the space available in the canal or foramen. Most patients recover spontaneously. Even people who have severe sciatica and large herniations usually improve over the first several weeks to months.

Physicians caring for such patients should try to prevent overtreating this self-limited symptom. Most patients respond well to a brief period of limitation of activity, anti-inflammatory medication, and gradual return to full activity. A physician's optimistic approach can go a long way toward minimizing the patient's fears and disability.

The minority of patients who are severely affected or who do not improve over the first 1 to 2 weeks may benefit from a short course of bed rest (not to exceed 3 days and rarely if ever to exceed 7 to 10 days) and assisted rehabilitation.

The severity of symptoms will usually determine the degree of limitation of activities. For some patients, general conditioning exercises, including abdominal and paraspinal muscle strengthening and stretching, are the mainstays of treatment.

Other treatments are widely used but have not been proved beneficial. These include traction, weight loss, graduated exercise programs, epidural steroids, trigger point injections, "back school," and passive physical therapy (ultrasound, diathermy, and hot packs).[9]

Some modalities are better substantiated in controlled studies than are others. These include analgesics, restricted activity, bed rest (which may not be beneficial if it's for less than 2 days), and transcutaneous electrical nerve stimulation (TENS).[9] However, Deyo et al.[10] have recently reported that TENS is no better than a sham stimulation in relief of low-back pain. The study included 145 subjects, 61 men and 84 women, aged 18 to 70.

In some studies, spinal manipulation promoted short-term pain relief for low-back pain[11] and helped in a few reported cases of sciatica.[12,13] However, careful controlled studies remain to be done in this area. Gallinaro and Cartesegna[14] report that acute disk herniation has occurred as a rare complication of spinal manipulation.

Although exercise has not been proven effective in controlling pain, it does enhance general conditioning and helps restore function—and restored function is the first step toward a return to work. Many authors[15,16] recommend general and specific spinal exercises after an initial period of rest to allow the inflamed sciatic nerve or nerve roots to recover sufficiently.

Some authors believe bed rest is not advisable. Instead they advocate training patients to find a "neutral spine" position of least pain, and then begin progressive exercises as tolerated. Such conditioning may rebuild trunk strength and improve the mechanics and efficiency of body movement.[17]

To Operate or Not to Operate?

Indications for surgery—and its effectiveness—are controversial. For example, Weber[18] compared surgically and nonsurgically treated patients and demonstrated that those who had surgery generally did better in the first year. After 4 years, however, the surgical group fared only slightly better than nonsurgical cohorts, and this difference was not statistically significant.

Nevertheless, it is clear that surgical decompression may substantially reduce morbidity among the small percentage of sciatica patients who get worse or simply do not improve with time. Patients who don't respond to nonoperative treatment may have relative spinal stenosis, which may require decompression at the time of diskectomy.[17]

In a recent report by Saal and Saal,[17] about 85% of 58 nonoperatively treated sciatica patients had an "excellent" or "good" recovery and returned to work in 3 to 5 months. Fifty percent of study subjects reported needing only 1 week of sick leave. However, for study subjects who had extruded disks, loss of work time was much greater for nonoperatively treated patients.

Indications for surgery among patients who have sciatica may be either absolute or relative. The two absolute indications are cauda equina syndrome, which is characterized by loss of bladder or bowel function (with or without a saddle distribution of anesthesia), and progressive neurologic deficit, characterized by increasing weakness in the affected dermatome or worsening foot drop. This latter indication is somewhat controversial. Patients who do not have absolute indications for surgical decompression should undertake 8 to 12 weeks of nonoperative therapy. Relative indications for surgery include continued symptoms after this 3-month trial of conservative treatment, as well as severe, persistent, intolerable pain that significantly interferes with daily living.

Patients who have significant weakness may not recover as well if treated surgically later than 3 months after the onset of symptoms. Patient selection is the most important factor in surgical success. Surgery is most successful for patients who have:

- Physical examinations positive for sciatica, including a positive SLR, a positive contralateral SLR, and weakness.

- Imaging studies that correlate with physical findings.

- Appropriate psychological score[19] determined as part of a standard preoperative workup for disk herniation patients.

- No significant psychosocial factors such as pending litigation, worker's compensation proceedings, financial incentive to remain injured, depression, prolonged narcotic use, or unsatisfactory prior back surgery.

Evaluating Surgical Options

When surgery is deemed to be the treatment of choice for a patient who has sciatica, several options are available.

Simple Diskectomy

This procedure requires the exposure of 2 to 3 vertebral levels. To expose the disk the surgeon removes 1 to 2 cm^2 of lamina above and below the herniation, then curettes the disk space to remove as much of the nucleus pulposus as possible. The procedure may involve foramenotomy, with removal of some of the inferior facet and medial pedicle.

Limited Diskectomy

This is similar to simple diskectomy, except the surgeon removes only the herniated portion of the disk, leaving the remainder of the disk intact. With carefully selected patients, the success rate for this procedure is about 90%.[20]

Microsurgical Lumbar Diskectomy

This procedure is performed through a limited incision, using an operating microscope. The initial results of the procedure may be similar to those of standard diskectomy.[21] Proponents report shorter hospital stays and less surgical trauma and scarring. Critics note the difficulty in adequately decompressing lateral recess stenosis with such a limited approach. Others[22] consider stenosis a contraindication. Fager[23] reports a higher rate of intraoperative complications such as dural tears and diskitis with this procedure (compared to standard simple diskectomy).

Percutaneous Diskectomy

Like microsurgical lumbar diskectomy, this is a controversial procedure. Some authors report a 75% success rate or higher,[24] while critics report that among patients who qualify for it (those who have contained disk protrusions, not extruded or sequestered), the recovery rate with no surgical intervention is also 75%.[17,18] At best, this procedure is most suited to the L4-L5 disk space. Sequestered disks and spinal stenosis are relative contraindications for this procedure.

Chymopapain

In a double-blind study,[25] treatment with chymopapain was successful in about 65% to 75% of cases. These data indicate chymopapain is superior to placebo, but treatment with it can have devastating, though rare, complications such as anaphylaxis, disk infection, epidural adhesions, or transverse myelitis. For this reason, chymopapain nucleolysis has not been commonly performed in recent years.

Prompt Relief

Active people often seek medical care for shooting pain in their backs or legs. The ability to determine whether a patient's pain is radicular or referred enables the physician to distinguish mechanical low-back and leg pain from sciatica, the painful symptom of lumbar disk herniation. With the diagnosis in hand, the physician can promptly and effectively treat patients who have sciatica, choosing from a variety of treatment options.

References

1. Pearce JM: Lasegue's sign, letter; *Lancet* 1989;1(8635):436.

2. Christodoulides AN: Ipsilateral sciatica on femoral nerve stretch test is pathognomonic of an L4/5 disk protrusion. *J Bone Joint Surg* (Br) 1989;71(1):88-89.

3. Forristall RM, Marsh HO, Pay NT: Magnetic resonance imaging and contrast CT of the lumbar spine: comparison of diagnostic methods and correlation with surgical findings. *Spine* 1988;13(9):1049-1054.

4. Brown MD: Current approach to diagnosis of low back pain and sciatica. Presented at the AAOS Inst Course, Lect #118, Las Vegas, Nevada, Feb 10,1989.

5. Frocrain L, Duvauferrier R, Husson JL et al. Recurrent postoperative sciatica: evaluation with MR imaging and enhanced CT. *Radiology* 1989;170(2):531-533.

6. Hueftle MG, Modic MT, Ross JS, et al. Lumbar spine: postoperative MR imaging with Gd-DTPA. *Radiology* 1988;167(3): 817-824.

7. Weinreb JC, Wolbarsht LB, Cohen JM, et al. Prevalence of lumbosacral intervertebral disk abnormalities on MR images in pregnant and asymptomatic nonpregnant women. *Radiology* 1989;170(1 pt 1):125-128.

8. Spengler DM: Chapman's Operative Orthopedics: Lumbar Disk Herniation, Philadelphia, JB Lippincott Co, 1988.

9. Walter OP, et al. Lumbar spine: scientific approach to the assessment and management of activity-related spinal disorders: report of the Quebec Task Force on Spinal Disorders, *Spine* Euro Ed [suppl 1] 1987;12:7S.

10. Deyo RA, Walsh NE, Martin DC, et al. A controlled trial of transcutaneous electrical nerve stimulation (TENS) and exercise for chronic low back pain. *N Engl J Med* 1990;322(23): 1627-1634.

11. Haldeman S: Spinal manipulative therapy: a status report. *Clin Orthop* 1983;Oct(179):62-70.

12. Quon JA, Cassidy JD, O'Connor SM, et al. Lumbar intervertebral disk herniation: treatment by rotational manipulation. *J Manipulative Physiol Ther* 1989;12(3):220-227.

13. Kuo PP: Loh ZC: Treatment of lumbar intervertebral disk protrusions by manipulation. *Clin Orthop* 1987; Feb(215):47-55.

14. Gallinaro P, Cartesegna M: Three cases of lumbar disk rupture and one of cauda equina associated with spinal manipulation (chiropraxis), letter. *Lancet* 1983;1(8321):411.

15. Bell GR, Rothman RH: The conservative treatment of sciatica. *Spine* 1984;9(1):54-56.

16. Fast A: Low back disorders: conservative management. *Arch Phys Med Rehabil* 1988;69(10):880-891.

17. Saal JA, Saal JS: Nonoperative treatment of herniated lumbar intervertebral disk with radiculopathy: an outcome study. *Spine* 1989;14(4):431-437.

18. Weber H: Lumbar disk herniation: a controlled, prospective study with ten years of observation. *Spine* 1983;8(2):131-140.

19. Spengler DM, Ouellette EA, Battie M, et al. Elective diskec-
    tomy for herniation of a lumbar disk: additional experience
    with an objective method. *J Bone Joint Surg* (Am)
    1990;72(2):230-237.

20. Spengler DM: Lumbar diskectomy. Results with limited disk
    excision and selective foraminotomy. *Spine* 1982;7(6):604-607.

21. Silvers HR: Microsurgical versus standard lumbar diskec-
    tomy. *Neurosurgery* 1988;22(5):837-841.

22. Eismont FJ, Currier B: Surgical management of lumbar inter-
    vertebral-disk disease. *J Bone Joint Surg* (Am) 1989;71(8):
    1266-1271.

23. Fager CA: Lumbar microdiskectomy: a contrary opinion. *Clin
    Neuosurg* 1986;33:419-456.

24. Gill K, Blumenthal S: Clinical experience with automated per-
    cutaneous diskectomy: the Nucleotome System. *Orthopedics*
    1991;14(7):757-760.

25. Dabezies EJ, Langford K, Morris J, et al. Safety and efficacy
    of chymopapain (Discase) in the treatment of sciatica due to a
    herniated nucleus pulposus: results of a randomized, double-
    blind study. *Spine* 1988:13(5):561-565.

*—by Alexander A. Davis, DC, MD
and Eugene J. Carragee, MD*

Dr Davis is a resident in the Division of Orthopaedic Surgery at
Stanford University Medical Center in Stanford, California. Dr
Carragee is director of the Orthopaedic Spine Center and an assis-
tant professor of orthopedic surgery at Stanford University School of
Medicine.

Chapter 8

Spina Bifida

Definition

Spina Bifida means cleft spine, which is an incomplete closure in the spinal column. In general, the three types of spina bifida (from mild to severe) are:

1. Spina Bifida Occulta: There is an opening in one or more of the vertebrae (bones) of the spinal column without apparent damage to the spinal cord.

2. Meningocele: The meninges, or protective covering around the spinal cord, has pushed out through the opening in the vertebrae in a sac called the "meningocele." However, the spinal cord remains intact. This form can be repaired with little or no damage to the nerve pathways.

3. Myelomeningocele: This is the most severe form of spina bifida, in which a portion of the spinal cord itself protrudes through the back. In some cases, sacs are covered with skin; in others, tissue and nerves are exposed. Generally, people use the terms "spina bifida" and "myelomeningocele" interchangeably.

National Information Center for Children and Youth with Disabilities, FS12, December 1995.

Incidence

Approximately 40% of all Americans may have spina bifida occulta, but because they experience little or no symptoms, very few of them ever know that they have it. The other two types of spina bifida, meningocele and myelomeningocele, are known collectively as "spina bifida manifesta," and occur in approximately one out of every thousand births. Of these infants born with "spina bifida manifesta," about 4% have the meningocele form, while about 96% have myelomeningocele form.

Characteristics

The effects of myelomeningocele, the most serious form of spina bifida, may include muscle weakness or paralysis below the area of the spine where the incomplete closure (or cleft) occurs, loss of sensation below the cleft, and loss of bowel and bladder control. In addition, fluid may build up and cause an accumulation of fluid in the brain (a condition known as hydrocephalus). A large percentage (70%-90%) of children born with myelomeningocele have hydrocephalus. Hydrocephalus is controlled by a surgical procedure called "shunting," which relieves the fluid buildup in the brain. If a drain (shunt) is not implanted, the pressure buildup can cause brain damage, seizures, or blindness. Hydrocephalus may occur without spina bifida, but the two conditions often occur together.

Educational Implications

Although spina bifida is relatively common, until recently most children born with a myelomeningocele died shortly after birth. Now that surgery to drain spinal fluid and protect children against hydrocephalus can be performed in the first 48 hours of life, children with myelomeningocele are much more likely to live. Quite often, however, they must have a series of operations throughout their childhood. School programs should be flexible to accommodate these special needs.

Many children with myelomeningocele need training to learn to manage their bowel and bladder functions. Some require catheterization, or the insertion of a tube to permit passage of urine.

The courts have held that clean, intermittent catheterization is necessary to help the child benefit from and have access to special education and related services. A successful bladder management program can be incorporated into the regular school day. Many children learn to catheterize themselves at a very early age.

In some cases, children with spina bifida who also have a history of hydrocephalus experience learning problems. They may have difficulty with paying attention, expressing or understanding language, and grasping reading and math. Early intervention with children who experience learning problems can help considerably to prepare them for school.

Mainstreaming, or successful integration of a child with spina bifida into a school attended by nondisabled young people, sometimes requires changes in school equipment or the curriculum. Although student placement should be in the least restrictive environment the day-to-day school pattern also should be as "normal" as possible. In adapting the school setting for the child with spina bifida, architectural factors should be considered. Section 504 of the Rehabilitation Act of 1973 requires that programs receiving federal funds make their facilities accessible. This can occur through structural changes (for example, adding elevators or ramps) or through schedule or location changes (for example, offering a course on the ground floor).

Children with myelomeningocele need to learn mobility skills, and often require the aid of crutches, braces, or wheelchairs. It is important that all members of the school team and the parents understand the child's physical capabilities and limitations. Physical disabilities like spina bifida can have profound effects on a child's emotional and social development. To promote personal growth, families and teachers should encourage children, within the limits of safety and health, to be independent and to participate in activities with their nondisabled classmates.

Resources

Bloom, B.A., & Seljeskog, E.S. (1988). *A parent's guide to spina bifida*. Minneapolis, MN: University of Minnesota Press. (Telephone: 1-800-388-3863.)

McLone, D. (1994). *An introduction to spina bifida*. Washington, DC: Spina Bifida Association of America. (See address below.)

Rowley-Kelly, F.L., & Reigel, D.H. (Eds.). (1993). *Teaching the student with spina bifida*. Baltimore, MD: Paul H. Brookes. (Telephone: 1-800-638-3775.)

Spina Bifida Association of America. (1994). *Publications list* Washington, DC: Author. (See address below.)

Organizations

Spina Bifida Association of America
4590 MacArthur Boulevard, Suite 250
Washington, DC 20007
(202) 944-3285
(800) 621-3141 (Toll Free)

March of Dimes Birth Defects Foundation
1275 Mamaroneck Avenue
White Plains, NY 10605
(914) 428-7100

National Center for Education in Maternal and Child Health
2070 Chain Bridge Road, Suite 450
Vienna, VA 22182-2536
(703) 821-8955, Ext. 254 or 265

National Easter Seal Society
230 West Monroe Street, Suite 1800
Chicago, IL 60606
(312) 726-6200
(800) 221-6827 (Toll Free)

National Rehabilitation Information Center (NARIC)
8455 Colesville Road, Suite 935
Silver Spring, MD 20910-3319
(301) 588-9284
(800) 227-0216 (Toll Free)

[More information on Spina Bifida can be found in a forthcoming volume of Omnigraphics' *Health Reference Series* focused on congenital disorders.]

Chapter 9

Scoliosis

When Laura Bradbard was 12, her mother noticed a lump on her back and was concerned it might be a tumor.

"It was my rib cage rotating," Bradbard says today, 38 and working as a secretary in Rockville, Md. "The lump was my shoulder blade and ribs protruding out the back. X-rays showed my spine was growing sideways, curving in the shape of an 'S.' The doctor said I should do something about it before it got worse."

Sideways curvature of the spine of 11 degrees or more is known as scoliosis. Bradbard's spine was off-center 36 degrees.

Bradbard has scoliosis—in her case, it's called "idiopathic," which means the cause is unknown. Some 80 percent of patients have this variety. Other cases are due to birth defects, spinal cord injuries, and nerve and muscle diseases such as muscular dystrophy.

Who Gets Scoliosis?

Showing up during the growth spurt at ages 10 to 15, scoliosis strikes 2 to 3 percent of adolescents. For unknown reasons, it affects more girls than boys—an inequality of about 3.6 to 1 overall, but 10 to 1 when curves are 30 degrees or more.

Very mild scoliosis curves, under 20 degrees, are nothing to worry about, doctors say. Even 20-degree curves sometimes improve on their own, with only 1 in 5 worsening, and only 3 in 1,000 worsening enough to need treatment.

"Correcting the Curved Spine of Scoliosis," *FDA Consumer*, July-August 1994.

When curvature gets worse, the spine twists on its center, slowly pulling the rib cage out of normal position. One side of the rib cage becomes higher at the back and sticks out. The ribs inside the curve scrunch together as those outside the curve spread apart. Although most scoliosis curves are "S" shaped like Bradbard's, some resemble a long "C."

"As a curve approaches 60 degrees," says Martin Yahiro, M.D., "the distorted rib cage restricts expansion of the lungs, causing breathing problems." Yahiro is an orthopedist (specialist in bone disorders) at the Food and Drug Administration's Center for Devices and Radiological Health, which regulates scoliosis treatment devices.

Why some scoliosis curves worsen and others don't is unknown. The larger the curve and the younger the patient when it's discovered, the greater the chance it will worsen, Yahiro says.

Curve Watch

Often, the first clue that scoliosis is developing is an uneven skirt hemline or a difference in pant-leg length. Other early warning signs, which might resemble poor posture to an untrained eye, include a hip or shoulder higher than the other, protruding shoulder blade, or tilted head.

After a thorough examination to rule out other problems, the orthopedist diagnoses scoliosis and orders one or more x-rays (see "X-Ray Safety") to determine the type and extent of the curve. (A person with scoliosis may also have other abnormal curvatures, which can be detected by x-ray and treated along with the scoliosis. If the normal rounding of the back is too great, the condition is called "hyperkyphosis." If the normal forward curving in the lower back is too great, the condition is called "hyperlordosis.")

The American Academy of Pediatrics recommends screening for scoliosis during routine doctor visits at ages 10, 12, 14, and 16. The American Academy of Orthopaedic Surgeons and the Scoliosis Research Society recommend screening girls at 10 and 12 and boys once at 13 or 14. Many states have scoliosis screening programs in schools.

Tailored Treatment

Decisions about scoliosis treatment depend on the person's age, gender, general health, and potential for growth, as well as severity and location of the curve.

For a very mild curve, the doctor may only advise monitoring check-ups, with x-rays to detect worsening, every three or four months or maybe once a year.

Even moderate curves of 25 to 40 degrees may not warrant treatment, Yahiro says. "If an 18-year-old no longer growing has a 30-degree curve," he says, "I probably would do no more than monitor it. On the other hand, I'd immediately treat such a curve, and often a slighter one, in a 12-year-old just starting the growth spurt."

A severe curve of 40 to 50 degrees or more that's detected early, Yahiro says, would be expected to rapidly get much worse, so he would treat it even more aggressively.

Another important factor is the patient's attitude toward treatment. For instance, Yahiro says, a worsening 35-degree curve that could have been treated with bracing may, in fact, need surgery if the young person refuses to wear a brace.

Bracing for Prevention

A nonsurgical treatment for moderate curves (24 to 40 degrees) is a body brace. Not a cure, bracing is intended to check a curve until growth is completed. It can generally straighten a moderate curve. Unfortunately, as happened with Bradbard, some curves return after the brace is no longer worn.

Bradbard wore a full torso brace, formed from a cast modeled from her body. It consisted of a molded leather girdle, straps, and a neck ring to hold support bars in position. Together, these parts held Bradbard in a position that kept her rigid from chin to hips. Bolts and buckles permitted adjustments as she grew.

"I wore it day and night for 23 hours from eighth grade through 10th," she says, "only taking it off for gym and showers. After a time, it was just part of me. I played neighborhood baseball and basketball and rode a bike wearing it."

But Bradbard's inability to bend meant she couldn't look down, and she had to adjust for this. "I couldn't see the stairs when I was walking," she says, "and I had to carry a desk frame from class to class to hold my books up where I could see them. I had several frames that had belonged to an older girl in school who didn't need her brace anymore."

Today, molded braces are available that generally don't show under clothing because they fit close and only come up to the underarms. Although underarm braces are effective for lower chest and lower back curves, a full torso brace works best for a high chest curve. Getting a young person to wear a full brace continuously isn't always successful, says Yahiro, "so it's not used as much as it could be."

An alternative treatment is stimulation of muscles alongside the spine during sleep with an electrical muscle stimulator, attached by electrodes placed on the skin. FDA approved stimulators for scoliosis in 1986.

But doctors may not want to use this alternative. One study, sponsored by the Scoliosis Research Society, reported success with bracing, but not stimulation. The study was summarized in the fall-winter 1993 newsletter of the National Scoliosis Foundation, Inc.

Surgery

Of the 30,000 to 70,000 spinal surgery procedures done each year, "about a third are probably for severe scoliosis," says Mark Melkerson, who reviews the medical devices used in these procedures for FDA's orthopedic devices branch. "Depending on the patient's age," he says, "doctors usually start considering surgery when a curve exceeds 40 to 50 degrees, to prevent breathing problems."

The surgeon attaches steel rods to vertebrae at the top and bottom of the curve with hooks, screws or wires, fusing the vertebrae with bone fragments taken from the hips, ribs, or the spine itself. The healed fusions harden in a straightened position, leaving the rest of the spine flexible.

Afterwards, most patients need a brace for about six weeks.

"It usually takes three months for everything to fuse," Yahiro says. "Still, we don't say a fusion has failed until after a year."

Bradbard had corrective surgery five years ago. She'd gone back to the doctor complaining of back pain, and x-rays showed her curve had progressed to 52 degrees.

Since someone past adolescence is no longer growing, why would a scoliosis curve worsen?

Yahiro says that doctors don't yet have a complete answer, but they do know that when the spine is already severely curved, the person's weight is distributed across the abnormal curve. Over time, this stress may make the curve worse.

Before Bradbard's surgery, her right hip and ribs practically sat on each other, she says, so that she essentially had no waist. Afterwards, she suddenly was 2 inches taller, thanks to straightening with 8 inches of rods and a fused spine.

"For the longest time," she says, "I kept hitting my head when I'd get in or out of the car."

When corrective surgery is done *before* growth is completed, Yahiro says, the patient both gains height from the straightening and loses height from the fusions, which stop growth. The gain and loss tend to cancel each other out, he says.

Bradbard's recovery required two weeks in the hospital. But with help, she was sitting for short periods by the second day, and standing for short periods by the third. Unlike patients undergoing scoliosis surgery 15 years ago, Bradbard didn't have to lie in a body cast for months. She didn't even have to wear a brace, though it took a full year before muscle strength returned.

The lower end of her curve couldn't be corrected, or she wouldn't be able to bend at all. As a result, one leg is a quarter of an inch shorter, which she compensates for by wearing a heel lift in her shoe.

The corrective method her surgeon used is called Cotrel-Dubousset, one of several newer systems for attaching rods to the spine with hooks and screws. Researchers report Cotrel-Dubousset has less than 2 percent loss of correction, compared with 10 to 25 percent loss from the older (Harrington Rod) system. The older system allowed the hooks to rotate, so a body cast was needed to prevent their movement until fusion.

"With many of the newer systems," Melkerson says, "the hooks are rigidly fixed to resist rotation."

Like any surgery, a scoliosis operation can have complications, such as infection or a bad reaction to anesthesia. Additional risks, though rare, are possibly dislodging a hook, fracturing a fused vertebra, or damaging the spinal cord.

Someone facing possible scoliosis surgery should ask the doctor to explain how it will help and how it poses risks, which vary with the patient and method of surgery.

X-Ray Safety

When teenagers have scoliosis x-rays taken, they (or their parents) can help keep their radiation exposure as low as possible by asking whether exposure-reducing techniques are being used. This is especially important for young women, because developing breast tissue has increased sensitivity to radiation, and repeated exposure in adolescence can increase the risk of breast cancer later on.

In addition to the general practice of narrowing the x-ray beam to the spinal area, the techniques are:

93

- Attaching a special filter to the x-ray tube that absorbs much of the x-ray beam, reducing exposure by two to five times.

- Using a fast screen-film combination to reduce exposure by two to six times.

- Using breast shields that reduce radiation exposure to breast tissue by three to 10 times. These include the x-ray tube shield that shades the breasts; a lead vest or stole-like garment with a lead insert, worn if x-rays are taken with the patient facing the x-ray machine; or facing away from the x-ray machine so that the x-rays enter the body from behind, and the body shields the breasts.

- Combinations of these methods.

For More Information

American Academy of Orthopaedic Surgeons
6300 N. River Road
Rosemont, IL 60018-4262
(1-800) 346-2267

National Scoliosis Foundation, Inc.
72 Mt. Auburn St.
Watertown, MA 02172
(617) 926-0390

Scoliosis Research Society
6300 N. River Road, Suite 727
Rosemont, IL 60018-4226
(708) 698-1627

The Scoliosis Association, Inc.
P.O. Box 811705
Boca Raton, FL 33481-1705
(1-800) 800-0669

—by Dixie Farley

Dixie Farley is a staff writer for FDA Consumer.

Chapter 10

Degenerative Problems of the Back

What is a degenerative problem in the back?

Degeneration or deterioration of a part of the spine may result from a gradual wearing down of bone or soft connective tissue over time or from a reduction in the circulation of blood, which brings oxygen and other nutrients to the area. Degeneration is most likely to occur in the *disc* (cushion between the bones—vertebrae) or in the cartilage of the *facet joints* (joints between the vertebrae). When discs deteriorate, they can crack and slip outward (*herniate*), tear, or flatten causing excessive movement and irritation of the cartilage at the facet joints. One or more discs might actually flatten causing collapse of the vertebral column. The resulting narrowing of the spinal canal (*stenosis*) may cause pressure on the nerves that branch out from the spinal cord.

What causes degeneration?

As people age, various degrees of wear and tear in the spine may cause inflammation. This may be referred to as *degenerative arthritis* or *spondylitis*. If the degeneration is mild, no symptoms may appear. However, arthritis may destroy cartilage in the spine and cause bone overgrowth (*spurs*).

A fact sheet produced by the National Institute of Arthritis and Musculoskeletal and Skin Diseases, August 1992.

Osteoporosis, a condition in which bones become porous and susceptible to fracture, is another degenerative disease frequently affecting the back, particularly in postmenopausal women.

Degeneration may also occur in younger people, such as ballet dancers or athletes, where required movements repeatedly place extreme pressure on one or more parts of the spine. A curvature of the spine (*scoliosis*) that is developmental and often detected during childhood or adolescence, may cause the vertebral joints to move in abnormal ways leading to later degeneration.

What are the symptoms of degenerative spinal problems?

A frequent symptom of degeneration is an aching back. In many cases of arthritis, pain that is felt in the morning upon arising from sleep improves throughout the day with activity. Because the nerves that branch out from the spinal cord conduct impulses to all parts of the body, pressure on one or more nerves may cause pain that radiates into the hip and down the leg (*sciatica*) or tingling or numbness of an arm or leg. In more serious cases, there may be interference with bowel and bladder function, or, if nerves in the neck are compressed, difficulty speaking or respiratory problems.

How are degenerative changes in the spine detected?

There are several imaging tests that can help doctors diagnose degenerative changes in the spine. These include plain film radiographs (*x-rays*), CT scan, magnetic resonance imaging, and discography.

In a *CT scan*, combined use of a computer and x-rays passed through the body at different angles produces clear cross-sectional images of the tissues being examined.

Magnetic resonance imaging (MRI) is another diagnostic technique that provides cross-sectional images. Rather than using x-rays, powerful magnetic fields and radio waves that stimulate atoms in the body's tissues permit a computer to create an image of the tissue being examined.

In *discography*, a dye visible on x-ray films is injected into the spine. This procedure is seldom used.

What treatment might be prescribed?

Among the treatments that may be recommended are: bed rest lasting 2 or 3 days for sudden onset of pain (or longer if there is numbness in an extremity); nonsteroidal anti-inflammatory drugs (e.g., aspirin, ibuprofen, naproxen); application of heat or cold; and stretching and/or strengthening exercises that improve the condition of the muscles of the back, abdomen, and thighs. Exercises are thought to improve nutrition to the vertebral joints and prevent scarring of tissues around inflamed joints. When major arthritic conditions are suspected, stronger anti-inflammatory medicines (e.g., cortisone injections) may be prescribed.

In cases of severe degeneration where there is extensive pain and involvement of the nervous system, surgery may be necessary. During the operation, one or more of the *vertebral laminae* (bony arches of the vertebrae) are usually removed and the bones above and below the joints involved are sometimes fused together to provide stability. If there is bony overgrowth due to deposits of calcium, these growths or spurs are usually removed.

Chapter 11

Spinal Stenosis

Back pain may be one of life's great equalizers; at some point virtually everyone experiences it. For most, back pain is simply the result of lifting too much or pushing too hard—a pulled or strained muscle. But for others the cause is more complex: an arthritis-related condition called spinal stenosis. Spinal stenosis can bring long-term difficulties and some tough decision-making for doctors and their patients.

Because the initial symptom of spinal stenosis is back pain, the condition may at first be difficult to diagnose. The host of symptoms that often follow can make it difficult to treat. In fact, the search for an ideal treatment, as well as for answers about why women may be offered different treatment choices from men, are at the heart of current medical controversy about this painful and often debilitating condition.

Although this is not the definitive story on spinal stenosis, it should give you some answers—and perhaps it can serve as a basis for discussion with your physician.

The Spine: Support and Sensitivity

Our spines are marvels of structural engineering, able to hold our bodies at ramrod attention, yet supple enough to curve forward into a slump or double over in a backbend. Our spines absorb the subtle shock of each step we take, and they also tolerate it when we try a

Arthritis Today, May-June 1995; reprinted with permission.

bounce or two on a pogo stick or attempt the graceful sway that keeps a Hula Hoop spinning. Yet over the years, the price of all this wear and tear comes due.

"As we get older, disks in the spine degenerate. When this happens, the joints in the posterior part are subject to greater loads or pressure," explains Jeffrey Katz, MD, a rheumatologist at Brigham and Women's Hospital in Boston. These joints develop osteoarthritic changes; simultaneously, soft tissues in the spine, particularly the ligaments, may degenerate.

"Degenerative arthritic changes in the spine are normal in everybody," says Dr. Katz, "but for some people the changes are more accelerated or severe. In some they cause compression of nerve roots that run inside the spine. And that produces symptoms."

Our spines give us feedback about these changes because the vertebrae house the spinal cord, a rope of nerves extending for a foot and a half downward from the brain. The word "stenosis" refers to narrowing, and what's become more narrow is the canal protecting those exquisitely sensitive nerves. "This puts pressure on nerve roots, causing pain," says Dr. Katz.

Accumulated Wear

Spinal stenosis results from a lifetime of wear, so symptoms may develop gradually over the years. They seldom become severe before the age of 50. While the most common signal is low back pain, this might indicate a host of other problems—everything from muscle strain and poor posture to the presence of an infection. Thus, a physician's suspicions about spinal stenosis can be difficult to confirm. Other symptoms, which may or may not be present, include pain or numbness in the legs and—because compression in the spinal cord can affect nearby bodily systems—constipation or urinary incontinence.

Once a diagnosis is made, pain medications, including nonsteroidal anti-inflammatory drugs, offer a first line of defense. Some patients also benefit from physical therapy or use of a walker to support the body's weight. Yet for some 30,000 people in the U.S. each year, the pain becomes so significant that these measures don't do the job. For these people, the choice is surgery.

The most typical procedure is known as laminectomy, requiring an incision to reveal the bony arches of the vertebrae. The surgeon then cleans out the accumulated debris that is pressing on the nerves. Because surgical decompression is a major procedure, recovery can require a few days in bed as well as avoidance of heavy lifting for several weeks. Nonetheless, most people tolerate it well. Most also find that the surgery works, relieving their pain and allowing them to resume activities.

Second Surgeries

But not everyone is so lucky. For some, the pain persists. For others, discomfort returns within a year or two. According to one study, these problems are more likely in people who have other physical problems, such as cardiac or pulmonary disease or rheumatoid arthritis. It's not uncommon for such individuals to undergo surgery again.

It's hard to predict just who will benefit most from laminectomy, and that difficulty is what has helped fuel controversy about what approach works best in the operating room. While a laminectomy alone may remove debris pressing on the nerve, an underlying instability of the spine—already weakened by arthritic changes—might require more extensive repair. That's why some patients undergo spinal fusion, a procedure that provides additional support by linking two or more vertebrae into a single unit.

This more extensive surgery joins the vertebrae with a plate or screws and may require a graft using a section of bone from the pelvis. Recovery demands as many as six weeks of bed rest, and some people temporarily need to wear plaster jackets until the fusion is complete. There is also the possibility that fused vertebrae may put greater strain on the rest of the spine, causing more pain later.

Studies are being conducted to determine which people with the condition need both procedures and which can benefit from only one. In addition, researchers may also soon take up another question about spinal stenosis—why women apparently wait longer than men to undergo surgery for it.

Gender Differences

Between 1989 and 1992 Dr. Katz studied the profiles of 98 women and 56 men undergoing laminectomy for the first time at Brigham and Women's Hospital in Boston and at the University of Vermont. He compared the severity of symptoms before surgery, as well as progress afterward. Dr. Katz found that by the time women underwent laminectomy, they had more pain and their ability to function had fallen lower.

"Women had much worse functional status than men prior to laminectomy," Dr. Katz concluded from his study, published in the journal *Arthritis and Rheumatism*. His results showed that, "Women were operated on at a more advanced stage in the course of their disease."

Because unrelated research has found women undergoing surgery at later stages for other conditions, particularly heart and kidney disease, Dr. Katz is concerned that women may also wait longer to get help for spinal stenosis. Despite this, surgery appears equally effective in providing relief for both sexes.

A number of reasons may be causing surgery to be delayed for women, Dr. Katz believes. For example, women may experience family and personal demands that prevent them from taking time out for treatment. On the other hand, there is the chance that physicians treat women less aggressively because they fear greater complications or believe that limited mobility presents fewer difficulties for women than for men.

"We suspect the striking differences in preoperative functional status are due to a combination of these mechanisms," Dr. Katz says. He hopes the various reasons women delay surgery can be explored in further studies.

Choices for Healthier Backs

In the meantime, people considering surgical decompression for back and leg pain should look into whether laminectomy alone is the most promising treatment option. If spinal instability is a problem, they may also need to undergo the more extensive procedure of spinal fusion.

As for those of us fortunate enough to have avoided low back pain so far, the message is clear: We need to be kind to our spines. While genetic differences may contribute to spinal stenosis, wear and tear also take their toll. Keeping abdominal and back muscles strong with appropriate exercises in middle age and in later years is as important as anything in reducing spinal problems. For the first 50 years of our lives, our spines forgive us almost every contortion we ask of them, letting us lift weight carelessly or spin and twist with the Lindy, the limbo or slam dancing. Yet sooner or later a bill can come in—stamped past-due and payable in pain.

— by Carol Orlock

Carol Orlock is a freelance writer in Seattle.

Chapter 12

Osteoporosis

Information about Osteoporosis

While its cause remains a mystery, scientists are learning more about treating and preventing osteoporosis, the most common disease affecting bone. Characterized by loss of bone density and strength, osteoporosis is associated with debilitating fractures, especially in people aged 45 and older.

As many as 24 million Americans, 80 percent of them women, now suffer from the condition, with more than 1.3 million osteoporosis-related fractures occurring annually.

With the "graying of America" as baby boomers age, the incidence of broken wrists and hips could skyrocket within the next couple of decades. Fortunately, research to identify treatments not only to arrest bone loss, but to reverse it, is starting to pay off.

This chapter includes "Osteoporosis Treatment Advances," *FDA Consumer*, April 1991; "Osteoporosis and Physical Activity," *Physical Activity and Fitness Research Digest* (Published quarterly by the President's Council on Physical Fitness and Sports), September 1995; "Osteoporosis: Improved Detection and Treatment," Reprinted with permission from *The Johns Hopkins Medical Letter Health After 50*, copyright MedLetter Associates, 1996; and "After the Vertebral Fracture in Osteoporoses," Osteoporosis and Related Bone Diseases—National Resource Center, 1150 17th Street, N.W., Suite 500, Washington, D.C. 20036-4603, March 1995; text used with permission of the National Osteoporosis Foundation.

Bone Basics

Although bones seem to be as lifeless as rocks, they are, in fact, composed of living tissue that is continually being broken down (or resorbed) and rebuilt, in a process called remodeling.

Bone is made from a protein framework—the osteoid matrix—into which calcium is deposited. About 99 percent of the calcium in the body is stored in the bones and teeth. Calcium not only makes bone hard, but also is involved in other essential functions, such as enabling the heart and other muscles to contract. Whenever dietary intake of calcium is insufficient to meet the body's needs, increased amounts are drawn from the bones to maintain a relatively constant supply in the bloodstream.

Complex chemical signals prompt bone cells known as osteoclasts to break down bone and others called osteoblasts to deposit bone. Calcitriol (a form of vitamin D), calcitonin (a thyroid hormone), parathyroid hormone, growth factors, and prostaglandins are among the substances that orchestrate bone remodeling.

It takes about 90 days for old bone to be resorbed and replaced by new bone; then the cycle begins anew. Bones continue to grow in strength and size until a person's mid-30s, when peak bone mass is attained.

After that, the rate of bone resorption exceeds the rate of deposition, resulting in decreased bone mass and density (osteoporosis is Latin for "porous bones").

"There are many factors involved, and it's hard to pinpoint why this imbalance occurs," says Chhanda Dutta, Ph.D., a pharmacologist with FDA's division of metabolism and endocrine drug products.

Who's At Risk?

According to one hypothesis, there are two types of primary osteoporosis. Type I occurs only in women, typically in the years immediately following menopause, from age 50 to 70. Dutta explains that Type I is related to decreased estrogen, and is characterized by rapid bone loss, especially in trabecular bones (vertebrae and flat bones, such as the pelvis). At greatest risk are thin, small-boned Caucasian or Asian women who have had a hysterectomy or reached natural menopause before age 45 and have a family history of the condition.

"Heredity is probably the most important factor," says Mona Calvo, Ph.D., a nutritionist in FDA's Center for Food Safety and Applied Nutrition. Thus, someone whose parents or grandparents have had the tell-tale signs, such as fracturing a hip after a minor fall, may be at greater risk of developing this type of osteoporosis.

Lifestyle factors that may contribute to or worsen Type I osteoporosis include low calcium intake, a sedentary lifestyle (weight-bearing exercise promotes bone deposition), cigarette smoking (heavy smokers have lower blood levels of estrogen), and excessive alcohol consumption (alcohol inhibits calcium absorption).

"While you don't have any control over heredity, you can attenuate your genetic legacy by focusing on those lifestyle risk factors you can do something about," advises Calvo.

Type II primary osteoporosis affects nearly half of all people over the age of 75. It's the only type of primary osteoporosis that men get; however, it's twice as common in women. According to Dutta, Type II is characterized by reduced osteoblast cell activity and decreased formation of bone. Loss occurs in both trabecular and cortical bones (hip and long bones such as those in the leg). Over the expected lifespan, women typically lose as much as 35 percent of cortical bone and up to half of trabecular bone; men, who have denser bones to begin with, lose only about 23 percent of cortical bone and 33 percent of trabecular bone. Experts say that everyone who lives long enough will develop Type II primary osteoporosis. But the extent of its severity is very individual. The same lifestyle factors that play a role in Type I primary osteoporosis can also cause an acceleration of bone loss in those with Type II.

Secondary osteoporosis may occur as a side effect of such drugs as corticosteroids and heparin. Hyperthyroidism, rheumatoid arthritis, kidney disease, and certain cancers such as lymphoma and leukemia are among the disorders that also contribute to secondary osteoporosis.

Diagnosis Important

Bone loss develops over the span of many years and is largely symptomless, though some women may experience chronic pain along the spine or muscle spasms in the back. Often, the first indication that a person has osteoporosis is a wrist or hip fracture or a compression fracture that causes the vertebrae in the upper back to collapse, curving the spine into the dowager's hump that has come to symbolize osteoporosis.

All told, 20 to 25 percent of postmenopausal women in this country are at risk of suffering an osteoporotic fracture. Such fractures cost some $10 billion each year in direct medical expenses such as hospitalization and home nursing care, as well as an incalculable amount in lost earnings.

Hip fractures, in particular, can have dire consequences: Up to 20 percent of victims will die, within a year of fracture, from such complications as pneumonia, blood clots in the lungs, and heart failure. Fewer than half of those who survive can walk unaided or return to their former level of activity. Some 300,000 Americans suffer osteoporosis-related hip fractures each year.

Medical technology has developed several methods to detect osteoporosis before fractures occur. With the noninvasive radiologic imaging techniques, photon absorptiometry and computed tomography, doctors can measure bone mass in the spine, wrist and hip.

"A fracture is the endpoint of the disease. If you can prevent a fracture by taking preventive measures, you can slow down progression of osteoporosis," explains Dutta. However, since scans to measure bone density are not currently reimbursed by most insurance companies and are not covered by Medicare, testing is currently reserved only for women at risk for osteoporosis rather than as a mass screening tool.

Prevention Through Diet

Osteoporosis is a complex condition, and researchers have been investigating a number of treatment approaches. However, prevention remains paramount.

"Calcium intake over lifetime really seems to matter, especially during periods of bone growth," says Linda Golden, M.D., a medical officer in FDA's division of metabolism endocrine drug products. "Starting in childhood, a diet adequate in calcium can maximize peak bone mass," she says.

Calvo agrees: "The more bone mass you have at maturity, the more you can lose before you will succumb to an osteoporotic fracture."

Health experts are divided over how much calcium is enough, and whether supplements are necessary. A consensus statement issued in October 1990 by a panel of experts at the Third International Symposium on Osteoporosis held in Copenhagen, Denmark, recommended a minimum intake of 800 milligrams of calcium daily for all adults. The year before, the U.S. National Academy of Sciences set the Recommended Dietary Allowances (RDA) for calcium at 1,200 mg daily for females from age 11 to 24 (the peak bone-forming years), dropping to 800 mg thereafter. Previously, the 1984 National Institutes of

Health Consensus Development Conference on Osteoporosis had concluded that all women should get 1,000 to 1,500 mg of calcium daily.

Why the discrepancies in recommendations? For a while, "everyone was gung-ho about calcium; the more calcium you could get in a woman, the better," says Calvo. "But enthusiasm waned when subsequent research showed that raising calcium intake was not effective in slowing bone loss in pre-menopausal women," she explains, citing a study of 25- to 34-year-old women showing that highest bone density was achieved with a daily calcium intake of 800 to 1,000 mg, and that exceeding this range did not appear to result in any additional benefit to bone. But older women may need to take in greater amounts of calcium because as a person ages, the body's ability to absorb calcium diminishes.

While nutritionists and medical experts recommend eating a calcium-rich diet during the crucial bone-forming years between adolescence and young adulthood, new evidence suggests that dietary intervention may be more effective in menopausal women than was previously thought. Increasing daily calcium intake to 800 mg can slow or prevent bone loss in post-menopausal women, according to a study reported in the September 1990 issue of *The New England Journal of Medicine*. In the study by researchers at Tufts University in Boston, 361 women aged 40 to 70 were divided according to whether their diets were high or low in calcium (400 mg daily was the dividing line). The subjects were given either a placebo or 500-mg doses of calcium supplements daily. Supplementation significantly retarded bone loss in those who had undergone menopause at least six years earlier and whose diets were very low in calcium.

Allowing that "this research shows that people with low calcium intake in their late menopausal years can benefit from taking supplements," Calvo nonetheless recommends that calcium intake come from dairy foods. "I'll bet that if the subjects in the Tufts study had received their calcium from dairy foods, they would have done even better because milk and milk products are naturally rich in vitamin D, which enhances calcium absorption. Dairy products also provide vitamins A and D, protein, magnesium, and phosphorus, which are also building blocks for bone."

The Tufts study also found that bone loss was more rapid during the first five years following menopause, and then slowed to a constant rate. This finding is consistent with other studies showing that dietary calcium had little effect in moderating the rate of bone loss immediately following menopause. Recognizing this, the consensus statement developed at the Third International Symposium on Osteoporosis termed estrogen therapy "the drug of choice for preventing bone loss in women after the menopause or in women with impaired ovarian function."

Estrogen Replacement

It has been known for some time that estrogen prevents osteoporosis-related fractures. Conjugated estrogens—a mixture of estrogens from natural sources—received FDA approval as a treatment for osteoporosis in 1988. More recently, a Swedish study reported in the *Annals of Internal Medicine* in September 1990 found that combined estrogen-progestin therapy may also have a protective effect in preserving bone and preventing fractures. The study reported that taking a combination of the female sex hormones estrogen and progestin at or soon after menopause can lower the risk of a broken hip during the next 10 years by 60 percent.

These new findings are encouraging because a debate has been raging for years about the safety of taking estrogen after menopause. While the hormone decreases the risk of osteoporosis and heart disease, with long-term use it may also increase the risk of breast and endometrial cancers. Recent research indicates that added progestin can lower the uterine cancer risk, but may also slightly increase a woman's chances of developing breast cancer.

"For post-menopausal women who have no contraindications, estrogen is the first line of treatment," says Golden. However, "estrogen only works for as long as you take it, and the protective effects wear off when you discontinue use—but the longer you're on it, the higher the cancer risk." Golden adds that each woman's profile of risk and benefit depends on individual circumstances, and that the decision whether to begin hormone replacement therapy rests with a woman and her doctor.

Other Possible Therapies

In clinical studies, calcitonin, a thyroid hormone that inhibits the breakdown of bone, has been reported to reduce back pain from compression fractures; however, the hormone has not yet been proven to prevent fractures. With long-term use, some women develop antibodies to calcitonin, rendering the drug ineffective. FDA has approved an injectable form of calcitonin for treating osteoporosis. The effectiveness of a nasal spray version is being studied.

Figure 12.1. Surprising Sources of Calcium. While the Tufts study indicates that older women whose diets are low in calcium can benefit from increasing their intake of the mineral, American women at any age do not seem eager to eat more calcium-rich foods. Many worry about the caloric and saturated fat content of dairy foods. To address this concern, food manufacturers have introduced low-fat—and, in some cases, nonfat—versions of just about every dairy food, from cottage cheese to ice cream.

But being good to your bones doesn't necessarily mean eating yogurt every day for the rest of your life. Many products contain calcium-based food additives, and the tap water in some parts of the country contains a fair amount of calcium. In addition, a lot of foods contain some calcium and, depending on the quantities eaten, they can be a significant source of the mineral. For example, several slices of bread can provide a healthy dose of calcium.

If you read labels carefully, you'll spot some unexpected sources of calcium. Here are just a few:

Food	Serving Size	Calcium	Calories	Fat
Sardines (in oil, with bones)	3 medium (3 oz)	370 mg	175	9 g
Cheese pizza	1 slice (1/8th of 15" pie)	220 mg	290	9 g
Macaroni & cheese	1 cup	200 mg	230	10 g
Oatmeal (instant, fortified)	1 packet	160 mg	105	4 g
Tomato soup (made w/milk)	1 cup	160 mg	160	6 g
Baked beans (w/pork & tomato sauce)	1 cup	140 mg	310	7 g
Tofu	1 piece (1 1/2" x 2 3/4" x 1")	100 mg	85	5 g
Hot cocoa	6 oz	90 mg	100	1 g
Pancakes (from mix)	1 4" pancake	30 mg	60	2 g
Wheat bread (enriched)	1 slice (18 per loaf)	30 mg	65	1 g

Source: Adapted from the "USDA Nutritive Value of Foods," *Home and Garden Bulletin*, No. 72.

Researchers are also investigating several non-hormonal therapies. Currently, the most promising is etidronate, a drug used in treating Paget's disease of bone (a condition characterized by an excessive bone turnover that results in new bone being dense but fragile).

In a study by the Emory University School of Medicine in Atlanta, and reported in the July 1990 issue of *The New England Journal of Medicine*, 429 postmenopausal women who had suffered one to four spinal fractures took either a placebo or etidronate for 14 days, followed by calcium supplementation for 76 days (to match the body's 90-day bone turnover cycle). Etidronate slowed the loss of bone resorption while the calcium helped build bone mass, resulting in a 4 to 5 percent increase in spinal bone density. The women on the drug-and-supplement regimen also suffered less than half the vertebral fractures as the group receiving the placebo. On the minus side, the study found neither evidence of improved bone mass in the wrist and hip, nor any indication that fractures at those sites could be prevented.

Sodium fluoride, another experimental treatment for osteoporosis-related spinal fractures, increased bone mass but did not prevent fractures in a Mayo Clinic study of 202 women 50 to 75 years old, reported in *The New England Journal of Medicine* in March 1990. The group treated with a combination of sodium fluoride and calcium had a 35 percent increase in spinal bone density. The new bone was structurally abnormal and weak, however. The number of spinal fractures was not significantly different between the treated and placebo groups. Furthermore, the treated group sustained more broken hips.

Although treatments being developed aim to stop bone loss and rebuild weak and brittle bones, none of them can undo the damage caused by hip or spinal compression fractures. Thus, while researchers are getting a better understanding of the factors that increase bone resorption—and can mitigate their action to some degree—a true cure for osteoporosis remains as elusive as the origins of the condition.

—by Ruth Papazian

Ruth Papazian is a freelance writer in New York City specializing in health and medicine.

Osteoporosis and Physical Activity

Physical activity has been proposed as one strategy to reduce fractures by increasing bone mass and by preventing falls through improved functional ability. Although the mechanism by which exercise increases bone mass is not clear, it likely influences bone directly through mechanical forces (loading) transferred to bone. Bone responds to changes in mechanical loading and the regulation of bone strength is a function of the loads to which the skeleton is exposed. The most striking examples of this adaptation are the reports which demonstrate marked bone loss in the absence of weight bearing activity, such as occurs in space travel and prolonged bedrest. Conversely, many reports have shown that bone mass among physically active individuals and athletes is significantly higher compared to their non-active and non-athletic counterparts. Some studies which have imposed significant mechanical forces via exercise intervention report positive effects on bone mass, although the magnitude of effect is much less impressive than would be predicted from studies on athletes and active individuals. Therefore, the ideal exercise program that maximizes bone response remains elusive. Evidence is accumulating to suggest, however, that exercise which increases muscle strength, mass, and power, may provide the best osteogenic stimulus. Activities of this type provide additional skeletal protection in the older adult by preventing falls, which are highly related to the incidence of fractures, particularly at the hip.

This review will serve to present the most recent literature in the field and provide recommendations for exercise design which may aid in fracture prevention. In this review, the terms "bone mass" and "bone mineral density (BMD)" will be used as synonyms.

Physical Activity and Bone Mass

Physical activity transmits loads to the skeleton in two ways: by muscle pull and by gravitational forces from weight bearing activity. It is generally assumed that a high level of activity corresponds to a high level of mechanical loading. However, despite the intensity of muscular activity associated with competitive swimming, studies comparing athletic groups have demonstrated that swimmers generally have BMD values lower than those of non-athletic controls. Therefore, activities that require full support of body weight (i.e., those that are performed on the feet) are recommended if skeletal response is a desired outcome of exercise participation. Sports with unilateral activity, such as tennis, continue to provide the best representation of the positive effects of exercise on bone in humans. These studies have demonstrated greater BMD in the dominant playing arm vs the nondominant arm across different age groups. However, most forms of activity are not as easily characterized by such specific, localized loading patterns.

Other indicators that physical activity exerts a positive influence on the skeleton is the finding that certain measures of physical fitness are correlated with BMD. Specifically, body composition and muscular strength exhibit positive associations with bone mass. Investigations of BMD and body composition have arisen out of the common finding that body weight is associated with bone density. Research has attempted to specify which aspect of body composition, lean (muscle) or fat mass, is the best predictor of bone mass. Muscle directly attaches to bone and may influence the skeletal system via this mechanism, while fat mass contributes to body weight in a nonspecific manner. It has been proposed that fat mass has the potential to increase circulating levels of estrogen, although this explanation for its beneficial influence on bone has yet to be established. Associations between both fat and lean mass and BMD have been demonstrated. Although fat mass has been associated with bone and can provide cushioning in the fall-prone elderly, there are known health problems associated with excess body fat (e.g., cardiovascular disease, type II diabetes). On the other hand, adequate muscle mass is necessary for optimal function throughout the lifespan and muscular atrophy that accompanies the aging process is associated with falling and fracture. Therefore it is prudent to recommend that a fracture prevention program include activities that encourage muscle mass development.

Mechanical forces are directly applied to bone by muscular attachments and individuals with high muscle strength are able to generate large forces during contraction. Thus, muscle strength is a measure of physical fitness which has been studied with respect to skeletal health. Research has shown that the relationship between muscle strength and bone demonstrates site-specificity. Strength of the hip muscles has been related to hip BMD, and grip strength has been associated with forearm BMD. The contribution of muscle strength to BMD in various cross-sectional studies has ranged from 9 to 38% in nonathletic adults. Since approximately 60-80% of bone mass is estimated to be genetically determined, the relationship between muscle strength and bone is not trivial and again points to the importance of the muscular system with respect to bone health.

Research has demonstrated that male and female athletes who participate in sports that require muscular strength and power (e.g., weight lifting, gymnastics, wrestling) exhibit higher bone mass than those whose sports involve primarily muscular endurance (e.g., distance running, triathlon). Information on the loading characteristics of various activities suggests that walking and slow running provide loads equal to or slightly higher than body weight alone at the spine. In comparison, forces at the spine have been estimated to be 5 to 6 times body weight while weight lifting. Jumping associated with gymnastics training may elicit forces as high as 10 to 12 times body weight.

The research on athletes and the size of the load for a specific sport suggests that the skeleton's response to mechanical loading depends on the magnitude of the force. In practical terms, the skeleton must encounter forces that are greater than those it experiences on a day-to-day basis. Even though walking is a weight-bearing activity, its ability to evoke a skeletal response is limited to the older adult who was previously bedridden and unable to ambulate for a period of time. On the other hand, one who performs activities of daily living without assistance will be in a weight bearing posture much of the day. For this person, walking as an exercise will not exceed the loading threshold of daily activities and therefore will not improve bone mass.

Exercise intervention studies have attempted to introduce various exercise programs in humans to determine the best exercise prescription for bone health. The results of these studies are equivocal. While some reports indicate that BMD increases slightly with exercise, some report no change or slight decreases. In order to detect changes in bone mass, an intervention must be several months in duration, depending on the age group and type of program (6 months minimum). Relative to other exercise interventions, these are long time intervals (e.g., muscular strength increases can be observed in 8 weeks). Over the life span, however, these time intervals are relatively short. This may be one reason why remarkable changes have not been observed within the time frame of training studies. In addition, the expected magnitude of skeletal response is much less than that observed in the muscular system. To illustrate, muscular strength improvements on the order of 50-100% during the course of a resistance training program are not unusual, especially if initial values were low. A 1.5% increase in bone mass over a period of 9 months is meaningful, since average rates of loss are approximately 0.5-1% per year. To date, most exercise studies have not designed their exercise training programs according to the principles of training. This may be the main reason why many studies have observed minimal or no training effects on the skeleton. The application of these principles to bone loading is outlined in Figure 12.2.

Specificity	Overload	Reversibility	Initial Values	Diminishing Returns
The impact of the training should be at the bone site of interest since loading seems to have a localized effect.	The training stimulus must include forces much greater than that afforded by habitual activity.	In the absence of the training stimulus, the positive effect on bone will be lost.	Individuals with low BMD will have the greatest potential to gain from increased mechanical loading.	Each individual's biological ceiling determines the extent of adaptation to the training.

Figure 12.2. *Principles of Training*

Prevention Strategies Throughout the Lifespan

Bone is a dynamic tissue that is constantly undergoing remodeling activity, a function of bone cells, during which old bone is removed and new bone is formed. The factors which determine the level of bone cell activity are mechanical loading, calcium intake, and reproductive hormones. Strategies to decrease risk for osteoporotic fracture should take these factors into consideration throughout the lifespan since bone mass in the older adult is a product of the amount of bone acquired during growth and subsequent rates of loss during adulthood.

Physical activity has been shown to be an important contributor to bone mass in children prior to adolescence. In addition, this group should have adequate calcium intake so that the necessary blocks for building bone mineral are present during growth. It has been proposed that young bone may be more responsive to mechanical loading than old bone. Given that approximately 60% of the final skeleton is acquired during adolescence, one preventive strategy is to maximize skeletal loading during this rapid phase of growth. It is also important to consider reproductive endocrine status at this time of life. The negative effects of abnormally low estrogen on BMD in amenorrheic women with a high volume of physical training and very low body weight (primarily distance running and ballet dancing) are well documented. These effects are even more dramatic in amenorrheic women with anorexia nervosa. Although there is little if any documentation in men, abnormally low testosterone levels are theoretically detrimental for bone.

Preventive strategies in adults are generally aimed at maintaining bone mass or reducing the rate of loss. However, recent studies on young adult women indicate that physical activity may play an important role with respect to the capacity to increase bone mass after growth has stopped (Recker, et al., 1992; Bassey & Ramsdale, 1994). Recker and colleagues observed increases in spine BMD over a period of 5 years in a large group of women in their twenties. The increases were related to self-selected physical activity patterns. Bassey and Ramsdale (1994) administered high and low impact exercise programs to young women for 6 months and observed BMD increases at the hip in the high impact group only. The authors note that small improvements in bone mass in young to middle adulthood may result in quite significant reductions in risk for osteoporotic fracture in later years. It is important to note that BMD increases with physical activity are likely to be most dramatic in young adulthood when bone appears to be more responsive to mechanical loading. In addition, loading characteristics must be substantial, as demonstrated by the high impact activity administered by Bassey and Ramsdale (1994) which included jumping. Adequate calcium intake and maintenance of normal circulating levels of reproductive hormones are still important factors for optimal bone health in adulthood. However, since growth has ceased, recommendations for calcium intake are slightly lower than in adolescence.

Older adults face multiple challenges with advancing age. Age-related reductions in bone mass, muscle strength and power, and postural stability make this group at highest risk for fracture. Impaired musculoskeletal function and dynamic balance associated with aging and disuse ultimately result in decreased mobility. In addition, these declines in musculoskeletal function have been associated with an increase in falls and incidence of hip fracture. Vandervoort, et al. (1990) report that once function has declined to the point where mobility is significantly reduced, older individuals may refuse to ambulate due to a fear of falling, which is the beginning of a downward spiral which ultimately results in loss of independence. This situation, in which very few physical attempts are made, leads to marked reductions in strength and power of the lower extremities which have specifically been linked to fall risk. Although bone mass is a major risk factor for osteoporosis, falls and their severity are highly related to fractures in the elderly. In fact, 90% of all hip fractures occur with a fall.

Falls are caused by many different factors. Epidemiological research has consistently found that lower limb strength, reaction time, sensory impairment, and postural instability are important risk factors for falls. Greenspan, et al. (1994) have proposed that not all falls are potentially injurious and that fall severity in combination with bone mass at the hip are the two primary determinants of hip fracture in ambulatory elderly. Specifically, those who fall to the side and have no ability to alter fall direction or speed of impact and land directly on the hip, are more likely to fracture, particularly if BMD at that site is low. The link of muscular strength and power to fall risk is most logically in the stabilization and control required for voluntary movements as well as for the ability to recover from a stumble. One study determined that leg extensor (quadriceps) power in older men and women was the best predictor of functional performance.

Strategies to prevent fracture in older adults must target bone mass as well as factors associated with falls. Several studies have observed beneficial effects of weight training in older populations including increased bone mass, muscular strength, power, dynamic balance, and functional independence. Thus, this may be the best choice of exercise training at this stage in the lifespan. Most research has focused on machine-based training (e.g., Universal Gym, Nautilus), which requires a seated posture for lower body exercises. While this isolates muscle groups in the legs, it effectively reduces loads at the hip and does not require postural control and balance. To encourage optimal function in a standing posture, older adults should be encouraged to perform exercises such as stepping and rising from a chair. These exercises target muscle groups and actions which are important for everyday function. While it may seem dangerous for older adults to engage in this type of training, resistance training has proven successful in nursing home residents, even among quite old adults. The benefits of participation clearly outweigh the risks of immobility, decreased function and increased likelihood of falls and fracture.

Summary and Conclusions

Exercise may benefit the skeleton and reduce osteoporosis and fracture risk in the following ways: 1) increase bone mass up to and through adolescence which will result in higher BMD levels across the lifespan; 2) improve and maintain bone density during early adulthood; and, 3) reduce or slow the rate of age-related loss during middle and older age. In order to have an effect on bone, exercise must be different from daily activities, that is, an overload must be applied to the skeleton. It is important to remember that physical activity has not been shown to offset the transient increase in bone loss resulting from estrogen deficiency that is observed in the first 5-7 years past menopause. Although still uncertain, the gap is beginning to narrow with respect to the types and amount of activities which confer the best osteogenic stimulus. Participation in activities of high load and low repetitions which increase muscle strength and power may ultimately prove to be the most beneficial to bone mass. Research to quantify forces from activities that promote strength and power will substantiate these predictions and the models should be evaluated in populations at different stages of skeletal development.

The importance of building lower extremity strength and cardiovascular health cannot be overemphasized with respect to fall prevention and general health. Low bone mass is a primary risk factor for fractures, with 90% of hip fractures occurring as the result of a fall. Perhaps the most significant benefit of participation in exercise relates to improvements in neuromuscular function. Sound neuromuscular function is essential for both static and dynamic postural stability. The ability to avoid an obstacle, recover from a stumble or alter the direction of a fall may significantly reduce fall severity. Muscle mass, strength, and power decline with age, particularly in the lower extremities and this has been attributed, in part, to a decrease in physical activity. As a result, it is more difficult for the elderly to perform activities of daily living, particularly ambulation. Resistance training programs have demonstrated significant improvement in neuromuscular function in the elderly through the tenth decade, which translates to reduced risk of fall-related fractures.

Osteoporosis: Improved Detection and Treatment

Until recently, only two approved treatments were available: estrogen (appropriate only for women), and injectable calcitonin (Calcimar, Miacalcin). Many physicians also use another drug called etidronate (Didronel), although it is approved by the Food and Drug Administration only for a less-common bone condition called Paget's disease.

None of these treatments is ideal. Estrogen and calcitonin are hormones with many systemic effects—some of them beneficial, others undesirable. Etidronate belongs to a man-made group of drugs called bisphosphonates, which act only on bone. Although it may slow bone loss, it may also offset any net gain by reducing the rate of new bone formation.

Fortunately, patients now have two new, approved options: alendronate (Fosamax), a cousin of etidronate; and a nasal spray form of calcitonin. Other treatments may soon be on the way. These drugs provide alternatives for patients who can't take estrogen or choose not to, and they improve on the safety and effectiveness of previous treatments. But because the early stages of osteoporosis are silent, doctors face a difficult dilemma: how to diagnose the condition so that treatment can begin *before* bones weaken and break.

Densitometry (a safe, non-invasive imaging study) can help determine whether treatment is required. But the technique is still relatively unknown, expensive, and not widely available. "Densitometry is where mammography was about 15 years ago," says Dr. Ethel S. Siris, an endocrinologist at Columbia-Presbyterian Medical Center in New York City. "Mammography became a standard screening tool for breast cancer only because many patients and doctors insisted that it be accepted." Densitometry is likely to be accepted in the same way because research is proving the technique to be both accurate and useful in patients at risk for osteoporosis.

Knowing more about when to consider densitometry and what treatment options are available should osteoporosis be detected can help reduce the risk of experiencing the debilitating fractures that often occur after age 70.

Detecting Osteoporosis

The gold standard for detecting osteoporosis is a form of densitometry, called dual energy x-ray absorptiometry (DEXA), which measures bone density based on how bone absorbs two sets of photons (atomic particles with no electrical charge) generated by an x-ray tube. Measurements are obtained at the wrist, hip, and lower spine. The equipment provides values for density as well as standard deviations, making it possible to estimate fracture risk.

DEXA takes between 15 and 45 minutes, depending on the age of the machine. The level of radiation exposure is so low that the technician can remain in the room. There are about 1,500 DEXA machines in the United States, most near major academic centers. The cost of the procedure ranges from $150 to $350. Insurance reimbursement is spotty and varies widely among carriers, states, and even regions within the same state. Medicare regulations are worth checking.

If DEXA is unavailable, three other techniques may suffice: single-photon absorptiometry, dual energy absorptiometry, and quantitative computed tomography. Like DEXA, these tests measure bone density based on photon activity. However, they are not as precise as DEXA.

Risk Factors and Prevention

The first step in preventing osteoporosis is to adopt diet and lifestyle practices that promote bone health. For postmenopausal women and older men, these include consuming 1,500 mg of calcium daily, exercising (walking and lifting light weights are recommended), avoiding excessive alcohol and caffeine consumption, and not smoking. For women past menopause, taking estrogen (when there is no contraindication) is the best prevention strategy. By age 65, most women lose about 35% of their bone mass. About half of that loss is related to declining estrogen. Studies show that two years of estrogen supplementation can increase bone mass by 1.6% in the hip, and that five years of supplementation can cut fracture risk in half.

When osteoporosis does occur, early diagnosis and treatment can reduce the risk of fractures. Postmenopausal women with any of the following risk factors should have an evaluation:

- white or Asian race;

- thin body type;

- family history of osteoporosis;

- early menopause (before age 45);

- smoking;

- a diet low in calcium, or excessive in alcohol consumption (more than two drinks a day) and caffeine intake (multiple cups of coffee or caffeinated beverages a day);

- a sedentary lifestyle.

Women who take estrogen can usually forego imaging because of estrogen's bone-protective qualities. Others may want to determine whether one of the new drug options is appropriate by considering densitometry, especially if the risk for osteoporosis is high.

Choosing the Best Treatment

Modest gains in bone density can significantly reduce fracture risk, and medication can help achieve this goal. While many experts believe that estrogen is still the treatment of choice, the following two options can be considered:

- **Calcitonin.** Like estrogen, calcitonin is a naturally occurring hormone, but most of its effects occur in the skeleton. The newly approved nasal spray is usually preferred over the injectable form because it's easier to use and it limits the nausea and flushing that frequently occur following an injection. Two years of daily treatment increases spine density by 3%. (There are no data for the hip.) Although rare, the major side effect is nasal irritation. Some patients report that calcitonin also relieves osteoporotic pain.

- **Alendronate.** Like etidronate, alendronate is a bisphosphonate. After three years of therapy, alendronate increases spinal density by about 8%, and hip density by about 7%. In studies, those who took alendronate had half the fracture rate than patients taking a dummy pill. In contrast, etidronate does not seem to increase bone mass at the hip, and it is not known whether it reduces fracture risk.

Calcitonin and alendronate inhibit the action of osteoclasts, cells that break down bone. Although the medications have not been tested against each other in double-blind, placebo-controlled trials, the available research supports their use if osteoporosis is confirmed and estrogen is not an option.

On the Horizon: Early Diagnosis, Individual Treatment

Over the next decade, diagnostic options and treatments may improve so much that physicians will be able to screen all older women and at-risk men for osteoporosis, and tailor therapy to individual needs. On the horizon are laboratory tests of the blood and urine to detect the biochemical markers of bone loss. One such procedure, the Osteomark urine test, was recently approved, but only as an aid for monitoring treatment. Promising new drugs include slow-release fluoride therapy, and certain growth hormones. Unlike the currently approved medications, these drugs stimulate the formation of new bone.

After the Vertebral Fracture in Osteoporoses

Osteoporotic fractures can result from a fall, the lifting of a heavy object, or a sudden twisting motion. Sometimes an activity which is not considered stressful or dangerous, such as bending over to pick up a newspaper, sneezing, turning a key in a lock, or receiving an affectionate hug can result in a fractured vertebra, a broken wrist, or cracked rib.

When Mr. Johnson, 72, broke 2 vertebrae, he had many questions about what to expect. Would there be a cast or a brace put on his back? How long would it be before he could resume gardening and his other hobbies? Mr. Johnson s doctor scheduled a special appointment with Mr. and Mrs. Johnson to answer their questions about what they could expect in the next several months. This is what he and his wife learned:

How long will it take for me to recover from these broken bones?

A fractured vertebra can take anywhere from 6 to 8 weeks for the bone to set, and up to 12 weeks to heal completely. But recovery from a vertebral fracture goes beyond healing the bone. Recovery becomes an ongoing process to enable you to regain strength and mobility, and to resume your daily activities.

Everyone experiences a slightly different recuperation. You may find your posture changing and have some nagging pain. This is because a vertebral fracture results in a deformity of the vertebra itself, which affects the muscles, tendons, ligaments, and nerves near the fractured bone. Fortunately, there are steps you can take to minimize these consequences of vertebral fracture.

Will I need surgery to correct the fracture?

No, surgery is not required with a vertebral fracture.

Will I have to stay in bed the whole time?

Bed rest for the first 2-3 days following a fracture is important. The body has suffered a trauma—a broken bone—and needs time and rest in order to heal. How long you stay in bed depends on how much pain you feel, and how long you can be up before your back starts hurting again. In general, we encourage people to be active as soon as pain permits.

During the healing period, you may find that you need help doing things you ordinarily do for yourself, like dressing, bathing, getting in and out of bed or chairs. It's okay to ask for help during this time. Just remember, you won't remain in this dependent condition if you give yourself time to heal, and take the proper steps toward recovery.

While it's important to rest after you've had a vertebral fracture, it is also important to get up and around as soon as you can. Bones and muscles respond well to movement and activity, and in the long run, you'll improve more quickly if you are able to slowly ease back into your usual routine. If you have access to a pool, walking in the water is a great way to maintain and use your muscles without putting stress on the bone which is healing.

What medications will I be taking now?

You will be given pain medication and a different medication to prevent further bone loss so you'll be less likely to fracture again. For pain control, we'll start you on simple, over-the-counter analgesics. We'll also use heating pads, ice packs, and gentle massage to alleviate the pain. If the pain does not subside with these methods, you may be given prescription pain-killers. The duration and intensity of pain is different for every person, and often depends on how many vertebral fractures one has had.

To prevent further bone loss, you will most likely take calcitonin, which is a medication used for the treatment of osteoporosis in women and men. Women have another option: they can take estrogen. Fortunately, there are several drugs for osteoporosis treatment currently being researched.

Calcitonin is a naturally occurring hormone involved in calcium regulation and bone metabolism. It helps prevent bone loss and has been known to have an analgesic or pain-killing effect. It is currently administered by injection only, although a nasal spray form is under investigation. Once you are feeling better, the nurse will teach you how to give yourself the injections.

I will also want you to be sure to get 1,500 mg per day of calcium, and at least 400 IU of vitamin D each day.

Will osteoporosis cause my back to curve over? I would like to avoid developing stooped posture if I can.

The back curvature you refer to is called *kyphosis*. Kyphosis is the result of physical changes in the spine and adjacent muscles, tendons, and ligaments which occur after vertebral fractures. The degree of kyphosis varies with the number of fractures and muscle strength. To minimize the curvature, you will need to learn flexibility and strengthening exercises for your back and torso. I know a rehabilitation clinic with specialists in physical medicine and rehabilitation who can work with you on these exercises. You probably won't start with the therapeutic exercise for about two to four weeks after the fracture, depending on how you're feeling. You'll start out slowly at first—the therapy can be painful, but in the long run you will have the benefits of a stronger back, increased flexibility, and straighter posture.

Should I wear a back brace?

A back brace or support may be beneficial during the healing period for several reasons: 1) it helps the patient to avoid strenuous bending; 2) it provides some pain relief by supporting the spine; and 3) it helps reduce the degree of kyphosis. If a brace is used too much or for too long a time, the back muscles will weaken, which is actually worse for spinal osteoporosis because strong muscles help support the spine. Physical therapy, in the form of exercises to strengthen the back and torso, can be performed even while the individual is wearing the brace.

There are several different types of braces to choose from. If you find that your pain persists or if your posture starts to stoop drastically, we can fit you with the appropriate brace.

Another type of support you might find useful is a cane or walker. While you are recovering from the fracture, you may be a little unsteady on your feet and a cane or walker will give you better balance. Also, these devices distribute weight off of your spine, which can ease some of the pain you feel in the first few weeks.

Will I have to buy a special mattress to protect my back?

A very firm mattress is the best type for people with spinal osteoporosis. For comfort, you can cover it with synthetic sheepskin or an egg crate mattress pad. If you have a very soft mattress, you may have to buy a new one. But before you do that, try putting a piece of plywood on top of the box spring, beneath the mattress. This may provide the support your spine needs.

What kinds of changes will I have to make in my life? My wife and I have plans to do some traveling.

You will be able to resume nearly all of your normal activities, with minimal changes to your routine. You can still travel and garden. In fact, being active is beneficial to your health.

The changes you do have to make involve the way you move, and the safety of your environment. For example, no more bending from the waist to pick something up, you'll have to learn to bend your knees. Activities that require a twisting motion of the torso, such as golf, puts a heavy strain on the spine and should be avoided. And no lifting of anything heavier than a light bag of groceries, depending on the severity of the osteoporosis.

You should fall-proof your home to minimize the chances of tripping and falling. Be careful when taking medications that might make you dizzy, and be aware of the effects of alcohol on your balance.

I'm usually not the kind of person to talk about my troubles, but this osteoporosis is pretty serious and I'm worried about it. Is there a group of people I could get together with to discuss some of these changes?

Attending a support group is a great way to share information and discuss feelings as you learn to cope with these changes. The nurse can give you the name and phone number of the osteoporosis support group leader in the area. Many of my patients and their family members attend meetings regularly. Quite often a speaker comes to the meetings to present information on different aspects of osteoporosis prevention and treatment. I have spoken at a couple of the meetings myself.

Chapter 13

Syringomyelia

What is syringomyelia?

Syringomyelia (*sear-IN-go-my-EEL-ya*) is a disorder in which a cyst forms within the spinal cord. This cyst, called a *syrinx*, expands and elongates over time, destroying the center of the spinal cord. Since the spinal cord connects the brain to nerves in the extremities, this damage results in pain, weakness, and stiffness in the back, shoulders, arms, or legs. Other symptoms may include headaches and a loss of the ability to feel extremes of hot or cold, especially in the hands. Each patient experiences a different combination of symptoms.

Other, more common disorders share the early symptoms of syringomyelia. In the past, this has made diagnosis difficult. The advent of one outpatient test, however, called magnetic resonance imaging (MRI), has significantly increased the number of syringomyelia cases diagnosed in the beginning stages of the disorder.

About 21,000 American men and women have syringomyelia, with symptoms usually beginning in young adulthood. Signs of the disorder tend to develop slowly, although sudden onset may occur with coughing or straining. If not treated surgically, syringomyelia often leads to progressive weakness in the arms and legs, loss of hand sensation, and chronic, severe pain.

NIH Pub. No. 94-3780, August 1994.

What causes syringomyelia?

A watery, protective substance known as cerebrospinal fluid normally flows around the spinal cord and brain, transporting nutrients and waste products. It also serves to cushion the brain.

A number of medical conditions can cause an obstruction in the normal flow of cerebrospinal fluid, redirecting it into the spinal cord itself. For reasons that are only now becoming clear, this results in syrinx formation. Cerebrospinal fluid fills the syrinx. Pressure differences along the spine cause the fluid to move within the cyst. Physicians believe that it is this continual movement of fluid that results in cyst growth and further damage to the spinal cord.

What are the different forms of syringomyelia?

Generally, there are two forms of syringomyelia. In most cases, the disorder is related to a congenital abnormality of the brain called a *Chiari I malformation*, named after the physician who first characterized it. This malformation occurs during the development of the fetus and causes the lower part of the cerebellum to protrude from its normal location in the back of the head into the cervical or neck portion of the spinal canal. A syrinx may then develop in the cervical region of the spinal cord. Because of the relationship that was once thought to exist between the brain and spinal cord in this type of syringomyelia, physicians sometimes refer to it as *communicating syringomyelia*. Here, symptoms usually begin between the ages of 25 and 40 and may worsen with straining or any activity that causes cerebrospinal fluid pressure to fluctuate. Some patients, however, may have long periods of stability. Some patients with this form of the disorder also have *hydrocephalus*, in which cerebrospinal fluid accumulates in the skull, or a condition called *arachnoiditis*, in which a covering of the spinal cord—the arachnoid membrane—is inflamed.

The second major form of syringomyelia occurs as a complication of trauma, meningitis, hemorrhage, a tumor, or arachnoiditis. Here, the syrinx or cyst develops in a segment of the spinal cord damaged by one of these conditions. The syrinx then starts to expand. This is sometimes referred to as *noncommunicating syringomyelia*.

Symptoms may appear months or even years after the initial injury, starting with pain, weakness, and sensory impairment originating at the site of trauma.

The primary symptom of post-traumatic syringomyelia is pain, which may spread upward from the site of injury. Symptoms, such as pain, numbness, weakness, and disruption in temperature sensation, may be limited to one side of the body. Syringomyelia can also adversely affect sweating, sexual function, and, later, bladder and bowel control.

Some cases of syringomyelia are familial, although this is rare. In addition, one form of the disorder involves a part of the brain called the brainstem. The brainstem controls many of our vital functions, such as respiration and heartbeat. When syrinxes affect the brainstem, the condition is called *syringobulbia*.

How is syringomyelia diagnosed?

Physicians now use magnetic resonance imaging (MRI) to diagnose syringomyelia. The MR imager takes pictures of body structures, such as the brain and spinal cord, in vivid detail. This test will show the syrinx in the spine or any other conditions, such as the presence of a tumor. MRI is safe, painless, and informative and has greatly improved the diagnosis of syringomyelia.

The physician may order additional tests to help confirm the diagnosis. One of these is called electromyography (EMG), which measures muscle weakness. The doctor may also wish to test cerebrospinal fluid pressure levels and to analyze the cerebrospinal fluid by performing a lumbar puncture. In addition, computed tomography (CT) scans of a patient's head may reveal the presence of tumors and other abnormalities such as hydrocephalus.

Like MRI and CT scans, another test, called a myelogram, takes x-ray-like pictures and requires a contrast medium or dye to do so. Since the introduction of MRI this test is rarely necessary to diagnose syringomyelia.

How is syringomyelia treated?

Surgery is usually recommended for syringomyelia patients. The main goal of surgery is to provide more space for the cerebellum (Chiari malformation) at the base of the skull and upper neck, without entering the brain or spinal cord. This results in flattening or disappearance of the primary cavity. If a tumor is causing syringomyelia, removal of the tumor is the treatment of choice and almost always eliminates the syrinx.

Surgery results in stabilization or modest improvement in symptoms for most patients. Delay in treatment may result in irreversible spinal cord injury. Recurrence of syringomyelia after surgery may make additional operations necessary; these may not be completely successful over the long term.

In some patients it may be necessary to drain the syrinx, which can be accomplished using a catheter, drainage tubes, and valves. This system is also known as a shunt. Shunts are used in both the communicating and noncommunicating forms of the disorder. First, the surgeon must locate the syrinx. Then, the shunt is placed into it with the other end draining cerebrospinal fluid into a cavity, usually the abdomen. This type of shunt is called a *ventriculoperitoneal shunt* and is used in cases involving hydrocephalus. By draining syrinx fluid, a shunt can arrest the progression of symptoms and relieve pain, headache, and tightness. Without correction, symptoms generally continue.

The decision to use a shunt requires extensive discussion between doctor and patient, as this procedure carries with it the risk of injury to the spinal cord, infection, blockage, or hemorrhage and may not necessarily work for all patients.

In the case of trauma-related syringomyelia, the surgeon operates at the level of the initial injury. The cyst collapses at surgery but a tube or shunt is usually necessary to prevent re-expansion.

Drugs have no curative value as a treatment for syringomyelia. Radiation is used rarely and is of little benefit except in the presence of a tumor. In these cases, it can halt the extension of a cavity and may help to alleviate pain.

In the absence of symptoms, syringomyelia is usually not treated. In addition, a physician may recommend not treating the condition in patients of advanced age or in cases where there is no progression of symptoms. Whether treated or not, many patients will be told to avoid activities that involve straining.

What research is being done?

The precise causes of syringomyelia are still unknown. Scientists at the National Institute of Neurological Disorders and Stroke in Bethesda, Maryland, and at grantee institutions across the country continue to explore the mechanisms that lead to the formation of syrinxes in the spinal cord. For instance, Institute investigators have found that as the heart beats, syrinx fluid is forced downward. This finding suggests a role for the cardiovascular system in syringomyelia.

Surgical techniques are also being refined by the neurosurgical research community. In one treatment approach currently being evaluated, neurosurgeons perform a decompressive procedure where the dura mater, a tough membrane covering the cerebellum and spinal cord, is enlarged with a graft. Like altering a suit of clothing, this procedure expands the area around the cerebellum and spinal cord, thus improving the flow of cerebrospinal fluid and eliminating the syrinx.

It is also important to understand the role of birth defects in the development of hindbrain malformations that can lead to syringomyelia. Learning when these defects occur during the development of the fetus can help us understand this and similar disorders, and may lead to preventive treatment that can stop the formation of many birth abnormalities. Dietary supplements of folic acid during pregnancy have already been found to reduce the number of cases of certain birth defects.

Diagnostic technology is another area for continued research. Already, MRI has enabled scientists to see conditions in the spine, including syringomyelia, even before symptoms appear. A new technology, known as dynamic MRI, allows investigators to view spinal fluid pulsating within the syrinx. This research tool makes diagnosis easier and rules out the need for more invasive procedures such as myelography. CT scans allow physicians to see abnormalities in the brain, and other diagnostic tests have also improved greatly with the availability of new, non-toxic, contrast dyes. Patients can expect even better techniques to become available in the future from the research efforts of scientists today.

In addition, the National Institute of Neurological Disorders and Stroke (NINDS) sponsored a workshop on syringomyelia in June 1994. Leading experts from around the world convened in Washington, DC, to share their findings and help chart a course for future research on this important disorder. For a copy of the workshop summary, please contact the NINDS Office of Scientific and Health Reports at the address listed below.

Where can I go for more information?

The NINDS conducts and supports a wide range of research on neurological disorders, including pain and painful disorders such as syringomyelia. For more information on this and other neurological disorders, or on the Institute and its research programs, contact:

Office of Scientific and Health Reports
NIH Neurological Institute
P.O. Box 5801
Bethesda, Maryland 20824
(301) 496-5751
(800) 352-9424

The organization listed below provides printed information and assistance to syringomyelia patients and other interested individuals.

American Syringomyelia Alliance Project, Inc.
P.O. Box 1586
Longview, Texas 75606-1586
(903) 236-7079
800-ASAP-282

Several lay organizations are directly concerned with chronic pain. They are excellent sources of additional information, research updates, and specific help and referrals:

National Chronic Pain Outreach Association, Inc.
7979 Old Georgetown Road
Suite 100
Bethesda, Maryland 20814-2429
(301) 652-4948

American Chronic Pain Association
P.O. Box 850
Rocklin, California 95677
(916) 632-0922

The Chronic Pain Letter is a bimonthly review of new pain treatments, books, and resources for people who live with pain. For subscription information write:

Chronic Pain Letter
P.O. Box 1303
Old Chelsea Station
New York, New York 10011

The following national organizations are concerned with research, care, and treatment of spinal cord injury and other paralyzing or disabling conditions, and are sources of information, publications, and advice:

American Paralysis Association
500 Morris Avenue
Springfield, New Jersey 07081
(201) 379-2690
(800) 225-0292

National Spinal Cord Injury Association
545 Concord Avenue
Suite 29
Cambridge, Massachusetts 02138
(617) 935-2722
(800) 962-9629

Paralyzed Veterans of America
National Office
801 18th Street, NW
Washington, DC 20006
(202) 872-1300

Spinal Cord Society
Wendell Road
Fergus Falls, Minnesota 56537
(218) 739-5252
(218) 739-5262

Additional information about Chiari malformation may be available from:

Spina Bifida Association of America
4590 MacArthur Boulevard, NW
Suite 250
Washington, DC 20007
(202) 944-3285
(800) 621-3141

March of Dimes Birth Defects Foundation
1275 Mamaroneck Avenue
White Plains, New York 10605
(914) 428-7100

National Organization for Rare Disorders (NORD)
P.O. Box 8923
New Fairfield, Connecticut 06812-8923
(203) 746-6518
(800) 999-6673

Additional information about arachnoiditis is available from:

Arachnoiditis Information and Support Network
P.O. Box 1166
Ballwin, Missouri 63022
(314) 394-5741

Chapter 14

Spondylitis

What Does "Ankylosing Spondylitis" Mean?

"Spondylitis" means inflammation involving joints of the spine and is derived from the Greek word for vertebra (spondylos) and inflammation (itis). As the inflammation subsides, healing takes place during which the bone grows out from both sides of the joint, eventually surrounding it completely. The joint is then unable to move, and this stiffening is called "ankylosis."

Formation of the Spine

To understand the disease, we can take a closer look at the spine. The spine is made up of 24 vertebrae and 110 joints. The three main sections of vertebrae—the cervical, thoracic, and lumbar—differ somewhat in their form and their natural curvature. The cervical, or neck, vertebrae are the most mobile. In the thoracic section, each vertebra has a rib attached by joints on each side of it. Below the lumbar section is the sacrum, which sits like a keystone in the ring of bone which forms the pelvis. The joints between the sides of the sacrum and the pelvis, called the sacroiliac joints, are the starting points for ankylosing spondylitis.

A *Guidebook for Patients* (1994), and excerpts from *Straight Talk on Spondylitis* (1992), Spondylitis Association of America; reprinted with permission.

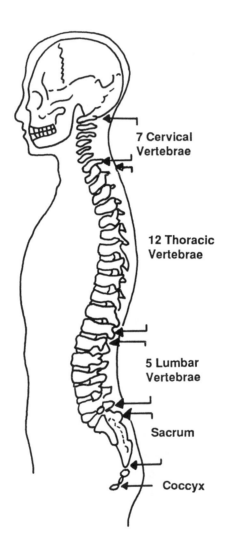

Figure 14.1. *The human spine.*

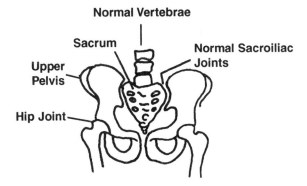

Figure 14.2. *This drawing shows the sacroiliac joints and the joints between each vertebra as they look before the disease, when they are normal. Hip joints can also be affected, but this is less common. Occasionally, hip surgery is recommended to restore movement in the affected joint.*

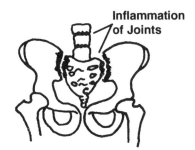

Figure 14.3.*In the early stages of the disease, changes begin to take place in the sacrum and upper pelvis. Here we also see evidence of changes in the joints between the vertebrae*

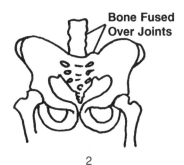

Figure 14.4. *In the advanced stage, the sacroiliac joints are fused, and the joints between the vertebrae have also grown together by bony changes. This produces the effect sometimes known as "bamboo spine."*

2

What Causes Ankylosing Spondylitis?

The cause of ankylosing spondylitis is not known, but there have been some important developments in our understanding of this condition over the last few years. What is known is that it is about three hundred times more common in people who inherit a certain *white* cell blood group numbered HLA B27 than in those who do not inherit this group. This white cell group is not related to the red cell blood groups, which are important in blood transfusions.

Who Gets Ankylosing Spondylitis?

For a long time we have known that this back complaint "runs in families." The link with the *white* cell blood groups confirms this and will be discussed later in this chapter. Typically, the disease affects young men. However, we know that the illness occurs in women as well. Many people go through their lives with back complaints that are never really diagnosed as ankylosing spondylitis. We know now how important it is to recognize the condition early, because treatment is usually very helpful and the patient benefits from early diagnosis and, therefore, early treatment.

What Is the Difference Between Ankylosing Spondylitis and Other Back Ailments?

Back troubles are some of the most common complaints seen in a doctors office. In each year, 2% of a general practitioner's patients consult him with backache. Although most patients with back pain do not have ankylosing spondylitis, the doctor must recognize the different nature of the back problem in each patient. The most common back ailment is "back strain," which may occur at any age. A "slipped disk" is another example. In older patients degenerative, or wear-and-tear, problems commonly affect the back.

When a patient goes to the doctor with backache, the doctor must decide whether the problem is an *inflammatory* arthritis, that is, ankylosing spondylitis, or one of the common mechanical back problems. The treatment is different. The diagnosis is made by listening to the symptoms and examining the patient. The doctor may perform certain blood tests and examine X-ray films of the back. We will discuss these points separately.

What Are the Symptoms of Ankylosing Spondylitis?

Symptoms of ankylosing spondylitis that help distinguish it from mechanical causes of back pain are:

* slow (insidious) onset over weeks rather than hours
* age of onset around 20 or 25 years, rather than any age
* early morning stiffness and pain
* persistence for more than 3 months (rather than coming on in attacks)
* improvement with exercise, worse with rest (the opposite is true with mechanical problems)

Although we have been talking about a disease of the spine, pain is not always confined to the back. Some patients have chest pain which is worse on deep breathing, and felt around the ribs. This chest pain does not come from the heart but from the joints between the ribs and the backbone. Many patients complain of a shut-in feeling in the chest because it is difficult to move the ribs fully with deep breathing. However, the lungs can continue to work because the diaphragm is not affected.

When ankylosing spondylitis begins, it usually causes an ache felt in the buttocks and, possibly, down the backs of the thighs and in the lower part of the back. One side is commonly more painful than the other. This pain arises from the sacroiliac joints. The morning stiffness which is so characteristic of the condition wears off during the day. Many patients find that pain wakes them in the early morning, and if they get up and walk around, the discomfort settles. Patients may also experience the pain and stiffness after a prolonged period of sitting, as, for example, in a cinema or on a long car ride.

Ankylosing spondylitis in its early stages may cause considerable pain, but effective treatment is available to relieve this, even though the discomfort is not always eliminated. Later the disease becomes much less active, or even totally inactive. The stiffness is rarely a handicap, provided that the spine is in a good position. Most patients with ankylosing spondylitis are able to carry on with their work and lead a normal life.

A few patients in the early stages of ankylosing spondylitis feel generally ill. In other words, they feel tired and miserable and may lose weight. It is not uncommon for them to be treated for depression. Some people may never have anything more than a series of mild aches and pains coming on and lasting for several months, never troubling them greatly. This seems to be more common in women with the disease. At this stage the disease can either clear up or it may go on to cause stiffening higher up the back, or in the neck.

Limb Joints

Sometimes, either at the start or later, ankylosing spondylitis may affect joints other than in the spine. The shoulders, hips, knees, ankles, and feet are the most commonly affected. The effect on these joints is similar to the effect on the spine; there may well be a period of aching in the joint, perhaps with some swelling, but treatment relieves these symptoms and they settle down. Ultimately, there may be some restriction in the movement of the affected joints, but with proper treatment and active exercises from the start, the disability is slight. In particular, the hip joint must not be allowed to stiffen in a bent position.

Enthesopathies (trouble spots)

Tender places may sometimes develop in bones that are not part of the spine. One of these is the heel bone, making it uncomfortable to stand on a hard floor, and another is the bone of the "seat" (ischium), making hard chairs unpleasant.

Does Ankylosing Spondylitis Only Affect the Joints of the Back and Limbs?

No. Other parts of the body may be affected. For example, attacks of inflammation of the eye occur in about 1 patient out of 7 sometime during their lives. These attacks are due to iritis, or inflammation in the colored part of the eye (the iris). A painful red eye should be reported to the doctor without delay, or permanent damage might occur. If the doctor is not available, then the patient should go directly to a hospital emergency room or ophthalmology department.

Other rare complications, happening in less than 1 patient in 100, may occur. These include problems in the heart, lungs, and central nervous system. Treatment is available for all of them. Patients with ankylosing spondylitis are not any more at risk of getting heart attacks, strokes, or cancer than the general population. Colitis, or inflammation of the bowel, is associated with ankylosing spondylitis in some patients, as is a skin condition called psoriasis.

How Is Ankylosing Spondylitis Diagnosed?

Many patients have commented that their ankylosing spondylitis was not diagnosed until many months or years after their first symptoms began. There is no diagnostic test that the doctor can do at the onset of back pain, but the patient's symptoms, which differ from those of mechanical back pain, should alert the doctor to the diagnosis. Identification of the HLA B27 blood group alone would certainly not make the diagnosis, although it helps. At best, it may alert the doctor's attention to the fact that a patient may be developing ankylosing spondylitis.

The Physical Examination

The doctor will take a history and examine the back (looking for muscle spasm and noting posture and mobility) and then look at all the other parts of the body, searching for evidence of ankylosing spondylitis.

What Tests Will the Doctor Do?

The diagnosis of ankylosing spondylitis is confirmed from the X-ray. The characteristic changes are in the sacroiliac joints, but they may take some months to develop and may not be seen at the first consultation. The doctor will also probably test for anemia and do a test called the erythrocyte sedimentation rate (ESR), which tells how "active" the disease is.

What Is the End Result?

Ankylosing spondylitis takes a different course in different people and no two cases are exactly the same. The symptoms may come and go over long periods, but in the end ankylosing spondylitis almost always settles down. The lumbar spine usually becomes stiff, and the upper part of the back and the neck can stiffen as well.

It is for this reason that it is so important for patients to maintain a good posture. The worst disability that can follow ankylosing spondylitis is fixation of your back in a bent or stooped position. This used to be common but is now prevented by early diagnosis and treatment. Not every patient with ankylosing spondylitis who maintains a good posture and follows an exercise program will return to normal, but serious deformities can be prevented by these measures. The patient who stiffens in a bent position has difficulty in looking straight in front and compensates by straining other muscles and joints, which gives rise to more pain.

People with ankylosing spondylitis can often be acutely aware of their own appearance and how they might look different from other people. Most patients can come to terms with the problem, even though this may be difficult.

What Is the Treatment?

There is no cure for ankylosing spondylitis. The doctor aims to relieve the symptoms, improve spinal mobility where this has been lost, and allow you to follow a normal occupational and social life. Although with increasing age the disease tends to become less active, you should realize that the treatment must continue more or less forever. In particular, you must pay continuous attention to adequate posture, mobility, and exercises.

The patient and doctor alike play an active role in the management of this condition, usually with the help of a physical therapist. Occasional visits to the doctor will ensure that an adequate management program is being followed. Although the treatment section of this chapter is divided into separate sections for drug treatment, posture, physical therapy, and exercises, these aspects of treatment will vary with the individual patient.

As part of the treatment of ankylosing spondylitis, it is important that you, as the patient, take care of your health and posture. This includes not allowing yourself to become overweight or overtired from working overtime or taking on too many commitments. The motto for treatment which all patients should learn like a catechism is:

It is the doctor's job to relieve pain and the patient's job to keep exercising and maintain a good posture.

Principles of Treatment

- Take good care of your general health and pay attention to your diet.

- Persevere with exercises which are designed to maintain mobility and posture of the joints affected by the disease. You must maintain good posture while working, playing, and sleeping.

- Consult your doctor if you need relief from pain.

- Do not be afraid to take drugs to control pain. Once pain is controlled, a regular exercise program becomes possible and should help control pain so that drugs become less necessary.

- Cooperate with your doctor in getting periodic checks on your general health.

Your General Health

At times when ankylosing spondylitis is active, your health as a whole suffers; you may lose weight, get unusually tired, even depressed, or become anemic. At such times, in addition to treatment for the back, you will need extra rest and a good nourishing diet.

A good diet in this case is one giving you at least two helpings of protein food each day—meat or fish. Fruit and vegetables are sources of vitamins, and a pint of milk daily will give you a sufficient supply of calcium. If necessary, your doctor may give you iron tablets for anemia.

Drug Treatment

Although the disease cannot be cured, most of the trouble caused by it can be helped or prevented. In the first instance, the doctor will prescribe for you a drug that relieves pain and inflammation (anti-inflammatory drug). There is a wide range of anti-inflammatory drugs that are used to reduce or abolish the pain, give you a good night's sleep, and provide sufficient freedom from pain to take part in an active exercise program.

Many patients find that they require continuous treatment on a small maintenance dose of their drug. Some of the newer tablets are manufactured to remain effective within the patient throughout the night and into the first part of the day. If you cannot find a suitable tablet to last throughout the night, suppositories may be used. It is not necessary to give drugs by injection. None of the drugs used for ankylosing spondylitis is habit-forming (i.e., patients don't get addicted to them).

Posture

Since ankylosing spondylitis left untreated causes increasing flexion of the spine (the patient becomes progressively more stooped), every endeavor must be directed toward keeping as straight and erect as possible. It is rare for the spine to stiffen completely but, in case this might happen, you should do everything to ensure that it at least stiffens in an erect rather than a bent position.

Sitting posture. To maintain good posture while sitting, use a chair with a firm seat, straight back, and armrests. Firm padding on the seat and back will make you more comfortable. The seat of the chair should not be too long from front to back because this might make it difficult to place your lower spine into the base of the back of the chair. Don't sit for long in low soft chairs as this will result in bad posture and increased pain.

At work. Pay special attention to the position of your back when at work, so that you do not have to stoop. If you sit at a desk or bench, see that your seat is at the proper height and do not sit in one position for too long without moving your back. A job that allows a variety of movements—sitting, standing, and walking—is ideal. The most unsuitable work is that in which you stoop or crouch over a bench for hours at a time. If you have a heavy or tiring job, do not tackle other activities at home or elsewhere until you have had a break, lying flat for a time if necessary. It may also help if you can lie flat for 20 minutes at midday. At such times try to lie for part of the time face downward.

Car driving. If you ever have to make a long car journey, it is important to stop for 5 minutes every hour or so and get out of the car for a stretch. Pain and stiffness can distract your attention, which is so vital for your safety if you are driving.

Many patients with stiffness of the neck and other parts of their spine have difficulty backing into parking spaces or a garage because they cannot turn easily to look behind them. It is possible to fit special mirrors onto your car to help you. You should practice backing up using this new technique in an open area with some light wooden obstacles to act as markers. (A piece of broom handle stuck into the ground could serve this purpose.) Head rests are advised so that sudden deceleration injuries to the neck can be avoided. The stiff neck of an ankylosing spondylitis patient is more easily hurt than a normal neck. Disabled drivers permits may be appropriate if you can't walk very far, but this is a rare problem in ankylosing spondylitis.

Rest. If ankylosing spondylitis is very active and the stiffness very troublesome, a spell off from work or in the hospital may be necessary. This does not mean resting immobile, for this might hasten the stiffening of the spine. So even a spell of rest from work means that you will be encouraged to do exercises for your back and chest and limbs to keep them supple. When you are lying in bed it is important that you should be quite flat on your back and, also, some of the time you should practice lying on your face. "Prone lying," as it is called, is best done for 20 minutes before rising in the mornings, and 20 minutes before going to bed at night.

At first you may not be able to tolerate more than 5 minutes of prone lying at a time, or may even need a pillow under your chest, but with practice, as the spine relaxes, it will become easier. If you make a habit of this it will help prevent your back and hips from becoming bent. Although this period of prone lying may not be practical every day, at least some time devoted to it is better than nothing at all.

Your bed. The bed you sleep on should be firm and without sag. If you have a soft or sagging mattress, get a suitable board to put between the mattress and the bed frame. A sheet of plywood or chipboard 2' x 5' x 1/2" is ideal.

You will find that this bed is more comfortable to lie on than one that is too yielding. Afterward, when the painful active phase of spondylitis is past, it is important to keep a firm bed to prevent any tendency for spinal curvature to develop later.

Corsets and braces. In general, corsets and braces are of no value whatsoever, and indeed can make ankylosing spondylitis worse. It is better to develop your own muscles and retain a good posture by natural means. Very occasionally some form of bracing may be necessary, for example, after a back injury, but this decision should be made by a doctor who is experienced in treating patients with ankylosing spondylitis.

Physical Therapy

Probably, at some time, you will receive treatment from a physical therapist, and you should learn an exercise routine which you can do every day. The exercises will be tailored to your individual requirements and, for this purpose, you should attend a Physical Therapy Department for one or two sessions to learn your exercises. The physical therapist, however, may require a referral from a doctor, so in the first place you must approach your doctor.

Until you have a set of exercises of your own you should make a start right away by doing daily exercises. Some of these are shown below. You may not be able to do all of the exercises, but do what you can. Their purpose is to make you conscious of your posture, especially the position of your back, and to encourage free movement of certain joints, particularly shoulders and hips. It is important to keep your muscles strong, because reduced movement, even for a short time, allows them to become weaker and it may take a long time to build them up again.

Sporting activities. Many patients ask what sporting activities are suitable for them and the most ideal one is swimming, since it uses all the muscles and joints without jarring them. Regular swimming is something the whole family can enjoy.

Some young patients enjoy cross-country running or tennis. Contact sports are not ideal because the joints can get injured. Even golf has its drawbacks, because patients may spend long periods practicing putting, during which the spine is in continued flexion. Badminton can be beneficial and also squash when the disease is going through remission. Basketball and volleyball are excellent as they combine movement with stretching and jumping.

However, not all patients tolerate weight-bearing and jarring activities. Bicycling is a very beneficial form of exercise because it helps keep the joints active and gives more strength in the legs. It is also a good breathing exercise and helps the rib cage to continue in its expansion, provided that the handlebars are adjusted properly so that the rider is sitting tall.

Heat. In its various forms, heat will help to relieve the pain and stiffness. A hot bath before retiring, or a hot water bottle or electric blanket in your bed may be quite enough. It is not necessary to use special lamps.

Surgery. Surgery has only a small place in the treatment of ankylosing spondylitis. It is used in restoring movement to damaged hip joints (arthroplasty) and, rarely, in straightening the back or neck in patients who have become so bent over that they cannot look forward and are having difficulty in crossing the road.

Folk remedies. Do not be beguiled into buying expensive treatments whose effectiveness has not been medically proved. For patients with stiff necks, manipulation can be dangerous.

Physical Therapy: General Reminders

- Lie on your front on a firm surface for about 20 minutes every morning or evening.

- Repeat your deep breathing exercises at frequent intervals during the day.

- Beware of your posture—correct it constantly, not only during your exercise periods but during the day while standing, sitting, and walking.

- Do some of your exercises EVERY day.

Daily Exercises

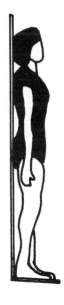

1. Standing with your heels and seat against a wall and keeping your chin in, push your head back toward the wall and keep it back for the count of 5, then relax. Repeat 10 times.

2. Sit on a firm chair, put your
    right hand across your chest
    and hold the side of the chair.
    Stretch your left arm out in
    front of you and then twist to
    the left, taking the arm hori-
    zontally as far behind you as
    possible, turning your head to
    look over the left shoulder.
    Hold this position, then push
    and turn a little further, hold
    that position and then return
    to facing forward. Repeat 3
    times with each arm.

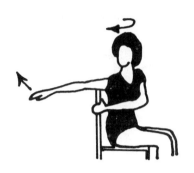

3. (a) Sit with your shoulders relaxed and chin drawn in, looking
    straight ahead. Bend your head sideways to bring your right
    ear toward your right shoulder, hold it there, make sure your
    shoulder muscles are still relaxed and bend a bit further, then
    return to straight. (As you do the side bending, the profile of
    your nose should remain in the same place, to make sure you
    don't turn your head.) Repeat to each side twice.

a

b

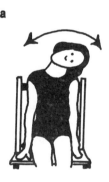
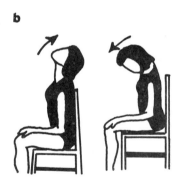

3. (b) Now tip your head back, looking up the wall and along the
    ceiling and bring it back to straight. Repeat

    Change to tipping your head forward as far as possible to get
    your chin touching your neck, and return to straight with chin
    pulled in. Repeat.

4. Lying on your back with knees bent up, lift up your hips, so your seat is off the floor and there is a straight line from shoulder to knees. Hold for the count of 5, and lower. Repeat 5 times.

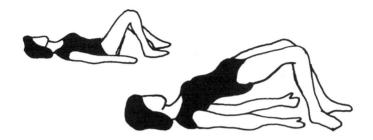

5. Lie on your front, head turned to one side, hands by your sides. (If necessary, you may put a pillow under your chest, but not your waist, in order to get comfortable.)

(a) Raise one leg off the ground, keeping your knee straight, 5 times each leg, making sure your thigh comes off the around.

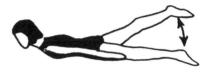

(b) Raise your head and shoulders off the ground as high as you can 10 times.

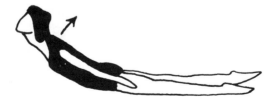

6. Kneeling on the floor on all fours, stretch the opposite arm and leg out parallel with the floor and hold for the count of 10. Lower and then repeat with other arm and leg. Repeat 5 times each side.

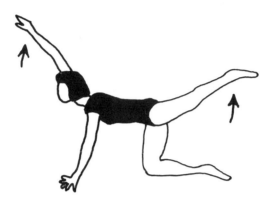

Breathing Exercises

7. Lie on your back, legs straight.

(a) Put your hands on your ribs at the sides of chest. Breathe in deeply through your nose and out through your mouth, pushing your ribs out against your hands as you breathe in. Repeat 10 times. (Remember, it is as important to breathe out fully as it is to breathe in deeply.)

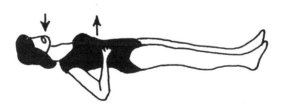

(b) Put your hands on the upper part of the front of your chest. Breathe in deeply through your nose and then breathe out as far as you can through your mouth. Push your ribs up against your hands as you breathe in. Repeat 10 times.

Other Topics

Ankylosing Spondylitis in the Family

In most populations of European origin, ankylosing spondylitis is virtually confined to those who inherit the white cell group HLA B27. This group occurs in 7% to 10% of the population. This means that virtually all people with ankylosing spondylitis will have this particular blood group. However, it is very important to note that the reverse is not true. There are far more people with the blood group who never get ankylosing spondylitis than those who do get it. Even in families where one member has ankylosing spondylitis, a brother or sister can have the blood group and never get the disease.

The chances of your children developing ankylosing spondylitis are quite low, not more than 5 in 100, compared with 95 out of 100 chances of producing normal healthy children. Even of this 5% who get the disease, probably only 1 in 5 will get the condition severely enough to interfere with a normal life. Parents with ankylosing spondylitis sometimes ask if they should have their children blood-grouped to see which ones have HLA B27. The answer at present is that this should not be done since there is no way of knowing which child with this blood group would get the disease. If there comes a time when we are able to prevent ankylosing spondylitis, then it would be important to find out which children carried the HLA B27 blood group, so that they could be protected from the disease.

Ankylosing Spondylitis in Men vs. Women

Until recently, ankylosing spondylitis was considered to be much more common in men than women. We now have evidence to suggest that women, too, frequently develop the disease. It does seem that some women have a very mild form of the condition which may not, in fact, be easy to detect.

Pregnancy and Sex

Ankylosing spondylitis does not usually interfere with normal love-making, unless the hips are affected, in which case the modern operation of hip arthroplasty may help considerably in freeing hip movement. The Arthritis Foundation has published a booklet entitled "Living & Loving: Information About Sex" which is obtainable by writing to The Arthritis Foundation, 1314 Spring Street NW, Atlanta, Georgia 30309.

Pregnancy in women with ankylosing spondylitis holds no particular hazard for the mother and baby, but in contrast with some other forms of rheumatism the spondylitis does not quiet down during pregnancy. The babies are usually born by the normal route, but occasionally it is necessary to have a Caesarean operation if the hip joints become very rigid.

Some Questions We Knew You'd Ask!

What about Other Means of Relieving Pain?

Before trying anything new, it is best to visit the doctor for a current evaluation. Perhaps the dosage of type of medicine needs to be changed. Or, your doctor may send you to a physical therapist for additional treatments, including one or more from the list below. Although these treatment modalities can help relieve pain, they should not be substituted for your daily routine of medication, exercise, posture, etc.

Except for the moist heat and ice packs, the others are generally costly and non of them can be counted on to relieve pain. Some companies have developed less expensive, portable home electrical stimulating unites. You may want to request a loaner for trial or to rent one rather than to purchase it.

- moist heat, such as a hot tub or Jacuzzi; or a hot pack, such as a hydrocollator moist pad (boiled in water) or a Thermophore (electric moist-like heating pad for topical application).

- ice packs, to reduce acute inflammation and swelling.

- transcutaneous nerve-stimulator (TNS or TENS), which sends an electrical current through electrodes taped adjacent to the painful areas to help block nerve transmission of pain. Two similar machines are the electro-acuscope and neuroprobe which act as types of electrical acupuncture.

- electric muscle simulators cause repeated muscle contractions to fatigue muscles in painful spasm and help cause them to relax.

- Other means of providing temporary relief are acupuncture (needles), acupressure (fingers), and massages.

What about Nutrition?

In recent years many "alternative" diets have gained popularity among some arthritis patients. The proponents of these diets promise results, but carefully controlled medical experiments have not validated the claims made for special foods or dietary supplements in the treatment of spondylitis. If you're interested in trying one of these non-traditional diets, be cautions, as they may not include adequate amounts of some nutrients.

Like the general population, spondylitis patients need all the essential nutrients. Your diet should include a wide variety of fruits, vegetables, breads, grains, cereals, meats, poultry and fish. some patients report feeling better when they restrict some items (such as fats) and/or emphasize others (such as roughage). If it works for you stay with it; just be sure it is not at the expense of essential nutrients.

Several spondylitis patients have expressed concern that a high intake of calcium may be related to bone fusion. There is absolutely no evidence to support this. Adequate daily amounts of calcium, phosphorous, magnesium, and other nutrients are important in maintaining health and preventing the brittle bone disease, osteoporosis. Spondylitis patients, and women in general, are known to be at higher risk for developing osteoporosis; so, calcium intake should not be curtailed. Always check with your physician before adding calcium supplements to your diet.

Iron and Vitamin C supplements have been advocated by some, but scientific research has not confirmed any special benefit in treating spondylitis. Iron may be necessary, however, to counteract a side effect of some NSAIDs (anemia from mild intestinal blood loss).

Spondylitis patients should take care to maintain their ideal body weight. Spondylitis can cause weight loss in some, adding to the feeling of fatigue and reduced resistance to disease. These patients will need to increase their intake of nutritious foods. consulting with your physician or a registered dietitian (R.D.) will help you in establishing a calorie goal and practical diet plan. The overweight patient should be advised that excessive weight puts an increased pressure on the spine and adversely affects weight-bearing joints like the hips and knees. These patients need to follow a program to ensure a safe, steady and permanent weight loss.

What about Braces and Corsets?

Corsets or braces are usually counterproductive. As was noted earlier, the best way to ensure good posture is by strengthening the muscles in the opposite direction of the flexion. The use of either a corset or brace will keep the back and/or neck upright; however, the muscles around those joints will become weakened from non-use. Thus, when the device is removed, the muscles will not be strong enough to support the area unless you conscientiously and consistently perform prescribed exercises to counteract the weakening effect of bracing.

What about Health Insurance?

At the time of this writing, adequate health insurance provision is a critical national issue. A large percentage of Americans are without insurance and have little or no chance of getting any.

Having spondylitis can add to problems in getting health insurance. The diagnosis alone may lead to denial of insurance without any concern of how mild your disease might be. The difficulty is the "pre-existing condition clause" that insurance companies write into policies. The policy might be limited in one or more ways. It might exclude or restrict payment for any costs related to the condition. It might impose a waiting period of six months to a year or more, during which no costs related to spondylitis will be paid. it might impose a nigh deductible, or an increased premium. Or, it might exclude coverage—denying health insurance altogether.

What can you do? First, if you already have insurance, do not cancel the policy or let your coverage lapse unless you have already been accepted by another insurance company. If your insurance is through your employer, be aware that if you change jobs or stop working, you are at risk of losing your insurance. Fortunately, a law known as COBRA, allows you to keep your group health benefits for up to 18 months after you leave the job. You must pay the premiums, but costs are held to no more than two percent above regular group rates.

If you need insurance, look for coverage through a group, such as a union, trade association or professional organization.

Before signing a policy, read the complete document. Ask questions. Make sure you understand what is covered, and what is not covered. If an agent says something is covered, ask to see where in the policy it is stated—make sure it is in writing.

Don't be tempted to make a false statement or leave something out of your application. Fill it out truthfully and completely. If later the insurance company finds your application misleading, it may refuse to pay your claims.

Don't give up. Sometimes, sheer persistence can pay off—the squeaky wheel gets more oil. Furthermore, legislators are being increasingly pressured to improve the situation and new laws can make a difference.

What about Surgery?

Basically, surgery is the last line of defense. Most common is hip replacement, which can be very helpful in reducing pain and increasing function. One rare, but unique, post-operative problem in spondylitis is that occasionally new bone grows over the hip replacement and new ankylosis of the joint occurs. Less common surgeries are the more recently developed knee and shoulder replacements; they involve a longer rehabilitation period than the hip operation, and the results tend to be less favorable. Finally, the surgeon may operate on the spine to correct deformity. This is a more risky surgery and is only used in extreme cases.

No matter what kind of surgery you may require (appendectomy, hysterectomy, etc.), always remember to tell the anesthetist prior to surgery if you have involvement of the neck in case an airway has to be passed down your throat.

For More Information

The Spondylitis Association of America (SAA), a national non-profit organization founded in 1983, is a leading information source for patients, their families and physicians in the United States. The SAA mission is to help people affected by ankylosing spondylitis and related diseases to lead productive lives, familiarize health care professionals with early symptoms and appropriate treatments, and increase the funding of medical research to discover the cause and develop a cure.

For more information about the Spondylitis Association of America or to obtain a list of SAA publications, contact:

Spondylitis Association of America
14827 Ventura Boulevard, Suite 119
Sherman Oaks, CA 91403
(818) 981-1616
(818) 981-9826 fax
(800) 777-8189 toll-free

Chapter 15

Spinal Cord Tumors

Introduction

The diagnosis of a brain or spinal cord tumor often comes as a shock, leaving confusion, uncertainty, fear, or even anger in its wake. After the diagnosis, a physician's explanation can fall on ears deafened by this blow. Although it cannot substitute for the advice and expertise of a physician, this chapter is designed to convey the latest research information on the diagnosis, course, and possible treatment of various brain and spinal cord tumors, so that patients and their families have the information they need to become active participants in their treatment.

What Are Brain and Spinal Cord Tumors?

Brain and spinal cord tumors are abnormal growths of tissue found inside the skull or the bony spinal column. The word *tumor* is used to describe both abnormal growths that are new (*neoplasms*) and those present at birth (*congenital tumors*). This chapter will focus primarily on neoplasms.

No matter where they are located in the body, tumors are usually classed as *benign* (or noncancerous) if the cells that make up the growth are similar to other normal cells, grow relatively slowly, and are confined to one location. Tumors are called *malignant* (or cancerous)

Brain and Spinal Cord Tumors NIH Pub. No. 93-504, March 1993.

when the cells are very different from normal cells, grow relatively quickly, and can spread easily to other locations.

In most parts of the body, benign tumors are not particularly harmful. This is not necessarily true in the brain and spinal cord, which are the primary components of the central nervous system (CNS). Because the CNS is housed within rigid, bony quarters (that is, the skull and spinal column), any abnormal growth can place pressure on sensitive tissues and impair function. Also, any tumor located near vital brain structures or sensitive spinal cord nerves can seriously threaten health. A benign tumor growing next to an important blood vessel in the brain does not have to grow very large before it can block blood flow. Or, if a benign tumor is found deep inside the brain, surgery to remove it may be very risky because of the chances of damaging vital brain centers. On the other hand, a tumor located near the brain's surface can often be removed surgically.

An important difference between malignant tumors in the CNS and those elsewhere in the body lies with their potential to spread. While malignant cells elsewhere in the body can easily seed tumors inside the brain and spinal cord, malignant CNS tumors rarely spread out to other body parts. Laboratory and clinical investigators are exploring such unusual characteristics of CNS tumors because these unique properties may suggest new strategies to prevent or treat them.

What Causes These Tumors?

When newly formed tumors begin within the brain or spinal cord, they are called *primary tumors*. Primary CNS tumors rarely grow from neurons—nerve cells that perform the nervous system's important functions—because once neurons are mature they no longer divide and multiply. Instead, most tumors are caused by out-of-control growth among cells that surround and support neurons. Primary CNS tumors—such as gliomas and meningiomas—are named by the types of cells they contain, their location, or both. The appendix at the end of this chapter describes many types of primary CNS tumors, as well as other tumor-related conditions.

In a small number of individuals, primary tumors may result from specific genetic diseases—such as neurofibromatosis and tuberous sclerosis—or exposure to radiation or cancer-causing chemicals. Although smoking, alcohol consumption, and certain dietary habits are associated with some types of cancers, they have not been linked to primary brain and spinal cord tumors.

In fact, the cause of most primary brain and spinal cord tumors—and most cancers—remains a mystery. Scientists do not know exactly why and how cells in the nervous system or elsewhere in the body lose their normal identity as nerve, blood, skin, or other cell types and grow uncontrollably. Research scientists are looking for clues to this process with the goals of learning why and how cancer begins and developing new tools to stop it. Some of the possible causes under investigation include viruses and defective genes. Also, there is increasing interest in learning about the possible role played by environmental factors, such as chemicals and new technologies.

Metastatic tumors are caused by cancerous cells that shed from tumors in other parts of the body, travel through the bloodstream, burrow through the blood vessel walls, latch onto tissue, and spawn new tumors inside the brain or spinal cord.

For every four people who have cancer that has spread within the body, one develops metastasis within the CNS. The top two culprits that lead to these secondary CNS tumors are lung and breast cancer. Other, less frequent causes of CNS metastases include kidney (renal) cancer, lymphoma (a cancer affecting immune cells), prostate cancer, and melanoma, a form of skin cancer.

Brain and spinal cord tumors are not contagious or, at this time, preventable.

How Many People Have These Tumors?

Research studies suggest that new brain tumors arise in more than 40,000 Americans each year. About half of these tumors are primary, and the remainder are metastatic.

Individuals of any age can develop a brain tumor. In fact, they are the second most common cause of cancer-related death in people up to the age of 35, with a slight peak in occurrence among children between the ages of 6 and 9. However, brain tumors are most common among middle-aged and older adults. People in their 60s face the highest risk—each year 1 of every 5,000 people in this age group develops a brain tumor.

Spinal cord tumors are less common than brain tumors. About 10,000 Americans develop primary or metastatic spinal cord tumors each year. Although spinal cord tumors affect people of all ages, they are most common in young and middle-aged adults.

By studying the epidemiology of CNS tumors, scientists can learn if different tumors are more common at certain ages or in certain people. This information, in turn, may reveal environmental factors that are linked to tumors, connections between tumors and other disorders, or patterns of tumor occurrence, all of which offer clues about why tumors develop.

What Are the Symptoms?

Brain and spinal cord tumors cause many diverse symptoms, which can make detection tricky. Whatever specific symptoms a patient has, the symptoms generally develop slowly and worsen over time.

Brain Tumors

A 3.5-pound wrinkled mass of tissue, the brain orchestrates behavior, movement, feeling, and sensation. It controls automatic functions like breathing and heartbeat. Many of these important functions are controlled by specialized brain areas. For example, the brain's left and right hemispheres jointly control hearing and vision; the front part of each hemisphere controls voluntary movements, like writing, for the opposite side of the body; and the brain stem is responsible for basic life-sustaining functions, including blood pressure, heartbeat, and breathing.

As a result, brain tumors can cause a bewildering array of symptoms depending on their size, type, and location. Certain symptoms are quite specific because they result from damage to particular brain areas. Other, more general symptoms are triggered by increased pressure within the skull as the growing tumor encroaches on the brain's limited space or blocks the flow of *cerebrospinal fluid* (fluid that bathes the brain and spinal cord). Some of the more common symptoms of a brain tumor include:

Headaches. More than half of people with brain tumors experience headaches. Because the skull cannot expand, the growing mass places pressure on pain-sensitive areas. The headaches recur, often at irregular periods, and can last several minutes or hours. They may worsen when coughing, changing posture, or straining. As the tumor grows, headaches often last longer, become more frequent, and grow more severe.

Seizures. The abnormal tissue found in a brain tumor can disrupt the normal flow of electricity through which brain cells communicate.

The resulting bursts of electrical activity cause seizures with a variety of symptoms, such as convulsions, loss of consciousness, or loss of bladder control. Seizures that first start in adulthood (in a patient who has not been in an accident or had an illness that causes seizures) are a key warning sign of brain tumors. Sometimes, seizures are the only sign of a slowly growing brain tumor.

Nausea and vomiting. Increased pressure within the skull can cause nausea and vomiting. These symptoms sometimes accompany headaches.

Vision or hearing problems. Increased intracranial pressure can also decrease blood flow in the eye and trigger swelling of the optic nerve, which in turn causes blurred vision, double vision, or partial visual loss. Tumors growing on or near sensory nerves often trigger visual or hearing disturbances, such as ringing or buzzing sounds, abnormal eye movements or crossed eyes, and partial or total loss of vision or hearing. Tumors that grow in the brain's occipital lobe, which interprets visual images, may also cause partial vision loss.

Behavioral and cognitive symptoms. Because they strike at the core of the individual's identity, changes in behavior and personality can be the most frightening and devastating symptoms of a brain tumor. These symptoms usually occur when the tumor is located in the brain's cerebral hemispheres, which are responsible, in part, for personality, communication, thinking, behavior, and other vital functions. Examples include problems with speech, language, thinking, and memory, or psychotic episodes and changes in personality.

Motor problems. When tumors affect brain areas responsible for command of body movement, they can cause motor symptoms, including weakness or paralysis, lack of coordination, or trouble with walking. Often, muscle weakness or paralysis affects only one side of the body.

Balance problems. Brain tumors that disrupt the normal control of equilibrium can cause dizziness or difficulty with balance.

Spinal Cord Tumors

The spinal cord is, in part, like a living telephone cable. Lying protected inside the bony spine, it contains bundles of nerves that carry messages between the brain and the body's nerves, such as instructions from the brain to move an arm or information from the skin that signals pain. A tumor that forms on or near the spinal cord can disrupt this communication. Often, these tumors exert pressure on the spinal cord or the nerves that exit from it; sometimes, they restrict the cord's supply of blood. Common symptoms that result from this include:

Pain. Normally, the spinal cord carries important warnings about pain from the body's nerves to the brain. By putting pressure on the spinal cord, a tumor can trigger these circuits and cause pain that feels as if it is coming from various parts of the body. This pain is often constant, sometimes severe, and can have a burning or aching quality.

Sensory changes. Many people with spinal cord tumors suffer a loss of sensation. This usually takes the form of numbness and decreased skin sensitivity to temperature.

Motor problems. Since the nerves control the muscles, tumors that affect nerve communication can trigger a number of muscle-related symptoms. Early symptoms include muscle weakness; *spasticity* in which the muscles stay stiffly contracted; and impaired bladder and/or bowel control. If untreated, symptoms may worsen to include muscle wasting and paralysis. In addition, some people develop an abnormal walking rhythm known as *ataxia*.

The parts of the body affected by these symptoms vary with tumor location along the spinal cord. In general, symptoms strike body areas at the same level or at a level below that of the tumor. For example, a tumor midway along the spinal cord (in the thoracic spine) can cause pain that spreads over the chest in a girdle-shaped pattern and gets worse when the individual coughs, sneezes, or lies down. A tumor that grows in the top fourth of the spinal column (or cervical spine) can cause pain that seems to come from the neck or arms. And a tumor that grows in the lower spine (or lumbar spine) can trigger back or leg pain.

In some cases, one or more tumors extend over several sections of the spinal cord. This results in symptoms that are spread over various parts of the body. Sometimes sensory symptoms occur in a patchy, confusing pattern in which some parts of the body are unaffected even though they lie between affected areas.

160

Doctors divide spinal cord tumors into three major groups based on where they are found. Extradural tumors grow between the bony spinal canal and the tough membrane called *dura mater* that protects the spinal cord. Tumors inside the dura (intradural tumors) are further divided into those outside the spinal cord (extramedullary tumors) and those inside the spinal cord (intramedullary tumors).

How Are CNS Tumors Diagnosed?

Research has made major strides in the ability to detect and diagnose CNS tumors. When a doctor suspects a brain or spinal cord tumor because of a patient's medical history and symptoms he or she can turn to a number of specialized tests and techniques to confirm the diagnosis. However, the first test is often a traditional neurological exam. A neurological exam checks:

Eye movement, eye reflexes, and pupil reaction. For example, the doctor can shine a pen light into the eye to see if the pupil contracts normally or ask the patient to follow a moving object, such as a finger.

Reflexes. Tests like tapping below the knee with a rubber hammer can identify changes in reflexes.

Hearing. Using a tuning fork, the physician can cheek for changes in hearing.

Sensation. The doctor can use something sharp like a pin to test the sense of touch.

Movement. Problems with movement are often tested by asking the patient to move his or her tongue, head, or facial muscles—as in smiling—and to perform tasks with the arms and legs.

Balance and coordination. Typical tests include maintaining balance with the eyes closed, walking heel-to-toe in a straight line or touching the nose with the eyes closed.

The next step in diagnosing brain tumors often involves X-rays or special imaging techniques and laboratory tests that can detect the presence of a tumor and provide clues about its location and type.

Imaging and X-rays

Special imaging techniques developed through recent research, especially *computed tomography* (CT) and *magnetic resonance imaging* (MRI), have dramatically improved the diagnosis of CNS tumors in recent years. In many cases, these scans can detect the presence of a tumor even if it is less than half an inch across.

CT uses a sophisticated X-ray machine and a computer to create a detailed picture of the body's tissues and structures. Often, doctors will inject a special dye into the patient before performing a CT scan. The dye, also called contrast material, makes it easier to see abnormal tissue. A CT scan often gives doctors a good idea of where the tumor is located in the brain or spinal cord and can sometimes help them determine the tumor's type. It can also help doctors detect swelling, bleeding, and other associated conditions. In addition, CT scans can help doctors check the results of treatment and watch for tumor recurrence.

MRI is a relatively new imaging technique that is rapidly gaining widespread use in diagnosing CNS tumors. This technique uses a magnetic field and radio waves, rather than X-rays, and can often distinguish more accurately between healthy and diseased tissue. MRI gives better pictures of tumors located near bone than CT, does not use radiation as CT does, and provides pictures from various angles that can enable doctors to construct a three-dimensional image of the tumor.

A third imaging technique called *positron emission tomography* (PET) provides a picture of brain activity rather than structure by measuring levels of injected glucose (sugar) that has been labelled with a radioactive tracer. Glucose is used by the brain for energy. Detectors placed around the head can spot the labelled glucose, and a computer uses the pattern of glucose distribution to form an image of the brain. Since malignant tissue uses more glucose than normal, it shows up on the scan as brighter or lighter than surrounding tissue. Currently, PET is not widely used in tumor diagnosis, in part because the technique requires very elaborate, expensive equipment, including a cyclotron to create the radioactive glucose.

Although it is not widely used for diagnosis now that CT and MRI scans are possible, *angiography* continues to help doctors distinguish certain types of brain tumors and make decisions about surgery. In angiography, doctors inject dye into a major blood vessel, usually one of the large arteries in the neck. This dye deflects X-rays and makes it possible for doctors to see the network of blood vessels by taking a series of X-ray pictures as the dye flows through the brain. Since some tumors have a characteristic pattern of blood vessels and blood flow, the pictures can provide clues about the tumor's type. Information from angiography can also tell physicians if a tumor is located close to important, normal blood vessels that must be avoided during surgery.

Widespread use of CT and MRI has also largely displaced use of traditional X-rays for diagnosis of brain and spinal cord tumors, since X-rays do not provide very useful images of brain tissue. They are occasionally helpful when tumors cause changes in the skull or spinal cord or when they contain tiny deposits of bone-like material made of calcium.

Physicians may also use a specialized X-ray technique, called a *myelogram*, when diagnosing spinal cord tumors. In myelography, a special dye that absorbs X-rays is injected into the spinal cord. This dye outlines the spinal cord but will not pass through a tumor. The resulting X-ray picture shows a dark area or narrowing that reveals the tumor's location.

Laboratory Tests

Laboratory tests commonly used include the *electroencephalogram* (or EEG) and *lumbar puncture*, also known as the spinal tap. The EEG uses special patches placed on the scalp or fine needles placed in the brain to record electrical currents inside the brain. This recording can help the doctor see telltale patterns in the brain's electrical activity that suggest a brain tumor. Repeated EEG recordings can be particularly helpful in deciding if an abnormality in brain activity is getting worse.

In lumbar puncture, doctors obtain a small sample of cerebrospinal fluid. This fluid can be examined for abnormal cells or unusual levels of various compounds that suggest a brain or spinal cord tumor.

In the future, diagnosis of brain tumors should grow more accurate as additional techniques—including new ways to image the CNS and advanced laboratory tests—are developed through basic laboratory studies and clinical research.

What is a Biopsy and How is it Used?

A *biopsy* is a surgical procedure in which a small sample of tissue is taken from the suspected tumor, often during surgery aimed at removing as much tumor as possible.

A biopsy gives doctors the clues they need to specifically diagnose the type of tumor. By examining the sample under a microscope, the pathologist—a physician who specializes in understanding how disease affects the body's tissues—can tell what kinds of cells are in a tumor. Pathologists also look carefully for certain changes that signal cancer. These signs include abnormal growths or changes in the cell membranes and telltale problems in the cell nuclei, which normally control cell characteristics and growth. For example, cancerous cells may grow small finger-like projections on their normally smooth surface or have extra nuclei.

Using this information, the pathologist provides a diagnosis of the tumor type. The tumor may also be classified as benign or malignant and given a numbered score that reflects how malignant it is. This score can help doctors determine how to treat a tumor and predict the likely outcome, or *prognosis*, for the patient.

Although biopsy has long been a mainstay of brain tumor diagnosis, it is still an important research area. Scientists continue to look for better ways to identify and classify types of abnormal cells in order to improve the accuracy of prognosis and provide the best possible information for treatment decisions.

How Are Brain and Spinal Cord Tumors Treated?

The three most commonly used treatments—surgery, radiation, and chemotherapy—are largely the result of recent research. For some patients, doctors may suggest a new treatment still being tested. In any ease, the doctor will recommend a treatment or a combination of treatments based on the tumor's location and type, any previous treatment the patient may have received, and the patient's medical history and general health.

Surgery

Surgery to remove as much tumor as possible is usually the first step in treating an *accessible tumor*—that is, a tumor that can be removed without unacceptable risk of neurological damage. Fortunately, research has led to advances in neurosurgery that make it possible for doctors to reach many tumors that were previously considered inaccessible. These new techniques and tools equip neurosurgeons to operate in the tight, vulnerable confines of the CNS. Some recently developed approaches in use in the operating room include:

Microsurgery. In this widely used technique, the surgeon looks through a high-powered microscope to get a magnified view of the operating area. This makes it easier to see—and remove—tumor tissue while sparing surrounding healthy tissue.

Stereotactic procedures. In these procedures, a computer uses information from CT or MRI to create a three-dimensional map of the operation site. The computer uses the map to help the surgeon guide special, computer-assisted tools. This makes it possible for surgeons to approach certain difficult-to-reach tumors with greater precision. Many procedures can be performed using this approach, including biopsy, certain types of surgery, and planting radiation pellets in a tumor.

Lasers. Lasers release a beam of concentrated light energy that can destroy tissue. Lasers are occasionally helpful for tasks traditionally performed with a scalpel. For example, surgeons can use a laser to remove an entire tumor. Or, once most of a tumor is removed through surgery, they can destroy remaining tumor tissue with the laser's intense beam of energy.

Ultrasonic aspirators. Ultrasonic aspirators use sound waves to vibrate tumors and break them up. Like a vacuum, the aspirator then sucks up the tumor fragments.

Evoked potentials. Doctors use this test during surgery to determine the role of specific nerves and thus avoid damage. In this technique, small electrodes are used to stimulate a nerve so its electrical response, or evoked potential, can be measured.

Shunts. Shunts are flexible tubes used to reroute and drain fluid. Doctors sometimes insert a shunt into the brain when a tumor blocks the flow of cerebrospinal fluid and causes *hydrocephalus*. Shunting of the fluid can relieve headaches, nausea, and other symptoms caused by too much pressure inside the skull.

Surgery may be the beginning and end of treatment if the biopsy shows a benign tumor. If the tumor is malignant, however, doctors often recommend additional treatment following surgery, including radiation, chemotherapy, or experimental treatments. Sometimes, if a tumor is very large, radiation is used before surgery to reduce the tumor's size.

An *inaccessible or inoperable tumor* is one that cannot be removed surgically because of the risk of severe nervous system damage. These tumors are frequently located deep within the brain or near vital structures such as the brain stem—the part of the brain that controls many crucial functions including breathing and heart rate. Malignant, multiple tumors may also be inoperable. Doctors treat most malignant, inaccessible, or inoperable CNS tumors with radiation and/or chemotherapy.

Among patients who have metastatic CNS tumors, doctors usually focus on treating the original cancer first. However, when a metastatic tumor causes serious disability or pain, doctors may recommend surgery or other treatments to reduce symptoms even if the original cancer has not been controlled.

Radiation Therapy

In radiation therapy, the tumor is bombarded with beams of energy that kill tumor cells. Traditional radiation therapy delivers radiation from outside the patient's body, usually begins a week or two after surgery, and continues for about 6 weeks. The dosage is fairly uniform throughout the treated areas, making it especially useful for tumors that are large or have infiltrated into surrounding tissue.

However, when traditional radiation therapy is given to the brain, it may also cause damage to healthy tissue. Depending on the type of tumor, doctors may be able to choose a modified form of radiation therapy to help prevent this and to improve the effectiveness of treatment. Modifying therapy can be as simple as changing the dosage schedule and amount of radiation that a patient receives. For example, an approach called hyperfractionation uses smaller, more frequent doses. Neurological investigators are also testing several other, more complex techniques to improve radiation therapy.

Chemotherapy

Chemotherapy uses tumor-killing drugs that are given orally or injected into the bloodstream. Because not all tumors are vulnerable to the same anticancer drugs, doctors often use a combination of drugs for chemotherapy.

Chemotherapeutic drugs generally kill cells that are growing or dividing. This property makes them more deadly to malignant tissue, which contains a high proportion of growing and dividing cells, than to most normal cells. It also causes some of the side effects that can accompany chemotherapy—such as skin reactions, hair loss, or digestive problems—because a high proportion of these normal cell types are also growing and dividing at any given time. The drugs most commonly used for CNS tumors are known by the initials BCNU (sometimes called carmustine) and CCNU (or lomustine). Research scientists are also testing many promising drugs to learn if they can improve treatment for brain and spinal cord tumors and reduce side effects.

Other Drugs

Tumors, surgery, and radiation therapy can all result in swelling inside the CNS. Doctors may prescribe steroids for short or long periods to reduce this swelling. Examples of such drugs include dexamethasone, methylprednisolone, and prednisone.

Whether new treatment approaches involve surgery, radiation therapy, chemotherapy, or completely new avenues to treating CNS tumors, carefully planned clinical trials of new and experimental therapies are vital for identifying promising treatments and learning the best applications of current therapies. Experimental treatments, in turn, would not be possible without research by basic and clinical scientists who identify new approaches.

Where Should Patients Go for Treatment?

Brain and spinal cord tumors are often difficult to diagnose, and surgery to remove them demands great skill. Experience, therefore, is probably the most important factor in choosing among physicians. Brain and spinal cord tumors are also relatively rare. Many physicians see only a few patients with CNS tumors each year. Others, however, have made treating brain and spinal cord tumors their specialty. Patients should consider how many patients a physician treats each year. Because many patients are understandably perplexed or frightened by a CNS tumor diagnosis, it is also important that they choose a physician who will answer questions and describe treatment options clearly and fully.

Patients should also learn what techniques and tools are available at the physician's hospital. Teaching hospitals affiliated with a medical college or university are more likely to be involved in research and, thus, have the equipment and specialists necessary to offer experimental treatments. Finally, if a patient is dissatisfied with a physician or a physician's recommendations, he or she may wish to seek another opinion.

The voluntary organizations listed on the pocket card at the back of this publication may be able to help in locating physicians who specialize in treating brain tumors, as well as provide information about CNS tumors.

What Research Is Being Done?

Scientists are attacking CNS tumors through biomedical research to improve medical understanding and treatment. CNS tumor research ranges from bench-side studies on the origins and characteristics of tumors to bed-side studies that test new tumor-killing drugs and other innovative treatments. Much of this work is supported by the National Institute of Neurological Disorders and Stroke (NINDS) and by the National Cancer Institute (NCI), as well as other agencies within the Federal Government, non-profit groups, and private institutions.

Some key areas of brain tumor research include:

Brachytherapy. In brachytherapy, which is also known as interstitial radiation, doctors implant small radioactive pellets directly into the tumor. The pellets may be left in permanently or for a few days, weeks, or months. This technique can deliver a large dose of radiation to the tumor while minimizing radiation of normal tissue. Through research, scientists thus far have found that brachytherapy is most useful for small tumors that are difficult to remove surgically. Research scientists continue to examine whether this technique can help patients with other tumor types as well.

Drugs and techniques for chemotherapy. Dozens of new chemotherapeutic drugs are in various stages of development. Scientists are testing these drugs in animals and patients to determine what side effects they cause, what doses are appropriate, and whether they can improve survival and recovery. Patients interested in up-to-date information on current trials are encouraged to contact the resources listed at the end of this chapter.

Scientists are also working to overcome an obstacle to effective chemotherapy for brain and spinal cord tumors—*the blood-brain barrier*. The blood-brain barrier—an elaborate meshwork of fine blood vessels and cells that filters blood reaching the CNS—normally helps protect the sensitive tissues of the CNS from potentially dangerous compounds in the bloodstream and changes in its environment. But the blood-brain barrier also stymies many efforts to deliver anticancer drugs that may help patients with CNS tumors. Investigators are testing drugs, such as the chemical leukotriene, that may help open the barrier. If these drugs prove useful and safe in animal models and humans, then physicians would be equipped to test promising anticancer drugs that normally cannot cross the blood-brain barrier.

Another experimental path aimed at improving drug delivery into the CNS is called interstitial chemotherapy. In this technique, doctors place disc-shaped wafers soaked with chemotherapeutic drugs directly into tumor tissue. This technique may help physicians increase the dose of life-prolonging drugs while limiting side effects—since less of the drug spreads elsewhere in the body. Most trials of this technique currently involve patients with recurrent gliomas.

Drugs to improve radiation therapy. Many scientists are testing the usefulness of drugs known as radiosensitizers that make tumor tissue more vulnerable to radiation. Early results with the two most commonly studied radiosensitizers, metronidazole and misonidazole, have been mixed; some trials suggest these drugs may improve survival in certain patients, while other trials have shown little benefit. In addition, other scientists are looking at whether another family of drugs known as barbiturates may improve radiation therapy by protecting normal brain tissue. Early studies have shown these sedating drugs can slow down the metabolism of healthy brain tissue, possibly shielding it from radiation damage.

Gamma knife. The gamma knife, used for a procedure known technically as stereotactic gamma knife radiosurgery, combines precise stereotactic guidance and a sharply focused beam of radiation energy to deliver a single, precise dose of radiation. Despite its name, the gamma knife does not require a surgical incision. Investigators using this tool have found it can help them reach and treat some small tumors that are not accessible through surgery.

Gene therapy. Gene therapy, an innovative approach to treating CNS cancer, is in the early stages of research in laboratories around the country. Genes are the blueprints the body's cells use to make proteins and other vital substances. In gene therapy, scientists insert a new gene into specific cells. In the case of gene therapy for brain tumors, this inserted gene could make the tumor cells sensitive to certain drugs, program the cancerous cells to self-destruct, or instruct them to manufacture substances that would slow their growth. Scientists are using tumor cells and animal models to learn how various genes, once introduced, hinder cancer growth and to identify the best methods for inserting new genes into tumor cells. Human trials are just beginning.

Hyperthermia. Tumors are more sensitive to heat than normal tissue, partly because they have less blood flow to cool them. Research scientists testing hyperthermia take advantage of this sensitivity by placing special heat-producing antennae into the tumor region after surgery. Most often, these antennae send out microwaves that raise the temperature in nearby tissues. Hyperthermia is a new treatment for tumors in the brain, and scientists are still testing its effectiveness. They are also looking at heat sources that may be more effective than microwaves, including electromagnetic energy and radio frequencies.

Immunotherapy. The body's immune system normally seeks out and destroys foreign tissue such as cancerous cells by detecting antigens, telltale proteins found on foreign cells that alert the body to the foreign cells' presence. Stimulated by the antigens, the body manufactures a variety of immune cells and special proteins called antibodies. These antibodies then latch onto the antigens, working as tiny flags that alert immune cells to attack and destroy the foreign cells. In immunotherapy—an exciting and very new field of CNS tumor research—scientists are looking for ways to duplicate or enhance the body's immune response to fight against brain and spinal cord cancer.

Some scientists are testing the effectiveness of giving the body's immune system a general boost. Much like the way coffee can stimulate the nervous system, certain naturally occurring body chemicals trigger immune cells to grow and divide. In numerous studies, researchers have supplied patients with extra amounts of immune stimulants, such as interleukin-2, in the hope that they will improve the body's ability to fight CNS cancer. However, this technique has produced mixed results. A second type of general immunotherapy involves removing immune cells from a patient, growing and activating these cells, and then returning them to the patient where they can work against the cancer. This approach has also yielded mixed results.

Another, still more recent approach in immunotherapy research specifically targets tumor cells using monoclonal antibodies. Like duplicate keys for the same lock, monoclonal antibodies are multiple copies of a single antibody; they fit one—and only one—antigen. Scientists are now producing monoclonal antibodies against tumor cell antigens and testing their usefulness. For example, scientists at the NINDS and elsewhere are linking these antibodies to toxins that can kill tumor cells. The armed monoclonal antibodies then function like guided missiles; they seek out the tumor cells with a matching antigen, bind to these tumor cells, and deliver their toxin. Early experiments with this therapy suggest it has more promise for treating widespread cancer cells than solid tumors. Studies are underway to corroborate these early results and to learn if this therapy has promise for other types of CNS tumors. Monoclonal antibodies may also prove helpful in improving brain tumor diagnosis, because they can be attached to special tracers to make tumor cells more visible.

Intraoperative ultrasound. This technique, which uses sound waves, provides the surgeon with an image of brain tissues during the operation. Ultrasound is less expensive and complex than other imaging techniques. Some scientists conducting research on intraoperative ultrasound have found the technique makes it easier for the surgeon to locate the outer edges of tumor tissue, which can be hard to find. Thus, this technique may help improve tumor surgery by increasing the amount of tumor that can be safely removed.

Oncogenes. The body contains a number of genes that are important in normal cell growth and development. Changes in some of these genes—which might be triggered by such events as exposure to chemicals or radiation—can transform them into dangerous, cancer-causing oncogenes. A number of oncogenes have already been found, and scientists continue to look for more. They are also working to identify specific events that can create oncogenes and to learn if there may be ways to prevent oncogenes from forming or to impair oncogene function in cancerous cells.

PET. Based on recent research, some scientists believe that PET scans offer important clues for diagnosis of brain tumors. For example, physicians sometimes have trouble detecting recurrent tumors with

CT or MRI scans. Recent studies have shown that PET may make it easier to detect recurrent brain tumors. Scientists are also examining whether PET can help physicians tell the difference between benign and malignant tumors before performing a biopsy or surgery.

Physiological mapping. Mapping brain functions has promise for improving the safety and effectiveness of brain tumor surgery, particularly among children with tumors in critical brain regions. In physiological mapping, the physician locates brain areas responsible for key functions, such as language or sensation. The surgeon then has a map to help avoid these critical areas, thus reducing the chance of serious complications.

Photodynamic therapy. Photodynamic therapy uses drugs that collect in tumor cells and can be turned on or activated by special light. The drugs may be given by injection or placed directly into the tumor during an initial surgery. In order to activate the tumor-killing drug, the physician must expose the tumor tissue to light during surgery. Thus far, this technique has been found useful only for small amounts of tumor tissue, although researchers continue the search for new light-sensitive drugs and better light sources that can penetrate tumors.

Tumor growth factors. Cancerous tumors are often rich in an array of substances, called growth factors, that enable them to grow and spread rapidly. In recent years, scientists have identified a number of these factors, including one that triggers growth of nerve tissue and another that stimulates blood vessels to grow. Many investigators continue the search for more such factors. Meanwhile, other researchers have begun testing antibodies that can block these factors. Early results in animals have shown that blocking growth factors with antibodies may help slow tumor growth, suggesting this research arena could lead to new therapies for brain tumors.

Although many new approaches to treatment thus appear promising, it is important to remember that all potential therapies must stand the tests of well-designed, carefully controlled clinical trials and long-term follow-up of treated patients before any conclusions can be drawn about their safety or effectiveness.

Past research has led to improved tumor treatments and techniques, providing longer survival and richer lives for many CNS tumor patients. Current research promises to generate further improvements.

In the years ahead, physicians and patients can look forward to new forms of therapy developed through an understanding of the unique traits of CNS tumors.

What Can I Do to Help?

The NINDS and the National Institute of Mental Health jointly support two national brain specimen banks. These banks supply research scientists around the world with nervous system tissue from patients with neurological and psychiatric disorders. They need tissue from patients with CNS tumors so that scientists can study and understand these tumors. Those who may be interested in donating should write to:

Dr. Wallace W. Tourtellotte, Director
Human Neurospecimen Bank
VA Wadsworth Medical Center
Wilshire and Sawtelle Blvds.
Los Angeles, CA 90073
(310) 824-4307

Dr. Edward D. Bird, Director
Brain Tissue Bank, Mailman Research Center
McLean Hospital
115 Mill Street
Belmont, MA 02178
1-800-BRAIN-BANK (1-800-272-4622)
(617) 855-2400

Where Can I Find More Information?

The NINDS is the Federal Government's leading supporter of biomedical research on nervous system disorders, including brain and spinal cord tumors. The NINDS conducts research on brain tumors in its own laboratories at the National Institutes of Health (NIH) in Bethesda, MD, and supports research at institutions worldwide. The Institute also sponsors an active public information program. Other NINDS publications that may be of interest to those concerned about brain and spinal cord tumors include "Epilepsy: Hope Through Research" and the fact sheets "Neurofibromatosis" and "Tuberous Sclerosis."

The Institute's address and phone number, as well as information on other organizations that offer various services to those affected by brain and spinal cord tumors, are provided in the information resources section at the end of this chapter.

Appendix

Primary CNS Tumors and Tumor-Related Conditions

Chordomas. Chordomas, which are more common in people in their 20s and 30s, develop from remnants of the flexible spine-like structure that forms and dissolves early in fetal development and is later replaced by the spinal cord. Although these tumors are often slow-growing, they can metastasize or recur after treatment. They are usually treated with a combination of surgery and radiation.

Craniopharyngiomas. Craniopharyngiomas are brain tumors that usually affect infants and children. Like chordomas, they develop from cells left over from early fetal development. Craniopharyngiomas are often located near the brain's pituitary gland, a gland that releases chemicals important for the body's growth and metabolism. Treatment for these tumors usually includes surgery and, in some patients, radiation therapy.

Gliomas. About half of all primary brain tumors and about one-fifth of all primary spinal cord tumors are gliomas, meaning that they grow from glial cells. Within the brain, gliomas usually occur in the cerebral hemispheres but may also strike other areas, especially the optic nerve, the brain stem, and, particularly among children, the cerebellum. Gliomas are classified into several groups because there are different kinds of glial cells.

Astrocytomas. These are the most common type of glioma. They develop from star-shaped glial cells called astrocytes. Doctors will often assign one of three grades to an astrocytoma following biopsy. The types of graded astrocytomas include:

- *Well-differentiated*: Also known as low-grade astrocytomas or grade I astrocytomas, these tumors contain cells that are relatively normal and are less malignant than the other two grades. They grow relatively slowly and may sometimes be completely removed through surgery. However, even well-differentiated astrocytomas are life-threatening if they are inaccessible.

- *Anaplastic*: Anaplastic astrocytomas, also called mid-grade astrocytomas or grade II astrocytomas, grow more rapidly than well-differentiated astrocytomas and contain cells with some malignant traits. Surgery followed by radiation and, sometimes, chemotherapy is used to treat anaplastic astrocytomas.

- *Glioblastoma multiforme*: These tumors, sometimes called high-grade or grade III astrocytomas, grow rapidly, invade nearby tissue, and contain cells that are very malignant. Glioblastoma multiforme are among the most common and devastating primary brain tumors that strike adults. Doctors usually treat glioblastomas with surgery followed by radiation therapy and, sometimes, chemotherapy.

Ependymomas. Ependymomas usually affect children and develop from cells that line both the hollow cavities of the brain and the canal containing the spinal cord. About 85 percent of ependymomas are benign. Treatment usually includes surgery followed by radiation therapy. Chemotherapy is sometimes used, especially for recurrent tumors.

Oligodendrogliomas. These tumors, which develop from glial cells called oligodendroglia, represent about 5 percent of all gliomas. They occur most often in young adults, within the brain's cerebral hemispheres. Doctors often treat these tumors with surgery followed by radiation therapy.

Ganglioneuromas. The rarest form of glioma, these tumors contain both glial cells and mature neurons. They grow relatively slowly and may occur in the brain or spinal cord. These tumors are usually treated with surgery.

Mixed gliomas. Mixed gliomas contain more than one type of glial cell, usually astrocytes and other glial cell types. Treatment focuses on the most malignant cell type found within the tumor.

Brain stem gliomas. Named by their location at the base of the brain rather than the cells they contain, brain stem gliomas are most common in children and young adults. Surgery is not usually used to treat brain stem gliomas because of their vulnerable location. Radiation therapy sometimes helps to reduce symptoms and improve survival by slowing tumor growth.

Optic nerve gliomas. These tumors are found on or near the nerves that travel between the eye and brain vision centers and are particularly common in individuals who have neurofibromatosis. Treatment usually includes surgery or radiation.

Meningiomas. Meningiomas are tumors that develop from the thin membranes, or *meninges*, that cover the brain and spinal cord. Meningiomas account for about 15 percent of all brain tumors and about 25 percent of all primary spinal cord tumors. They affect people of all ages, but are most common among those in their 40s. Meningiomas usually grow slowly, generally do not invade surrounding normal tissue, and rarely spread to other parts of the CNS or body. Surgery is the preferred treatment for accessible meningiomas and is more successful for these tumors than for most tumor types.

Pineal Tumors. Tumors in the pineal gland, a small structure deep within the brain, account for about 1 percent of brain tumors. When possible, physicians will begin treatment with surgery or perform a biopsy to confirm the tumor type. They may also recommend radiation or chemotherapy, or both, for malignant pineal tumors. The three most common types of pineal region tumors are gliomas, germ cell tumors, and pineal cell tumors.

Pituitary Tumors. The pituitary gland, a small oval-shaped structure located at the base of the brain, releases several chemical messengers known as hormones, which help control the body's other glands and influence the body's growth, metabolism, and maturation. Tumors that affect the pituitary gland, also called pituitary adenomas, account for about 10 percent of brain tumors. Doctors classify pituitary tumors into two groups—secreting and non-secreting. Secreting tumors release unusually high levels of pituitary hormones, triggering a constellation of symptoms, which can include impotence, abnormal body growth, Cushing's syndrome, or hyperthyroidism depending on which hormone is involved. Surgery or the drug bromocriptine is used to treat most pituitary tumors.

Primitive Neuroectodermal Tumors. Primitive neuroectodermal tumors (PNETs) usually affect children and young adults. Their name reflects the belief, held by many scientists, that these tumors spring from primitive cells left over from early development of the nervous system. PNETs are usually very malignant, growing rapidly and spreading easily within the brain and spinal cord. In rare cases, they cause cancer outside the CNS.

Medulloblastomas, the most common PNET, represent more than 25 percent of all childhood brain tumors. Other, more rare PNETs include neuroblastomas, pineoblastomas, medulloepitheliomas, ependymoblastomas, and polar spongioblastomas. Because their malignant cells often spread in a scattered, patchy pattern, PNETs are difficult to remove totally through surgery. Doctors usually remove as much tumor as possible with surgery, then prescribe high doses of radiation and, in some cases, chemotherapy.

Schwannomas. These tumors arise from the cells that form a protective sheath around the body's nerve fibers. They are usually benign and are surgically removed when possible. One of the more common forms of schwannoma affects the eighth cranial nerve, which contains nerve cells important for balance and hearing. Also known as vestibular schwannomas or acoustic neuromas, these tumors may grow on one or both sides of the brain.

Vascular Tumors. These rare, noncancerous tumors arise from the blood vessels of the brain and spinal cord. The most common vascular tumor is the hemangioblastoma, which is linked in a small number of people to a genetic disorder called Von Hippel-Lindau disease. Hemangioblastomas do not usually spread, and doctors typically treat them with surgery.

Information Resources

NIH Neurological Institute
P.O. Box 5801
Bethesda, MD 20824
(301) 496-5751 or 1-800-352-9424

The National Institute of Neurological Disorders and Stroke, a component of the National Institutes of Health, is the leading Federal supporter of research on disorders of the brain and nervous system. The Institute also sponsors an active public information program and can answer questions about diagnosis, treatment, and research related to brain and spinal cord tumors.

Office of Cancer Communications
National Cancer Institute
Building 31, Room 10A-24
Bethesda, MD 20892
1-800-4-CANCER (1-800-422-6237)

The NCI, also a part of the NIH and the primary Federal supporter of cancer-related biomedical research, offers a variety of publications and a toll-free cancer information service.

Private organizations that offer information include the following:

American Brain Tumor Association
2720 River Road, Suite 146
Des Plaines, IL 60018
(708) 827-9910 or 1-800-886-2282

This association provides referrals and information and publishes a newsletter and brochures on various tumor types and treatments.

American Cancer Society
1599 Clifton Road, N.E.
Atlanta, GA 30329
1-800-ACS-2345 (1-800-227-2345)

The ACS supports research, conducts educational programs, and offers patient and family services.

Brain Tumor Information Service
(312) 684-1400

This 24-hour service provides information on diagnosis and treatment for patients and families.

The Brain Tumor Society
60 Leo Birmingham Parkway
Boston, MA 02135-1116
(617) 783-0340

The society distributes information, publishes a newsletter, and provides referrals to resources, as well as sponsoring research, a patient-family telephone network, and professional education programs.

The Children's Brain Tumor Foundation
35 Alpine Lane
Chappaqua, NY 10514
(914) 238-1656

The foundation funds research and professional training, sponsors support groups, publishes a newsletter, and provides services for children with brain tumors and their families.

National Brain Tumor Foundation
323 Geary Street, Suite 510
San Francisco, CA 94102
(415) 296-0404
1-800-93-4-CURE (1-800-934-2873)

The foundation sponsors support groups and offers a variety of publications, including a newsletter, a booklet for newly diagnosed tumor patients, and a guide to employment, support groups, insurance, and other resources. The foundation also offers audiocassettes of their annual brain tumor conference.

Written by Frances Taylor,
Office of Scientific and Health Reports,
NINDS.

Chapter 16

Neck Pain and Disorders of the Cervical Spine

What is the cervical spine?

The spine consists of small bones, called vertebrae, that are linked in a column extending down the center of the back from the base of the head to the buttocks area. The cervical spine consists of the top seven vertebrae of the vertebral column. The top vertebra next to the base of the skull is called the atlas. The second vertebra is called the axis. These two vertebrae are different in shape and function from the other vertebrae of the spine. Discs which act as cushions rest between vertebrae and facilitate movement of the vertebral column. The spinal cord runs through a hollow channel in each vertebra, and nerves carrying impulses to all areas of the body branch off from the spinal cord between the vertebrae.

What are some causes of neck pain?

Neck pain may be caused by injury, postural strain on the neck, a variety of diseases, or pain radiating from another site, such as the jaw. In acute cervical sprains where the head is thrust forward and then backward on impact (whiplash), pain or spasm in the neck may begin up to 48 hours after the accident. Neck symptoms which are worse in the morning and improve during the day suggest an inflammatory disease, but may be simply due to a sleeping position that puts

A fact sheet prepared by the National Institute of Arthritis and Musculoskeletal and Skin Diseases, April, 1992.

the neck in an awkward position (bending backwards or sideways). Occupations that require repetitive or prolonged flexion, extension, or rotation of the neck may cause problems. Pain that is accentuated by coughing, sneezing, or jolting suggests a disc problem, such as a herniation (slipped disc). In the case of a disease, like arthritis, degenerative (deteriorating or eroding) changes and partial dislocation may result from destruction of bone, disc, cartilage, ligaments, and other soft tissue. This condition is known as spondylosis. Although uncommon, tumors and infections may also cause cervical problems.

What are some symptoms of cervical spine disorders?

The signs of a problem involving the cervical spine depend on the location, extent, and cause of the problem. Symptoms may be due to pressure on the spinal cord (myelopathy) or on the nerve roots as they extend from the cord (radiculopathy). The first signs are stiffness and/or pain in the neck. There may also be tingling or, in more severe cases, numbness of the hands, arms, and shoulders or tingling that radiates upward to the base of the head or down the back. Rarely, weakness or numbness may extend into the legs or feet, and there may be a loss of bowel or bladder function.

Eye, ear, nose, and throat symptoms are sometimes associated with cervical disease. Irritation of nerves that branch upward from the cervical spine may cause blurred vision that is altered by moving the neck, increased tearing, and pain at the back of the eye. A need to repeatedly clear the throat or difficulty speaking and the feeling of being unable to get enough breath may also be symptoms of nerve irritation in the neck. Heart palpitations and a rapid heart beat may result from hyperextension of the neck.

How are cervical problems diagnosed?

Physical examination is sometimes all that is needed to diagnose a cervical problem. Often, however, additional diagnostic techniques are used. An x-ray may be all that is needed to see an obvious problem in the cervical spine. Various diagnostic techniques may be used to determine the nature and extent of a cervical problem. These include myelography, CT scan, and/or MRI. Cervical discography may play a role in the management of patients with degenerative conditions when the diagnosis cannot be determined by the other tests. An injection for pain (analgesic) is sometimes used to determine the pain pattern (where the pain is most acute and where it radiates).

What are conservative treatments for neck pain?

The goal of therapy for cervical spine problems is to relieve pain and reverse any neurological problems. For minor neck stiffness, exercises that stretch the muscles in the neck, massage, and heat may be all that is necessary to relieve pain. When the cause of pain is more than a temporary stiffness, resolution of pain by these conservative measures may take weeks or months. Rigid or soft cervical collars may be suggested. Soft collars, unlike rigid ones, only partially constrain neck motion, but they do support the head and remind the person to limit motion. However, these collars rarely reverse neurologic symptoms associated with more severe conditions, such as a partial dislocation of a cervical vertebra. People whose pain or stiffness is due to inflammation, rather than structural damage, often respond to treatment with nonsteroidal anti-inflammatory drugs. Physical therapy treatments may include range of motion and strengthening exercises, heat, cold, ultrasound, cervical traction, and the use of cervical support pillows. Narrowing of the spinal canal or intervertebral foramina with pain spreading along nerve pathways may respond to corticosteroid (anti-inflammatory steroid) injection. Pain treatment centers play an important role in helping patients cope with chronic neck pain. In addition to the traditional treatments mentioned, many centers offer behavioral modification, biofeedback, acupuncture, and acupressure.

What surgery might be necessary to treat cervical problems?

Most people with neck problems can be effectively treated non-operatively. Except in cases of injury, surgical intervention should not be considered until the patient has undergone an adequate trial of non-operative management. People with progressive neurological deterioration (e.g., persistent numbness, weakness, and interference with movement) may be candidates for cervical surgery, as may those with severe and persistent neck pain, even in the absence of neurological symptoms. There are two basic surgical approaches to the cervical spine: anterior and posterior. Anterior procedures, in which an incision is made in the front of the neck, primarily include removal of the disc with or without fusion. (Fusion creates a bony bridge between two or more vertebrae.) When a fusion is performed, bone is usually taken from the patient's hip, but bone from a donor or other source outside the body might also be considered. Patients with disc herniations and central cord compression are most often candidates for the anterior approach. Posterior procedures include surgical removal of all or part of one or more of the bony arches of the vertebrae that surround the spinal cord to relieve pressure on the cord or nerve extending from it (called a laminectomy). Disc material may be removed at the same time.

What can be expected after surgery?

Following surgery a hard collar is usually placed around the neck, and this may be worn day and night for a few weeks. When the doctor feels the neck has healed sufficiently, the hard collar may be replaced by a soft one, and eventually, no collar will be needed. Because the muscles of the neck may become weakened with prolonged wear of a collar, these devices are worn no longer than necessary. After removal of the collar, exercises to strengthen the neck muscles may be prescribed to help restore a full range of motion to the neck.

What can be done to protect the neck from future problems?

Following are some of the steps a person can take to guard against neck problems:

- When at a desk, sit straight, rather than bending forward or leaning over work—place work material so that it is unnecessary to bend or turn your head to see it;

- Sit in a chair with arm rests;

- Hold a phone receiver in your hand, not handless supported on the shoulder by the head;

- Use a foot stool if you must reach into a high cupboard or shelf;

- Don't read or watch TV with the head propped forward on a pillow or arm of a sofa;

- When lying down, place a pillow under the head and neck in a position that keeps the neck straight.

Chapter 17

Spasmodic Torticollis

Hal first noticed a nagging ache in the base of his neck. Then the ache became a sharp pain after his weekly games of racquetball.

At first, he dismissed these as signs of his stressful sales job. Then came a frightening day on the freeway. Hal's neck muscles involuntarily contracted, forcing his head to the left and pulling his chin to his shoulder. As Hal eased off the road, the knew it was more than his job. He needed to see a doctor.

The diagnosis? Spasmodic torticollis (spaz-MOD-ik tor-tih KOL-is), which can cause involuntary head movements and pain. Also known as cervical dystonia, it affects about 83,000 Americans and has no known cause or cure.

Fortunately, the outlook for people with the disease is improving. Doctors are making strides in treatment, and growing public awareness is making it easier to get information and support.

A Debilitating Disorder

Spasmodic torticollis belongs to a group of neurological disorders called dystonias. Dystonias are sustained muscle contractions that can lead to abnormal posture and repetitive twisting movements.

Spasmodic torticollis is a focal dystonia, meaning it affects one part of your body—your neck. It can begin at any age, but usually starts

Reprinted from the July 1996 *Mayo Clinic Health Letter* with permission of Mayo Foundation for Medical Education and Research, Rochester, MN 55905. For subscription information, call 1-800-333-9037.

in your 30s or 40s. Initial signs and symptoms may be mild. They can include involuntary turning of your head, or slight tremors associated with neck and muscle pain.

The disease usually grows more pronounced and painful. Sometimes, it can disrupt your ability to work and lead an active lifestyle.

A Physical Disease

As recently as 30 years ago, many doctors considered spasmodic torticollis a psychological disorder. Today, it's recognized as a physical disease thought to result when nerve messages tell your neck muscles to contract at the wrong time.

The contractions may last for hours or even longer. They may also occur intermittently, causing shaking movements of your head.

Researchers suspect head injury or heredity may play a role in some cases. Mayo Clinic doctors are also investigating the role of your immune system.

Improving Treatments

Doctors may still prescribe muscle relaxants or other drugs, but these often aren't very effective. The most effective treatments are:

Botulinum Toxin (Botox)

Botulinum (BOCH-u-lin-um) toxin is a chemical made by the bacteria that cause food poisoning. Injected into affected muscles, it relaxes them. Injections must be repeated about every three months. About 70 percent of those with spasmodic torticollis report improvement of their symptoms and pain. The treatment may lose effectiveness if you develop antibodies to the toxin.

Selective Denervation Surgery

This procedure involves severing nerves to affected neck muscles, permanently weakening or paralyzing them. Only a few muscles are involved, so excessive weakness is typically not a problem. Only a few North American medical centers—one of which is Mayo—have extensive experience with this procedure. About 80 percent of those who've undergone the surgery report improvement.

Living an Active Lifestyle

Hal's doctor prescribed botulinum toxin. Hal also joined a local support group for the disorder. The result? He can now work full-time and still enjoy racquetball.

Not everyone with spasmodic torticollis responds as well. But if you have the disease, you can learn from Hal's experience. With the help of your doctor and support from family and friends, spasmodic torticollis shouldn't keep you from enjoying an active lifestyle.

Getting Support

The National Spasmodic Torticollis Association is a non-profit organization that provides information about the disease and helps those with it cope.

For more information, contact the National Spasmodic Torticollis Association, P.O. Box 476, Elm Grove, Wis., 53122-0476; phone (800) 487-8385.

Chapter 18

Stiff Neck:
An Occupational Hazard

Two common causes of neck pain are primarily job-related. Both respond well to nonpharmacologic intervention.

While low-back pain is widely recognized as a cause of work-related disability, more subtle occupational injuries to the neck may be overlooked. Two such injuries, tension neck syndrome and occipital cephalgia, are related primarily to poor posture and a lack of neck motion, particularly in sedentary jobs. Both are eminently treatable.

Tension Neck Syndrome

Tension neck syndrome, as its name implies, arises from increased cervical muscle tension. It is not usually connected to a specific episode of injury but results from maintaining a static, ergonomically incorrect posture for a prolonged period of time. Muscles that are used to maintain a static posture are not allowed to relax when necessary. Plumbers and others who must work in awkward positions are at risk, but the problem is most often reported by people who have desk jobs that allow little head and neck motion.

Symptoms

Tension neck syndrome produees stiffness, sometimes accompanied by a dull headache, and pains throughout the neck, often spreading

Patient Care, July 15,1995. Reprinted with permission of *Patient Care*. Copyright by Medical Economics.

to the upper thoracic regions. The levator scapulae and trapezius muscles are tender, with increased tension to palpation.

The patient may wake up feeling fine, but symptoms increase as the day progresses. At the end of the day, the patient is tired and looks forward to sleeping to help relax the neck tension. Radicular symptoms are usually absent, and the neurologic examination is normal. If a patient complains of tingling sensations in the upper extremities, consider a coexisting repetitive motion injury. (See "Radiation, repetitive motion, and other job hazards," *Patient Care*, October 15,1994, page 77.)

Plain cervical spine films are normal in younger patients. Older people may have osteoarthritic changes in the spine. It may be hard to determine whether the cause of pain is lack of motion due to static job posture, underlying degenerative changes, or a combination of both.

Treatment

The key to effective treatment is to recognize and identify the poor postures and recommend changes in workstations and work habits where possible. (For a patient information sheet that offers workstation suggestions, see *Patient Care*, October 15,1994, page 92.) Encourage patients to take brief stretching breaks every hour or so, including gentle range-of-motion exercises for the neck and shoulder. You can temporarily relieve symptoms with drugs, physical therapy, or manipulation, but pain and stiffness will inevitably return unless you have dealt with the ergonomic issues.

Occipital Cephalgia

Occipital cephalgia results from a "locking" of motion about the occipital-atlantal joints where the neck and skull meet. Like tension neck syndrome, it results from maintaining the neck in an awkward position. Common causes include watching television while lying on a couch with the head and neck propped up, prolonged tucking of a telephone beneath the chin, and extended work at a desk job with few shifts in position.

Symptoms

Occipital cephalgia is more likely to be an acute condition than is tension neck syndrome. The upper vertebral facet on either side of the atlas locks up (subluxes) and restricts motion against the occiput. This is not something that can be visualized on X-ray films.

Local tissue changes result in intensely tender, warm muscle spasm along the affected side of the occipital muscular triangle. This inflammatory-like reaction also affects the C-2 nerve-root and may cause associated radicular symptoms.

These patients come to you in pain. They look uncomfortable and typically describe intense local aching in the occipital-atlantal region, often associated with pain or numbness on the scalp. The phenomenon is well-localized and-tends to be unilateral. Palpation of the affected occipital-atlantal joint usually reproduces the symptoms.

Some patients report dizziness or light-headedness. Those with severe pain may experience headaches of migraine intensity, with migraine-like symptoms such as nausea and photosensitivity. As long as the pain persists, they have trouble sleeping and performing daily activities.

The natural history of untreated acute occipital cephalgia is a headache that can be intense for 1-3 days before gradually subsiding and resolving, usually within a week. Chronic occipital headaches are not uncommon, however, in workers whose job postures put them at risk.

Treatment

The goal of treatment is to gently relieve the locked subluxation at the occipital-atlantal joint as soon as possible, certainly before symptoms peak. Gentle mobilization of the occipital-atlantal joint in the office can provide almost instantaneous relief of pain, followed by relaxation of muscle spasm over the next few hours.

If you do not perform manipulation, you can try another technique. With the patient supine, sit at the head of the table and gently stretch the neck muscles to begin relaxation. With your hands under the patient's head, use your fingers to cup the occipital condyles on either side. Your fingertips will nestle in the sulcus inferior to the occiput. Have the patient relax the head and neck so that the head drops toward the table (your fingers acting like a fulcrum), and apply gentle traction toward the apex of the skull. Hold this position for a few minutes, and slowly try rotating the skull on the neck. This maneuver relaxes the patient and may enable the joint to slip back into place on its own.

Patients with chronic occipital cephalgia can help themselves at home by placing two tennis balls in the toe of a sock and securing it tightly so that the balls don't move. They then lie on a carpeted floor so that each condyle rests on one of the tennis balls and remain supine for as long as it takes the occipital muscles to relax.

Regardless of how reduction of the joint is accomplished, apply ice to the region for its analgesic and anti-inflammatory effects. If the joint cannot be reduced, consider the following:

- *Medication.* For mild to moderate pain, prescribe a rapid-acting nonsteroidal anti-inflammatory drug (NSAID) such as naproxen sodium, double-strength (Anaprox DS). For moderate to severe pain, use an IM injection of an NSAID such as ketorolac tromethamine (Toradol) followed by the drug in its oral form. If the pain is severe, you may want to prescribe a stronger narcotic analgesic for emergency use, particularly in the evenings to help the patient sleep. Muscle relaxants may also provide relief, especially for patients who are too uncomfortable to go about their daily activities and need to rest at home until the pain resolves.

- *Physical therapy.* Physical therapists can use soft-tissue relaxation techniques or try modalities such as high-voltage electrical stimulation to reduce local muscle spasm in the occipital-atlantal region. Standard cervical traction, sometimes used for cervical disk disease, will not help patients with occipital cephalgia and may be very uncomfortable. After the subluxation is reduced, the therapist will educate the patient on proper body posture and initiate a preventive exercise program.

- *Trigger point injections.* The occipital-atlantal joints respond well to trigger point injections of a local anesthetic, especially when pain is secondary to arthritis. Follow this with an application of ice.

—Jeffrey K. Pearson, DO

Jeffrey K. Pearson, DO, is in the private practice of family medicine at the Industrial & Sports Medical Center, San Marcos, Calif., and is a member of the *Patient Care* Board of Editors.

Part Three

Treatment and Rehabilitation

Chapter 19

Treatment for Acute Low Back Problems in Adults

Purpose and Scope

Low back problems affect virtually everyone at some time during their life. Surveys indicate a yearly prevalence of symptoms in 50 percent of working age adults; 15-20 percent seek medical care. Low back problems rank high among the reasons for physician office visits and are costly in terms of medical treatment, lost productivity, and nonmonetary costs such as diminished ability to perform or enjoy usual activities. In fact, for persons under age 45, low back problems are the most common cause of disability.

Acute low back problems are defined as activity intolerance due to lower back or back-related leg symptoms of less than 3 months' duration. About 90 percent of patients with acute low back problems spontaneously recover activity tolerance within 1 month. The approach to a new episode in a patient with a recurrent low back problem is similar to that of a new acute episode.

The findings and recommendations included in the *Clinical Practice Guideline* define a paradigm shift away from focusing care exclusively on the pain and toward helping patients improve activity tolerance. The intent of this *Quick Reference Guide* is to bring to life

Bigos S, Bowyer O, Braen G, et al. *Acute Low Back Problems in Adults.* Clinical Practice Guideline, Quick Reference Guide Number 14, Rockville, MD: U.S. Department of Health and Human Services, Public Health Service, Agency for Health Care Policy and Research, AHCPR Pub. No. 95-0643, December 1994.

this paradigm shift. The guide provides information on the detection of serious conditions that occasionally cause low back symptoms (conditions such as spinal fracture, tumor, infection, cauda equina syndrome, or non-spinal conditions). However, treatment of these conditions is beyond the scope of this guideline. In addition, the guideline does not address the care of patients younger than 18 years or those with chronic back problems (back-related activity limitations of greater than 3 months' duration).

Initial Assessment

- Seek potentially dangerous underlying conditions.

- In the absence of signs of dangerous conditions, there is no need for special studies since 90 percent of patients will recover spontaneously within 4 weeks.

A focused medical history and physical examination are sufficient to assess the patient with an acute or recurrent limitation due to low back symptoms of less than 4 weeks duration. Patient responses and findings on the history and physical examination, referred to as "red flags" (Figure 19.1), raise suspicion of serious underlying spinal conditions. Their absence rules out the need for special studies during the first 4 weeks of symptoms when spontaneous recovery is expected. The medical history and physical examination can also alert the clinician to non-spinal pathology (abdominal, pelvic, thoracic) that can present as low back symptoms. Acute low back symptoms can then be classified into one of three working categories:

- *Potentially serious spinal condition*—tumor, infection, spinal fracture, or a major neurologic compromise, such as cauda equina syndrome, suggested by a red flag.

- *Sciatica*—back-related lower limb symptoms suggesting lumbosacral nerve root compromise.

- *Nonspecific back symptoms*—occurring primarily in the back and suggesting neither nerve root compromise nor a serious underlying condition.

Possible fracture	Possible tumor or infection	Possible cauda equina syndrome
From medical history		
Major trauma, such as vehicle accident or fall from height. Minor trauma or even strenuous lifting (in older or potentially osteoporotic patient).	Age over 50 or under 20. History of cancer. Constitutional symptoms, such as recent fever or chills or unexplained weight loss. Risk factors for spinal infection: recent bacterial infection (e.g., urinary tract infection); IV drug abuse; or immune suppression (from steroids, transplant, or HIV). Pain that worsens when supine; severe nighttime pain.	Saddle anesthesia. Recent onset of bladder dysfunction, such as urinary retention, increased frequency, or overflow incontinence. Severe or progressive neurologic deficit in the lower extremity.
From physical examination		
		Unexpected laxity of the anal sphincter. Perianal/perineal sensory loss. Major motor weakness: quadriceps (knee extension weakness); ankle plantar flexors, evertors, and dorsiflexors (foot drop).

Figure 19.1. Red flags for potentially serious conditions.

Medical History

In addition to detecting serious conditions and categorizing back symptoms, the medical history establishes rapport between the clinician and patient. The patient's description of present symptoms and limitations, duration of symptoms, and history of previous episodes defines the problem. It also provides insight into concerns, expectations, and nonphysical (psychological and socioeconomic) issues that may alter the patient's response to treatment. Assessment tools such as pain drawings and visual analog pain-rating scales may help further document the patient's perceptions and progress.

A patient's estimate of personal activity intolerance due to low back symptoms contributes to the clinical assessment of the severity of the back problem, guides treatment, and establishes a baseline for recommending daily activities and evaluating progress.

Open-ended questions, such as those listed below, can gauge the need for further discussion or specific inquiries for more detailed information:

- **What are your symptoms?** Pain, numbness, weakness, stiffness? Located primarily in back, leg, or both? Constant or intermittent?

- **How do these symptoms limit you?** How long can you sit, stand, walk? How much weight can you lift?

- **When did the current limitations begin?** How long have your activities been limited? More than 4 weeks? Have you had similar episodes previously? Previous testing or treatment?

- **What do you hope we can accomplish during this visit?**

Physical Examination

Guided by the medical history, the physical examination includes:

- General observation of the patient.
- A regional back exam.
- Neurologic screening.
- Testing for sciatic nerve root tension.

The examination is mostly subjective since patient response or interpretation is required for all parts except reflex testing and circumferential measurements for atrophy.

Addressing Red Flags

Physical examination evidence of severe neurologic compromise that correlates with the medical history may indicate a need for immediate consultation. The examination may further modify suspicions of tumor, infection, or significant trauma. A medical history suggestive of non-spinal pathology mimicking a back problem may warrant examination of pulses, abdomen, pelvis, or other areas.

Observation and Regional Back Examination

Limping or coordination problems indicate the need for specific neurologic testing. Severe guarding of lumbar motion in all planes may support a suspected diagnosis of spinal infection, tumor, or fracture. However, given marked variations among persons with and without symptoms, range-of-motion measurements of the back are of limited value.

Vertebral point tenderness to palpation, when associated with other signs or symptoms, may be suggestive of but not specific for spinal fracture or infection. Palpable soft-tissue tenderness is, by itself, an even less specific or reliable finding.

Neurologic Screening

The neurologic examination can focus on a few tests that seek evidence of nerve root impairment, peripheral neuropathy, or spinal cord dysfunction. Over 90 percent of all clinically significant lower extremity radiculopathy due to disc herniation involves the L5 or S1 nerve root at the L4-5 or L5-S1 disc level. The clinical features of nerve root compression are summarized in Figure 19.2.

- *Testing for Muscle Strength.* The patient's inability to toe walk (calf muscles, mostly S1 nerve root), heel walk (ankle and toe dorsiflexor muscles, L5 and some L4 nerve roots), or do a single squat and rise (quadriceps muscles, mostly L4 nerve root) may indicate muscle weakness. Specific testing of the dorsiflexor muscles of the ankle or great toe (suggestive of L5 or some L4 nerve root dysfunction), hamstrings and ankle evertors (L5-S1), and toe flexors (S1) is also important.

- *Circumferential Measurements.* Muscle atrophy can be detected by circumferential measurements of the calf and thigh bilaterally. Differences of less than 2 cm in measurements of the two limbs at the same level may be a normal variation. Symmetrical muscle bulk and strength are expected unless the patient has a neurologic impairment or a history of lower extremity muscle or joint problem.

- *Reflexes.* The ankle jerk reflex tests mostly the S1 nerve root and the knee jerk reflex tests mostly the L4 nerve root; neither tests the L5 nerve root. The reliability of reflex testing can be diminished in the presence of adjacent joint or muscle problems. Up-going toes in response to stroking the plantar footpad (Babinski or plantar response) may indicate upper motor-neuron abnormalities (such as myelopathy or demyelinating disease) rather than a common low back problem.

- *Sensory Examination.* Testing light touch or pressure in the medial (L4), dorsal (L5), and lateral (S1) aspects of the foot (Figure 19.2) is usually sufficient for sensory screening.

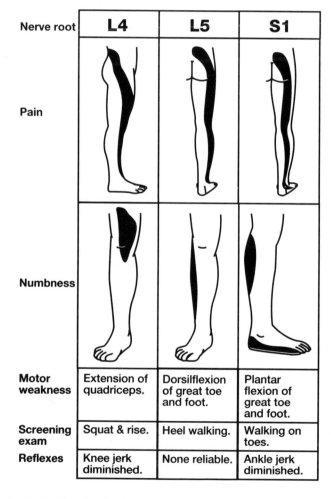

Nerve root	**L4**	**L5**	**S1**
Pain			
Numbness			
Motor weakness	Extension of quadriceps.	Dorsiflexion of great toe and foot.	Plantar flexion of great toe and foot.
Screening exam	Squat & rise.	Heel walking.	Walking on toes.
Reflexes	Knee jerk diminished.	None reliable.	Ankle jerk diminished.

Figure 19.2. Testing for lumbar nerve root compromise.

Clinical Tests for Sciatic Tension

The straight leg raising (SLR) test (Figure 19.3) can detect tension on the L5 and/or S1 nerve root. SLR may reproduce leg pain by stretching nerve roots irritated by a disc herniation.

Pain below the knee at less than 70 degrees of straight leg raising, aggravated by dorsiflexion of the ankle and relieved by ankle plantar

(1) Ask the patient to lie as straight as possible on a table in the supine position.

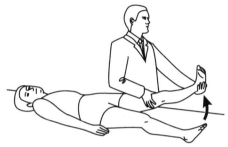

(2) With one hand placed above the knee of the leg being examined, exert enough firm pressure to keep the knee fully extended. Ask the patient to relax.

(3) With the other hand cupped under the heel, slowly raise the straight limb. Tell the patient, "If this bothers you, let me know, and I will stop."

4) Monitor for any movement of the pelvis before complaints are elicited. True sciatic tension should elicit complaints before the hamstrings are stretched enough to move the pelvis.

(5) Estimate the degree of leg elevation that elicits complaint from the patient. Then determine the most distal area of discomfort: back, hip, thigh, knee, or below the knee.

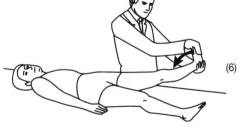

(6) While holding the leg at the limit of straight leg raising, dorsiflex the ankle. Note whether this aggravates the pain. Internal rotation of the limb can also increase the tension on the sciatic nerve roots.

Figure 19.3. *Instructions for the Straight Leg Raising (SLR) Test.*

flexion or external limb rotation, is most suggestive of tension on the L5 or S1 nerve root related to disc herniation. Reproducing back pain alone with SLR testing does not indicate significant nerve root tension.

Crossover pain occurs when straight raising of the patient's well limb elicits pain in the leg with sciatica. Crossover pain is a stronger indication of nerve root compression than pain elicited from raising the straight painful limb.

Sitting knee extension (Figure 19.4) can also test sciatic tension. The patient with significant nerve root irritation tends to complain or lean backward to reduce tension on the nerve.

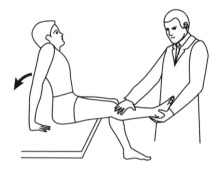

With the patient sitting on a table, both hip and knees flexed at 90 degrees, slowly extend the knee as if evaluating the patella or bottom of the foot. This maneuver stretches nerve roots as much as a moderate degree of supine SLR.

Figure 19.4. Instructions for sitting knee extension test.

Inconsistent Findings and Pain Behavior

The patient who embellishes a medical history, exaggerates pain drawings, or provides responses on physical examination inconsistent with known physiology can be particularly challenging. A strongly positive supine straight leg raising test without complaint on sitting knee extension and inconsistent responses on examination raise a suspicion that nonphysical factors may be affecting the patient's responses. "Pain behaviors" (verbal or nonverbal communication of distress or suffering) such as amplified grimacing, distorted gait or posture, moaning, and rubbing of painful body parts may also cloud medical issues and even evoke angry responses from the clinician.

Interpreting inconsistencies or pain behaviors as malingering does not benefit the patient or the clinician. It is more useful to view such behavior and inconsistencies as the patient's attempt to enlist the practitioner as an advocate, a plea for help. The patient could be trapped in a job where activity requirements are unrealistic relative to the person's age or health. In some cases, the patient may be negotiating with an insurer or be involved in legal actions. In patients with recurrent back problems, inconsistencies and amplifications may simply be habits learned during previous medical evaluations. In working with these patients, the clinician should attempt to identify any psychological or socioeconomic pressures that might be influenced in a positive manner. The overall goal should always be to facilitate the patient's recovery and avoid the development of chronic low back disability.

Initial Care

- Education and assurance.
- Patient comfort.
- Activity alterations.

Patient Education

If the initial assessment detects no serious condition, assure the patient that there is "no hint of a dangerous problem" and that "a rapid recovery can be expected." The need for education will vary among patients and during various stages of care. An obviously apprehensive patient may require a more detailed explanation. Patients with sciatica may have a longer expected recovery time than patients with nonspecific back symptoms and thus may need more education and reassurance. Any patient who does not recover within a few weeks may need more extensive education about back problems and the reassurance that special studies may be considered if recovery is slow.

Patient Comfort

Comfort is often a patient's first concern. Nonprescription analgesics will provide sufficient pain relief for most patients with acute low back symptoms. If treatment response is inadequate, as evidenced by continued symptoms and activity limitations, prescribed pharmaceuticals or physical methods may be added. Comorbid conditions, side effects, cost, and provider/patient preference should guide the clinician's choice of recommendations. Figure 19.6 summarizes comfort options.

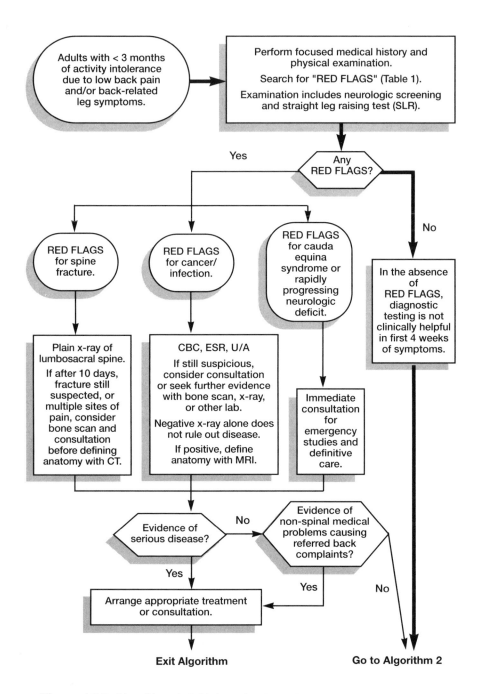

Figure 19.5. *Algorithm 1. Initial evaluation of acute low back problem.*

Recommended		
Nonprescription analgesics		
Acetaminophen (safest) NSAIDs (Aspirin,[1] Ibuprofen[1])		
Prescribed pharmaceutical methods	**Prescribed physical methods**	
Nonspecific low back symptoms and/or sciatica	Nonspecific low back symptoms	Sciatica
Other NSAIDs[1]	Manipulation (in place of medication or a shorter trial if combined with NSAIDs)	
Options		
Nonspecific low back symptoms and/or sciatica	Nonspecific low back symptoms	Sciatica
Muscle relaxants[2,3,4] Opioids[2,3,4]	Physical agents and modalities[2] (heat or cold modalities for home programs only) Shoe insoles[2]	Manipulation (in place of medication or a shorter trial if combined with NSAIDs) Physical agents and modalities[2] (heat or cold modalities for home programs only) Few days' rest[4] Shoe insoles[2]

[1] Aspirin and other NSAIDs are not recommended for use in combination with one another due to the risk of GI complications.
[2] Equivocal efficacy.
[3] Significant potential for producing drowsiness and debilitation; potential for dependency.
[4] Short course (few days only) for severe symptoms.

Figure 19.6. *Symptom control methods.*

Oral Pharmaceuticals

The safest effective medication for acute low back problems appears to be acetaminophen. Nonsteroidal anti-inflammatory drugs (NSAIDs), including aspirin and ibuprofen, are also effective although they can cause gastrointestinal irritation/ulceration or (less commonly) renal or allergic problems. Phenylbutazone is not recommended due to risks of bone marrow suppression. Acetaminophen may be used safely in combination with NSAIDs or other pharmacologic or physical therapeutics, especially in otherwise healthy patients.

Muscle relaxants seem no more effective than NSAIDs for treating patients with low back symptoms, and using them in combination with NSAIDs has no demonstrated benefit. Side effects including drowsiness have been reported in up to 30 percent of patients taking muscle relaxants.

Opioids appear no more effective than safer analgesics for managing low back symptoms. Opioids should be avoided if possible and, when chosen, used only for a short time. Poor patient tolerance and risks of drowsiness, decreased reaction time, clouded judgment, and potential misuse/dependence have been reported in up to 35 percent of patients. Patients should be warned of these potentially debilitating problems.

Physical Methods

- *Manipulation*, defined as manual loading of the spine using short or long leverage methods, is safe and effective for patients in the first month of acute low back symptoms without radiculopathy. For patients with symptoms lasting longer than 1 month, manipulation is probably safe but its efficacy is unproven. If manipulation has not resulted in symptomatic and functional improvement after 4 weeks, it should be stopped and the patient reevaluated.

- *Traction* applied to the spine has not been found effective for treating acute low back symptoms.

- *Physical modalities* such as *massage, diathermy, ultrasound, cutaneous laser treatment, biofeedback*, and *transcutaneous electrical nerve stimulation* (TENS) also have no proven efficacy in the treatment of acute low back symptoms. If requested, the clinician may wish to provide the patient with instructions on self-application of heat or cold therapy for temporary symptom relief.

- *Invasive techniques* such as *needle acupuncture* and *injection procedures* (injection of trigger points in the back; injection of facet joints; injection of steroids, lidocaine, or opioids in the epidural space) have no proven benefit in the treatment of acute low back symptoms.

- *Other miscellaneous therapies* have been evaluated. No evidence indicates that *shoe lifts* are effective in treating acute low back symptoms or limitations, especially when the difference in lower limb length is less than 2 cm. Shoe insoles are a safe and inexpensive option if requested by patients with low back symptoms who must stand for prolonged periods. Low back corsets and back belts, however, do not appear beneficial for treating acute low back symptoms.

Activity Alteration

To avoid both undue back irritation and debilitation from inactivity, recommendations for alternate activity can be helpful. Most patients will not require bed rest. Prolonged bed rest (more than 4 days) has potential debilitating effects, and its efficacy in the treatment of acute low back problems is unproven. Two to four days of bed rest are reserved for patients with the most severe limitations (due primarily to leg pain).

Avoiding undue back irritation. Activities and postures that increase stress on the back also tend to aggravate back symptoms. Patients limited by back symptoms can minimize the stress of lifting by keeping any lifted object close to the body at the level of the navel. Twisting, bending, and reaching while lifting also increase stress on the back. Sitting, although safe, may aggravate symptoms for some patients. Advise these patients to avoid prolonged sitting and to change position often. A soft support placed at the small of the back, armrests to support some body weight, and a slight recline of the chair back may make required sitting more comfortable.

Avoiding debilitation. Until the patient returns to normal activity, aerobic (endurance) conditioning exercise such as walking, stationary biking, swimming, and even light jogging may be recommended to help avoid debilitation from inactivity. An incremental, gradually increasing regimen of aerobic exercise (up to 20 to 30 minutes daily) can usually be started within the first 2 weeks of symptoms. Such conditioning activities have been found to stress the back no more than sitting for an equal time period on the side of the bed. Patients should be informed that exercise may increase symptoms slightly at first. If intolerable, some exercise alteration is usually helpful.

Conditioning exercises for trunk muscles are more mechanically stressful to the back than aerobic exercise. Such exercises are not recommended during the first few weeks of symptoms, although they may later help patients regain and maintain activity tolerance.

There is no evidence to indicate that back-specific exercise machines are effective for treating acute low back problems. Neither is there evidence that stretching of the back helps patients with acute symptoms.

Work Activities

When requested, clinicians may choose to offer specific instructions about activity at work for patients with acute limitations due to low back symptoms. The patient's age, general health, and perceptions of safe limits of sitting, standing, walking or lifting (noted on initial history) can help provide reasonable starting points for activity recommendations. Figure 19.7 provides a guide for recommendations about sitting and lifting. The clinician should make clear to patients and employers that:

• Even moderately heavy unassisted lifting may aggravate back symptoms.
• Any restrictions are intended to allow for spontaneous recovery or time to build activity tolerance through exercise.

Activity restrictions are prescribed for a short time period only, depending upon work requirements (no benefits apparent beyond 3 months).

	Symptoms					
	Severe →	Moderate →		Mild	→	None
Sitting[1]	20 min →	→	→	→	→	50 min
Unassisted lifting[2]						
Men	20 lbs →	20 lbs	→	60 lbs	→	80 lbs
Women	20 lbs →	20 lbs	→	35 lbs	→	40 lbs

[1]Without getting up and moving around.
[2]Modification of NIOSH Lifting Guidelines, 1981, 1993. Gradually increase unassisted lifting limits to 60 lbs (men) and 35 lbs (women) by 3 months even with continued symptoms. Instruct patient to limit twisting, bending, reaching while lifting and to hold lifted object as close to navel as possible.

Figure 19.7. Guidelines for sitting and unassisted lifting.

Initial visit

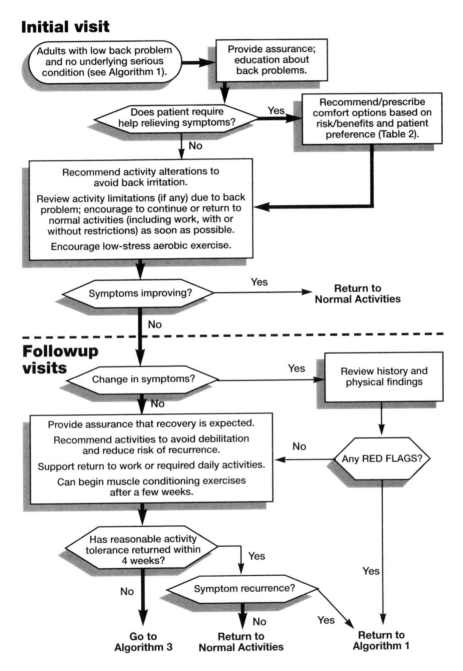

Figure 19.8. Algorithm 2. Treatment of acute low back problem on initial and followup visits.

Special Studies and Diagnostic Considerations

Routine testing (laboratory tests, plain x-rays of the lumbosacral spine) and imaging studies are not recommended during the first month of activity limitation due to back symptoms except when a red flag noted on history or examination raises suspicion of a dangerous low back or non-spinal condition. If a patient's limitations due to low back symptoms do not improve in 4 weeks, reassessment is recommended. After again reviewing the patient's activity limitations, history, and physical findings, the clinician may then consider further diagnostic studies, and discuss these with the patient.

Timing and Limits of Special Studies

Waiting 4 weeks before considering special tests allows 90 percent of patients to recover spontaneously and avoids unneeded procedures. This also reduces the potential confusion of falsely labeling age-related changes on imaging studies (commonly noted in patients older than 30 without back symptoms) as the cause of the acute symptoms. In the absence of either red flags or persistent activity limitations due to continuous limb symptoms, imaging studies (especially plain x-rays) rarely provide information that changes the clinical approach to the acute low back problem.

Selection of Special Studies

Prior to ordering imaging studies the clinician should have noted either of the following:

- The emergence of a red flag.
- Physiologic evidence of tissue insult or neurologic dysfunction.

Physiologic evidence may be in the form of definitive nerve findings on physical examination, electrodiagnostic studies (when evaluating sciatica), and a laboratory test or bone scan (when evaluating nonspecific low back symptoms). Unquestionable findings that identify specific nerve root compromise on the neurologic examination (see Figure 19.2) are sufficient physiologic evidence to warrant imaging. When the neurologic examination is less clear, however, further physiologic evidence of nerve root dysfunction should be considered before ordering an imaging study. Electromyography (EMG) including H-reflex tests may be useful to identify subtle focal neurologic dysfunction in patients with leg symptoms lasting longer than 3-4 weeks. Sensory evoked potentials (SEPs) may be added to the assessment if spinal stenosis or spinal cord myelopathy is suspected.

Laboratory tests such as erythrocyte sedimentation rate (ESR), complete blood count (CBC), and urinalysis (UA) can be useful to screen for nonspecific medical diseases (especially infection and tumor) of the low back. A bone scan can detect physiologic reactions to suspected spinal tumor, infection, or occult fracture.

Should physiologic evidence indicate tissue insult or nerve impairment, discuss with a consultant selection of an imaging test to define a potential anatomic cause (CT for bone, MRI for neural or other soft tissue). Anatomic definition is commonly needed to guide surgery or specific procedures. Selection of an imaging test should also take into consideration any patient allergies to contrast media (myelogram) or concerns about claustrophobia (MRI) and costs. A discussion with a specialist on selection of the most clinically valuable study can often assist the primary care clinician to avoid duplication. Figure 19.9

Technique	Identify physiologic insult	Define anatomic defect
History	+	+
Physical examination: Circumference measurements	+	+
Reflexes	++	++
Straight leg raising (SLR)	++	+
Crossed SLR	+++	++
Motor	++	++
Sensory	++	++
Laboratory studies (ESR, CBC, UA)	++	0
Bone scan[1]	+++	++
EMG/SEP	+++	++
X-ray[1]	0	+
CT[1]	0	++++[2]
MRI	0	++++[2]
Myelo-CT[1]	0	++++[2]
Myelography[1]	0	++++[2]

[1] Risk of complications (radiation, infection, etc.): highest for myelo-CT, second highest for myelography, and relatively less risk for bone scan, x-ray, and CT.

[2] False-positive diagnostic findings in up to 30 percent of people without symptoms at age 30.

Note: Number of plus signs indicates relative ability to identify or define.

Figure 19.9. Ability of different techniques to identify and define pathology.

211

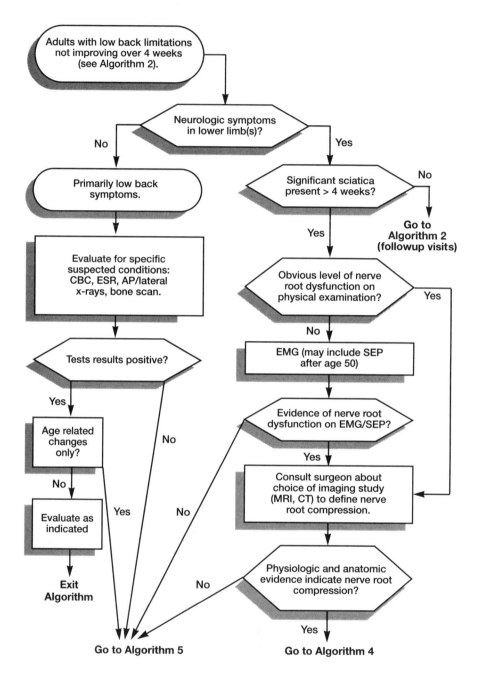

Figure 19.10. *Algorithm 3. Evaluation of the slow-to-recover patient (symptoms > 4 weeks).*

provides a general comparison of the abilities of different techniques to identify physiologic insult and define anatomic defects. Missing from the figure is discography, which is not recommended for assessing patients with acute low back symptoms.

In general, an imaging study may be an appropriate consideration for the patient whose limitations due to consistent symptoms have persisted for 1 month or more:

- When surgery is being considered for treatment of a specific detectable loss of neurologic function.
- To further evaluate potentially serious spinal pathology.

Reliance upon imaging studies alone to evaluate the source of low back symptoms, however, carries a significant risk of diagnostic confusion, given the possibility of falsely identifying a finding that was present before symptoms began.

Management Considerations After Special Studies

Definitive treatment for serious conditions (see Figure 19.1) detected by special studies is beyond the scope of this guideline. When special studies fail to define the exact cause of symptoms, however, no patient should receive an impression that the clinician thinks "nothing is wrong" or that the problem could be "in their head." Assure the patient that a clinical workup is highly successful in detecting serious conditions, but does not reveal the precise cause of most low back symptoms.

Surgical Considerations

Within the first 3 months of acute low back symptoms, surgery is considered only when serious spinal pathology or nerve root dysfunction obviously due to a herniated lumbar disc is detected. A disc herniation, characterized by protrusion of the central nucleus pulposus through a defect in the outer annulus fibrosis, may trap a nerve root causing irritation, leg symptoms and nerve root dysfunction. The presence of a herniated lumbar disc on an imaging study, however, does not necessarily imply nerve root dysfunction. Studies of asymptomatic adults commonly demonstrate intervertebral disc herniations that apparently do not entrap a nerve root or cause symptoms.

213

Therefore, nerve root decompression can be considered for a patient if all of the following criteria exist:

• Sciatica is both severe and disabling.

• Symptoms of sciatica persist without improvement for longer than 4 weeks or with extreme progression.

• There is strong physiologic evidence of dysfunction of a specific nerve root with intervertebral disc herniation confirmed at the corresponding level and side by findings on an imaging study.

Patients with acute low back pain alone, without findings of serious conditions or significant nerve root compression, rarely benefit from a surgical consultation.

Many patients with strong clinical findings of nerve root dysfunction due to disc herniation recover activity tolerance within 1 month; no evidence indicates that delaying surgery for this period worsens outcomes. With or without an operation, more than 80 percent of patients with obvious surgical indications eventually recover. Surgery seems to be a luxury for speeding recovery of patients with obvious surgical indications but benefits fewer than 40 percent of patients with questionable physiologic findings. Moreover, surgery increases the chance of future procedures with higher complication rates. Overall, the incidence of first-time disc surgery complications, including infection and bleeding, is less than 1 percent. The figure increases dramatically with older patients or repeated procedures.

Direct and indirect nerve root decompression for herniated discs. Direct methods of nerve root decompression include laminotomy (expansion of the interlaminar space for access to the nerve root and the offending disc fragments), microdiscectomy (laminotomy using a microscope), and laminectomy (total removal of laminae). Methods of indirect nerve root decompression include chemonucleolysis, the injection of chymopapain or other enzymes to dissolve the inner disc. Such chemical treatment methods are less efficacious than standard or microdiscectomy and have rare but serious complications. Any of these methods is preferable to percutaneous discectomy (indirect, mechanical disc removal through a lateral disc puncture).

Management of spinal stenosis. Usually resulting from soft tissue and bony encroachment of the spinal canal and nerve roots, spinal stenosis typically has a gradual onset and begins in older

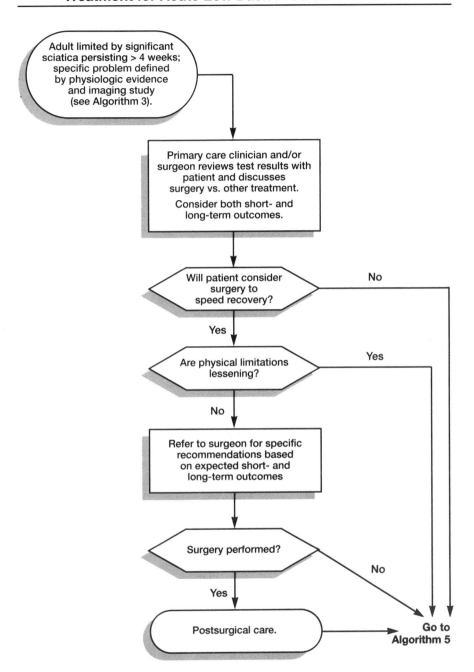

Figure 19.11. *Algorithm 4. Surgical considerations for patients with persistent sciatica.*

adults. It is characterized by nonspecific limb symptoms, called *neurogenic claudication* or *pseudoclaudication*, that interfere with the duration of comfortable standing and walking. The symptoms are commonly bilateral and rarely associated with strong focal findings on examination. Neurogenic claudication, however, can be confused or coexist with *vascular claudication*, in which leg pain also limits walking. The symptoms of vascular insufficiency can be relieved by simply standing still while relief of neurogenic claudication symptoms usually require the patient to flex the lumbar spine or sit.

The surgical treatment for spinal stenosis is usually complete laminectomy for posterior decompression. Offending soft tissue and osteophytes that encroach upon nerve roots in the central spinal canal and foramen are removed. Fusion may be considered to stabilize a degenerative spondylolisthesis with motion between the slipped vertebra and adjacent vertebrae. Elderly patients with spinal stenosis who tolerate their daily activities usually need no surgery unless they develop new signs of bowel or bladder dysfunction. Decisions on treatment should take into account the patient's preference, lifestyle, other medical problems, and risks of surgery. Surgery for spinal stenosis is rarely considered in the first 3 months of symptoms.

Except for cases of trauma-related spinal fracture or dislocation, fusion alone is not usually considered in the first 3 months following onset of low back symptoms.

Further Management Considerations

Following diagnostic or surgical procedures, the management of most patients becomes focused on improving physical conditioning through an incrementally increased exercise program. The goal of this program is to build activity tolerance and overcome individual limitations due to back symptoms. At this point in treatment, symptom control methods are only an adjunct to making prescribed exercises more tolerable.

- Begin with low-stress aerobic activities to improve general stamina (walking, riding a bicycle, swimming, and eventually jogging).

- Exercises to condition specific trunk muscles can be added a few weeks after. The back muscles may need to be in better condition than before the problem occurred. Otherwise, the back may continue to be painful and easily irritated by even mild activity.

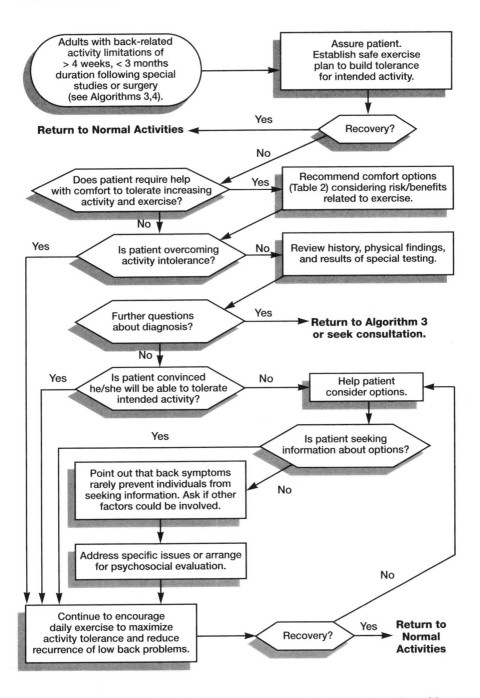

Figure 19.12. Algorithm 5. Further management of acute low back problem.

Following back surgery, recovery of activity tolerance may be delayed until protective muscles are conditioned well enough to compensate for any remaining structural changes.

- Finally, specific training to perform activities required at home or work can begin. The objective of this program is to increase the patient's tolerance in carrying out actual daily duties.

When patients demonstrate difficulty regaining the ability to tolerate the activities they are required (or would like) to do, the clinician may pose the following diagnostic and treatment questions:

- Could the patient have a serious, undetected medical condition? A careful review of the medical history and physical examination is warranted.

- Are the patient's activity goals realistic? Exploring briefly the patient's expectations, both short- and long-term, of being able to perform specific activities at home, work, or recreation may help the patient assess whether such activity levels are actually achievable.

- If for any reason the achievement of activity goals seems unlikely, what are the patient's remaining options? To answer this question, the patient is often required to gather specific information from family, friends, employers, or others. If, on followup visits, the patient has made no effort to gather such information, the clinician has the opportunity to point out that low back symptoms alone rarely prevent a patient from addressing questions so important to his or her future. This observation can lead to an open, nonjudgmental discussion of common but complicated psychosocial problems or other issues that often can interfere with a patient's recovery from low back problems. The clinician can then help the patient address or arrange further evaluation of any specific problem limiting the patient's progress. This can usually be accomplished as the patient continues, with the clinician's encouragement, to build activity tolerance through safe, simple exercises.

Chapter 20

Motion and Progress in Low-Back Pain

The cost of back pain in the United States has been estimated at $40 billion a year, including medical costs, lost wages, and compensation claims. Back pain is the leading cause of disability in persons younger than 45, and the third leading cause among those older than 45. The longer the pain and disability persist, the less likely a good outcome. Most patients recovering from an initial episode of acute low-back pain need rehabilitation to keep the pain and impairment from becoming chronic.

Patients who have no apparent underlying disease or neurologic involvement should usually begin active rehabilitation after approximately 2-4 months of conservative therapy. At this point, soft tissue damage should have healed, and surgery should have been safely ruled out. Rehabilitation that is started too early may be limited by the sequelae of initial injury, may actually be a hindrance to soft-tissue healing, and may add to the already significant time and cost of recovery.

After 4-6 months of conservative care, though, a comprehensive rehabilitation program becomes crucial to prevent deconditioning and the development of a chronic back pain syndrome. Programs of this nature now often involve either early reconditioning or work hardening—getting the patient accustomed to the movements he or she must use on the job. They are usually organized along the established back school or pain clinic formats or the newer functional restoration approach.

Patient Care, May 15, 1991. Reprinted with permission of *Patient Care*. Copyright by Medical Economics.

Candidates for an earlier, passive rehabilitation program include patients whose condition has not responded well to bed rest, analgesics, anti-inflammatory medications, heat, and muscle relaxants after at least two weeks. For these patients, such a program need involve only changes in life-style and simple exercise for back flexion and extension. Patients recovering from back surgery or automobile accidents and those with rheumatoid arthritis may be good candidates for comprehensive rehabilitation, although severe spinal injury following an automobile accident and certain kinds of back surgery would preclude anything but highly specialized programs.

As an interdisciplinary effort, rehabilitation may involve practitioners in any or all of these specialties: orthopedics, neurology, internal medicine, family practice, rheumatology, physiatrics, and psychology. However, referral to a rehabilitation center is not always necessary for patients with uncomplicated low-back pain, and most patients need not leave your care even when formal rehabilitation becomes necessary. Consider using the services of a physical therapist, occupational therapist, or back school and monitoring the patient's progress in monthly or biweekly office visits. The therapist or back school should be able to give you good estimates of costs and when the patient can expect to recover function.

Back schools, which can be associated with hospitals or operated independently, are usually supervised by physicians and taught by physical therapists who work closely with the patients. The schools are recommended for patients who do not need acute care but who must be educated about applying protective body mechanics to daily activities. Back schools sometimes ergometrically evaluate a patient's occupation and go as far as instructing patients who want to participate in sports. Patients may also learn pain control techniques, including detoxification from pain medications and behavior modification, which is sometimes necessary when pain and impairment have defined a life-style. These techniques are more often within the domain of the pain clinic, however.

Another important member of the rehabilitation team—perhaps the most important—is the patient's family. Sometimes family members cannot tolerate the patient's disability or will not work with him to regain function, leading to stressful intrafamily dynamics that hinder recovery. An overprotective family also works against the patient's recovery.

Expectation from a rehabilitation program must be realistic. The patient should understand that long-standing chronic pain will not be relieved overnight and that daily exercise is necessary to reverse the deconditioning caused by protracted immobility. This exercise will probably be associated with soreness, at least in the beginning. For most patients whose back pain has persisted more than two months or stems from recurrent injury, a combination of behavior modification and reconditioning or functional restoration is the best approach to working through discomfort and ultimately regaining fitness.

When choosing a comprehensive rehabilitation program, be it a work hardening program, a pain clinic, or a functional restoration program, there are important questions to ask, such as these:

- What is the rate of return to work or productivity? Reputable programs should be able to provide this information, perhaps even citing peer-reviewed publications.

- Does the program specify theme and cost limits? There should be some assurance that the patient will not be paying indefinitely for a service that may not be demonstrably effective.

- What options are available if the condition remains refractory after routine outpatient care? In more severe chronic pain that is nonresponsive to other procedures, some insurance companies will pay for reconditioning and inpatient rehabilitation at an approved center.

- How is the medical care system used after rehabilitation is completed? Is surgery done afterward? Is the patient sent to still other health professionals? Under what circumstances? The rehabilitation program should be coordinated or guided by a medical professional, either the primary care physician or a rehabilitation expert.

- Is the rehabilitation program open-ended or guided by quantifiable function measurements and the patient's own goals? Results are usually better when the patient has clear goals. If rehabilitation becomes protracted or disability is severe, quantification of lumbar motion and strength is important in determining exercise programs and therapy.

During the course of rehabilitation, specific modalities may supplement and enhance exercise. Over the years, thinking has changed about a number of them. Patients respond idiosyncratically to one or another method, and some degree of trial and error will usually be necessary before there is marked improvement.

Bracing and Taping

If a patient must return to work or activity before conservative therapy can bring about sufficient recovery, a fitted brace may be indicated. The patient with a brace should wear it for only a limited time to avoid deconditioning supporting muscles and should attend a rehabilitation program for training in exercises and posture. Fitted braces should have an uplift abdominal support, be long enough to contact the sacrum posteriorly, and limit thoracolumbar motion.

Taping is not recommended because it provides little support and may be painful, with removal possibly causing abrasions and bleeding skin ulcers.

Traction

Only partly in jest, experts refer to traction as a way to keep uncooperative patients in bed. Effecting any meaningful separation of vertebra requires the application of about a quarter to a third of a patient's body weight. Since this is extremely impractical and may have little therapeutic benefit, conventional traction in not usually indicated. Some experts recommend gravity traction for otherwise healthy persons recovering from acute low-back pain—they hang upside down from their knees using a specially constructed device that gives support without endangering leg circulation. This method has never been validated in a controlled study and is clearly contraindicated for anyone with hypertension or cardiovascular disease.

Acupuncture and Electrical Stimulation

Acupuncture can alleviate musculoskeletal pains, at least temporarily. Transcutaneous electrical nerve stimulation (TENS) may be effective in temporarily relieving pain, but it should be used only as part of a comprehensive rehabilitation program. The technique, which probably reduces the perception of pain, may be more effective in managing acute pain or exacerbations of chronic pain than in long-term syndromes. Although controlled trials are infrequent, one study of chronic low-back pain showed electroacupuncture to be more effective than TENS, and a recent controlled trial showed no benefit of TENS over placebo.

Superficial and Deep Heat

Hot tubs, whirlpool baths, and other forms of hydrotherapy have palliative value and may lessen the time a patient must take medications. Superficial dry heat from hot packs, hot water bottles, and other devices does not usually penetrate below the surface of the skin, but it can be applied with care if the patient finds it helpful or pleasant. Any deep changes in blood flow or muscle tension are usually reflexive.

Diathermy may also help patients feel better. Treatments should be administered by an experienced therapist. Microwave radiation or ultrasound should not be applied to the backs or viscera of pregnant patients, and ultrasound should be applied to the spine only with caution. Microwave irradiation can also cause skin burns from vaporized sweat droplets, and reflection over bone could result in undesirable high localized heat. Ultrasound devices can be focused well enough that facet joints could be treated without directly exposing the spinal cord to the ultrasound beam.

Stress Management

This is a crucial part of rehabilitating the patient with back pain, because controlling emotional responses to tension, conflicts, and circumstances that seem beyond his or her control can help reduce the perception of pain. In addition to the back pain itself, related problems tend to exacerbate the situation: Currently or previously injured body parts can become targets for stress, and most people who cannot work or function normally are likely to feel more tension than usual. Finally, family discord can create stress that will increase pain perception in the injured or pain-prone individual.

Early recognition and intercession can help reduce if not resolve much of this pressure, and back schools can often help patients learn to cope with emotional conflicts and pressures from job and family that are associated with pain and injury. It is also important to improve intrafamily dynamics surrounding the patient experiencing chronic pain and disability. By serving as an educator and counselor, the primary care physician or other trained practitioner can help the patient recognize the relationship between outside forces and his own physical discomfort. Always consider the impact of impairment within the family context: A young parent or breadwinner facing severe disability will probably be under more severe (and perhaps strongly internalized) stress than an older person, and a younger person may be under greater pressure to participate in family activities as well.

Rigorous scientific data on biofeedback in low-back pain rehabilitation are lacking. However, biofeedback within the context of a behavior modification program may help some patients control their reactions to pain, to life-style changes, and tension-producing situations. In anecdotal accounts, perhaps 10-20% of patients respond to biofeedback during rehabilitation.

Life-Style Changes

Paramount among the changes in a patient's life-style is a need to exercise constantly and maintain overall fitness. Specific causes of tension, conflict, and counterproductive emotional attitudes should be identified and dealt with. Encourage obese patients to achieve normal weight, smokers to quit, and sedentary people to become more active. Basic advice on how to lift, how to sit, and how to cope with situations beyond the patient's control (such as uncomfortable positions in automobile seats) can be helpful and is often available from a back school.

Other adjustments in the activities of daily living may be overemphasized and are often not warranted. Back pain is a prevalent but generally benign condition that does not cause disability in underdeveloped countries and was accorded far less significance before the advent of disk surgery. Its perceived importance in the United States today, real and chronic pain notwithstanding, may be a consequence of the current disability and compensation protocol requiring that the system legitimize a patient's pain and impairment. It may not be necessary or even desirable to adjust a life-style to conditions that in reality are not new.

When low-back pain persists through 2-4 months of passive and active conservative therapy, a more aggressive approach is usually indicated. Consider referring the patient for the sports medicine approach to back rehabilitation. This parallels the type of rehabilitation widely employed for musculoskeletal problems of the extremities.

Experience has shown by now that it is valid to expect an injured athlete to regain lost function—in other words, to go back to work—by building up stiff and atrophied joints through exercises that simulate the demands of the sport. Moreover, during rehabilitation the function of an injured knee or elbow can be compared with that of the uninjured joint both visually and objectively by measuring strength and range of motion.

But a person has only one back, so such comparisons are impossible and physical changes difficult to measure. And certainly, most people have not had baseline data established for comparison after a back injury. Subjective assessments are unreliable because so many factors—anxiety, depression, dependence, somatization, and the potential for secondary gain—can alter patients' perceptions. Finally, radiologic assessments do not correlate well with symptoms. For example, computed tomography has detected disk herniation and spinal stenosis in a significant number of asymptomatic persons.

The sports medicine approach makes it possible to compare an individual's mobility, strength, lifting capacity, and range of motion in different planes with data bases developed from studies of persons with healthy backs. These objective studies can be used to assess the patient's recovery at any point in the rehabilitation and to reassure him or her that despite pain and day-to-day frustration, his or her effort is succeeding.

To rehabilitate the back pain patient who has been incapacitated for several months, implement work simulation and work hardening. Work simulation is a reconditioning program designed to parallel the patients actual occupational activities as closely as possible. Motions and weight loads typical of one's job are used in conjunction with nonpharmacologic pain control measures to restore function.

Work hardening goes beyond the exercises and stretching of reconditioning programs in that it brings the entire body into activity, not just the painful or injured area. This is particularly useful when a patient's physical capabilities, relative to the requirements of the job, are borderline. Such a program need not be costly or long-term, and the sooner it is begun, the less reconditioning is necessary.

Work hardening should be highly individualized, depending on whether the patient's job is basically sedentary or may require strength and endurance. In work hardening, a therapist would actually supervise the patient in lifting, carrying, and manipulating bricks and concrete blocks. Static lifting capacity can be measured with a dynamometer (in fact, static-lift parameters are now incorporated into the safe practice guidelines of the National Institute for Occupational Safety and Health). Dynamic lifting can also be simulated, and lifting in three ranges—floor to waist, waist to shoulder, and shoulder to overhead—can be evaluated. Vibration as well as lifting is taken into account: medium lifting—11-23 kg (25-50 lb) repeatedly—when combined with two hours of vibration, as in truck driving or operating a jackhammer, becomes equivalent to heavy lifting (more than 23 kg).

A person's tolerance for sitting or standing for long periods can also be increased in a work hardening program. Usually, patients' own estimates of their ability to sit or stand in one position are lower than what is observed. A therapist can use a timed course, like an obstacle course, that simulates specific tasks with weights and such commonly available objects as vacuum cleaners to help the patient isolate movements and positions that require specific attention in a work hardening program.

The sports medicine approach differs from that of most back schools and pain clinics in its goal orientation and ability to quantify function. Back schools are inexpensive, and they help patients who are recovering, although somewhat slowly. But their lessons may be forgotten as function returns and pain lessens. In addition, back schools usually teach exercises that emphasize flexion rather than extensor strengthening, which is now known to be more important in rehabilitating patients with severe low-back problems.

Pain clinics, which try to alter a patient's perception about a subjective phenomenon, are often expensive and tend to focus on psychological characteristics. While back schools provide adequate education for the vast majority of patients who pass through them, and pain clinics play a major role in controlling many types of pain syndromes, none of these approaches has been shown to reduce the cost of low-back rehabilitation.

If all testing, diagnostic and therapeutic injections, educational approaches, and work hardening or simulation programs have been unsuccessful after 4-6 months, and if the patient is not a candidate for surgery, consider referring him or her to a specialized rehabilitation facility. Such programs try to help the patient achieve the highest possible level of activity, given his handicap or underlying impairment. Secondarily, they improve strength and mobility and thus decrease pain perception. The primary goal, therefore, is measurable, as are the outcome criteria, such as return to productivity and function.

Both physical and psychological components require attention, because by this late stage in rehabilitation patients are likely to develop a dependence on their own evolved responses to pain and disability that could become chronic. Patients with chronic low-back pain who have had a number of surgical procedures or who have been incapacitated for several years might also benefit from these programs.

Quantification of function becomes important once episodes of low-back pain become recurrent or chronic. Just as general and cardiovascular fitness require aerobic exercises, mobility and strength deficits should be addressed by exercising in the planes and directions where the deficits exist. The muscles that give the back its strength and mobility are the back extensor and oblique muscles, the abdominal muscles, the buttock and hip musculature, and the hamstrings.

Range-of-Motion Assessments

Determining lumbar range of motion can distinguish between intersegmental and hip mobility and can help evaluate the patient's effort in performing measured movements. For example, a patient whose spine is fused can still touch toes if the hamstrings are sufficiently supple. Comparing the ratio of true lumbar motion with hip motion will reveal voluntary guarding and symptom amplification.

Many rehabilitation centers use simple inclinometry to measure the patient's range of motion during sagittal and lateral bending. You can perform the same measurements in the office, using two inclinometers to correct for hip motion in the sagittal plane and for pelvic motion in the lateral. With one inclinometer over the sacrum parallel to the spine and the other bridging the spinous processes at T-12 and L-1, have the patient bend forward (flexion) and back (extension), holding the knees straight. The difference between upper and lower inclinometer readings, reflecting total motion minus hip motion, indicates lumbar sagittal motion. Left and right bending, with the same inclinometer placements to subtract out pelvic movement, yields a similar measurement of lateral motion.

Mobility deficits discovered in this way can be treated in large part by the Williams flexion and McKenzie extension exercises, combined with hamstring stretching. Unless the patient has significant psychological difficulty at this point in rehabilitation, the basic exercises can be done at home. A physical therapist may also be able to work with the patient on designing an individualized sequence of extension exercises, controlling symptoms through movements that incrementally eliminate peripheralization and increase centralization of pain. Implement other strengthening and stretching exercises according to the sports medicine approach, as appropriate. This would include work hardening if necessary.

The Effort Factor

Results of an inclinometric straight-leg-raising test compared with range-of-motion measurements indicate whether the patient is giving his best effort. Wide deviation between straight-leg raising and sacral hip motion indicates insufficient effort, due to either severe pain or symptom amplification. This comparison should not be made in the initial assessment of acute low-back pain or early in the recovery process, because soft-tissue injuries and muscle spasm will legitimately hamper movement. This assessment is appropriate only after complete medical healing has occurred and initial rehabilitation has proved unsuccessful.

Trunk Strength Measurements

Recent studies have demonstrated that patients with chronic low-back pain have significantly decreased trunk strength, with the extensor deficit being considerably greater than the flexor deficit. Moreover, torque levels decrease as trunk rotational speed increases in these patients. In normal subjects, torque is roughly constant at all rotational speeds. These data suggest that aggressive targeted exercise should be considered for patients who have been incapacitated for 4-6 months or do not seem to derive benefit from conventional rehabilitation programs. A sports medicine approach will strengthen muscles not isolated nor efficiently exercised by other means.

Pinpointing the strength of specific trunk muscles requires specialized, recently developed isokinetic equipment. Older static isometric lifting tests do not isolate the contributions of the trunk musculature from those of the arms and legs, which can be significant, and are not useful in measuring lift power through different planes. Isokinetic measurement make it possible to assess the strength of the functional thoracolumbar segment that transmits loads from the shoulder girdle to the pelvis by measuring torque at preselected speeds and in preselected directions.

Cardiovascular Fitness

The chronic inactivity that comes from a rehabilitation failure leads to an inevitable decline in cardiovascular fitness, although in those patients who are severely deconditioned, arm and leg fatigue may be the limiting factor in treadmill testing or bicycle ergometry. If aerobic exercise is not contraindicated for cardiovascular reasons, rehabilitation should include the kind of aerobic conditioning that would suit the patient's needs. This might include swimming (a shoulder girdle and cardiovascular exercise that does not strain the back), bicycling (a leg and arm cardiovascular exercise) using an exercise bicycle at home, or any other aerobic activity that can be easily monitored. Recommend exercises that the patient will enjoy enough to maintain on a regular basis.

Evaluating Success

Active rehabilitation programs have produced impressive results in returning patients to activity and employment. Although the subjectivity of pain, methodological variation in reported trials, and various other factors have made it difficult to assess management strategies for back pain, return to work is an unambiguous indication of success. The reported data on this outcome favor the aggressive approach described here.

Range of motion, effort factors, trunk strength, and aerobic fitness can be monitored for a patient in rehabilitation and compared with a data base, just as performance was evaluated initially. The ability to perform specific whole-body tasks such as lifting, climbing, bending, and stooping can be closely followed, with periodic quantitative or semiquantitative comparisons made. Patients respond well to objective data showing progress; such support helps them work through the pain of reconditioning.

—by Seymour Pedinoff DO,
Robert S. Pinals MD,
S. Andrew Schwartz MD,
and Dan M. Spengler MD

Chapter 21

General Information about Physical Therapy

Vast changes are occurring in the nation's health care delivery system. As part of this progressive trend, physical therapy, too, is changing. The physical therapy profession has kept pace with rapid advances in science and technology to provide the most effective patient treatment possible.

And the need for this care is growing. In the United States alone, physical therapists help hundreds of thousands of individuals daily to restore health, improve function, and alleviate pain.

Currently there are more than 80,000 physical therapists practicing in the United States. The demand for physical therapists' services will continue as the health care industry and payers of health care services focus on managed care, preventive health care programs, the health concerns of an aging population, and the pressing need for cost-effective health care. According to a 1994-95 report by the United States Department of Labor, Bureau of Labor Statistics, physical therapy is one of the leading health care professions.

Physical therapy was established during World War I with the inauguration of the Division of Special Hospitals and Physical Reconstruction by the Surgeon General's Office. Some 2,000 reconstruction aides restored function to persons with disabilities in army hospitals and to those with poliomyelitis.

Information in this chapter is taken from "Take a Look at Today's Physical Therapist" (1995) and "Put Your Health in the Hands of a Physical Therapist" (1995), publications of the American Physical Therapy Association; reprinted with permission.

Today, physical therapists provide health care services to patients of all ages and health conditions. They serve infants with birth defects to aid motor development and functional abilities; people with burns and wounds to prevent abnormal scarring and loss of movement; survivors of strokes to regain movement, function, and independent living; patients with cancer to regain strength and relieve discomfort; patients with low back problems to reduce pain and restore function; and patients with cardiac involvement to improve endurance and achieve independence. They also provide preventive exercise programs and programs to promote general health and fitness, postural improvement, and industrial safety and health.

Today's physical therapists serve a dynamic, comprehensive role in health care—improving and maintaining the quality of life for millions of Americans.

As clinicians, physical therapists:

- Examine patients
- Identify potential and existing problems
- Perform tests and measurements
- Perform evaluations
- Establish a diagnosis
- Determine a prognosis
- Provide interventions
- Evaluate the success of those interventions
- Modify treatment to effect the desired outcome
- Provide prevention and wellness (including health promotion) programs
- Consult
- Screen
- Educate
- Engage in critical inquiry
- Serve as administrators

The "Model Definition of Physical Therapy for State Practice Acts," adopted by the American Physical Therapy Association, states that physical therapy includes:

- Examining patients with impairments, functional limitations, and disability or other health-related conditions in order to determine a diagnosis, prognosis, and intervention.

- Alleviating impairments and functional limitations by designing, implementing, and modifying therapeutic interventions.

- Preventing injury, impairments, functional limitations, and disability, including the promotion and maintenance of fitness, health, and quality of life in people of all ages.

- Engaging in consultation, education and research

A Look at Patient Care

To initiate a program of physical therapy, the physical therapist examines the patient. This includes obtaining a patient history, performing relevant systems reviews, and selecting and administering specific tests and measurements to obtain data.

The physical therapist then performs an evaluation, making clinical judgments based on the data gathered during the examination.

Examination

During an examination, the physical therapist performs tests and measurements that provide information about the status of the musculoskeletal, neurological, pulmonary, and cardiovascular systems, and the individual's functional independence. Listed below are examples of six different types of examinations that a physical therapist might administer.

- **Motor Function Examinations** to assess an individual's ability to learn or demonstrate the skillful and efficient assumption, maintenance, modification, and control of voluntary postures and movement patterns.

- **Muscle Performance Examinations** to assess strength, power, and endurance, and to determine an individual's ability to produce movements that are prerequisites for functional activity.

- **Gait and Balance Examinations** to assess disturbances in gait and balance that may lead to decline of mobility and functional independence or an increased incidence of falls.

- **Neuromotor Development and Sensory Integration Examinations** to assess motor capabilities, including the acquisition and evolution of movement skills and abilities across the life span.

- **Aerobic Capacity or Endurance Examinations** to measure the ability to perform work or participate in activities over time, and to indicate the degree and severity of impairment and functional limitation.

- **Ventilation, Respiration, and Circulation Examinations** to assess whether the individual has an adequate ventilatory pump, oxygen uptake, and oxygen delivery system to perform activities of daily living, ambulation, and aerobic exercise.

Plan of Care

Based on the examination findings and diagnosis and prognosis, the physical therapist completes an evaluation and establishes a plan of care. The plan includes specific interventions designed to produce changes in the patient's condition in order to achieve the desired outcomes.

Intervention

Physical therapists use the following interventions to achieve patient treatment goals:

- Therapeutic exercises (including aerobic conditioning)

- Functional training in self care and home management (including activities of daily living and instrumental activities of daily living)

- Functional training in community or work reintegration (including activities of daily living and instrumental activities of daily living)

- Prescription, fabrication, and application of assistive, adaptive, supportive, and protective devices and equipment

- Manual therapy techniques (including joint mobilization and manipulation)

- Air way clearance techniques

- Debridement and wound care

- Physical agents and mechanical and thermal modalities

- Electrotherapeutic modalities

- Patient-related instruction

Patient-Related Instruction

Physical therapists use patient-related instruction to educate not only the patient but also families and other caregivers about the patient's current condition, treatment plan, and future transition to home, work, or community roles.

Common Conditions for Physical Therapy

Physical therapists treat the consequences of disease or injury by addressing impairments, functional limitations, and/or disabilities in patients. Some of the more common conditions for which physical therapists examine and provide intervention and treatment include the following:

- **Orthopedic conditions,** such as low back and neck pain, headaches, and osteoporosis.

- **Joint and soft-tissue injuries,** such as sprains and strains, hand injuries, fractures and dislocations, and pre- and post-surgical conditions.

- **Neurologic conditions,** such as stroke, traumatic brain injury, Parkinson's disease, cerebral palsy, peripheral nerve injury, and multiple sclerosis.

- **Connective tissue conditions,** such as burns, ulcers, wounds, and collagenous disorders.

- **Arthritic conditions,** including osteoarthritis and rheumatoid arthritis.

- **Systemic diseases,** such as cancer and AIDS/HIV infection.

- **Cardiopulmonary and circulatory conditions,** such as congestive heart failure, emphysema, chronic obstructive pulmonary disease, lymphedema, and peripheral vascular disease.

- **Workplace injuries,** such as carpal tunnel syndrome, cumulative trauma, and stress disorders.

- **Sports injuries,** such as overuse injuries and trauma in recreational and professional athletes.

What You Need to Know About Your Physical Therapist

Licensure. Physical therapists are professional health care providers who are licensed by the state in which they practice.

Education. Physical therapists enter the profession with either a baccalaureate or a post-baccalaureate degree, which consists of a total of four to six years of study in post-secondary education. They take courses that include basic and applied science, clinical sciences, social sciences, and research.

Specialization. Many physical therapists specialize in treating specific areas of the body such as the back, neck, knee, hand, or shoulder, or they may concentrate their practice on pre- and post-natal care, sports injuries, stroke rehabilitation, or one of many other areas of physical therapy. Physical therapists may also be certified by the American Board of Physical Therapy Specialties in seven specialty areas of physical therapy: orthopedics, sports, geriatrics, pediatrics, cardiopulmonary, neurology, and clinical electrophysiology.

Facilities. Physical therapists practice in hospitals, independent offices and clinics, private homes, public schools, rehabilitation centers, work site clinics, and many other settings.

Freedom of Choice. Some states require a referral from a physician before you can receive physical therapy. However, you always have the freedom to choose your own physical therapist. Although a physician may refer you to a physical therapy facility in which the physician has a financial interest, you are entitled to seek treatment from the physical therapist of your choice.

Insurance. Most insurance policies cover physical therapy services when provided by a physical therapist. Some policies require co-payments for some benefits. You should be familiar with what your policy does and does not pay.

Evaluation. Physical therapists evaluate your condition, set up a treatment program, answer your questions about your care, and keep a record of your progress. The objective of physical therapy is to treat and prevent disability and to relieve pain, increase your ability to function, and help you meet your treatment goals.

Goals. Your initial visit to a physical therapist consists of an evaluation including a review of your health history, a list of findings, a list of problems that can benefit from physical therapy, treatment goals, and a treatment plan and time table for achieving these goals.

A Team Approach. Physical therapists communicate with other health care providers involved in your treatment so that you receive comprehensive, quality care with the maximum outcome. You as the patient are a part of the team too, and your physical therapist will discuss your treatment and answer your questions about your program. To aid in recovery and maintain results, the physical therapist will also involve you in your plan of care.

Choosing a Physical Therapist. Feel free to ask a physical therapist questions. With the freedom to choose any physical therapist, you are the most qualified individual to determine which therapist can help you meet your goals.

Physical therapists who are members of the American Physical Therapy Association (APTA) pledge to comply with the Association's Code of Ethics and Guide for Professional Conduct. APTA members maintain and promote high standards in the provision of physical therapy services.

Consult your local telephone directory for a physical therapy facility near you, or write to APTA, PO Box 37257, Washington, DC 20013 for information about your APTA state chapter.

Chapter 22

Herniated Disk: New Laser Therapy Is More Efficient and Rapid than Standard Technique

The application of lasers is a new, efficient method to resolve the pain associated with herniated lumbar disk. The laser procedure utilizes both established techniques and advanced science; it is quicker and produces results that are comparable with or better than standard diskectomy.

The treatment of herniated disk has been evolving since 1908, when a complete laminectomy was first performed to resolve a patient's leg pain. Compared with today's laser therapy, laminectomy may seem excessive. However, at the turn of the century it was assumed that disks were ruptured by neoplastic growth.

During the ensuing decades, the mechanisms underlying herniation and the pain it causes came to be better understood. Now it is known that at approximately age 25, a deterioration begins in the annulus fibrosus. The annulus fibrosus is the fibrous ring that makes up the outer portion of the disk; inside the ring is a pulpy material called the nucleus pulposus. Both normal deterioration and trauma make the annulus fibrosus susceptible to stress tears. Nucleus pulposus can "leak" through a tear in the annulus and exert pressure on spinal ligaments and adjacent root nerves.

The Mechanisms of Laser Therapy

Laser light travels in a single wave length (frequency) whose peaks and troughs are synchronous (see Bailin P. Laser therapy: Its mechanisms and applications to clinical practice. *Modern Medicine* 1988;56[9]:52-9). These characteristics serve to contain and concentrate the beam's energy. When laser energy is absorbed by a receptive substance, it converts to heat and vaporizes the substance.

Two factors determine how well a laser can vaporize a substance: the frequency of its light and the target substance's sensitivity to that frequency. These factors also help determine which type of laser is best suited for a particular patient.

The four principal types of surgical laser are argon, carbon dioxide (CO_2), neodymium:yttrium aluminum garnet (Nd:YAG), and potassium titanyl phosphate (KTP). Of the four, the only type recommended for lumbar surgery is KTP.

The KTP laser strikes a balance between the CO_2 and Nd:YAG lasers. It can be directed at target tissue with optical fibers. More important, its light is readily absorbed and converted to heat by the matrix of protein-bound chondroitin sulfate, hyaluronic acid, keratin sulfate, and water that makes up the nucleus pulposus. The KTP laser can vaporize nucleus material without damaging adjacent material or tissue.

The Procedure

Laser therapy requires only a local anesthetic. The approach to the disc is planned with the help of computed tomography and/or magnetic resonance imaging. Using fluoroscopy to image the region, the surgeon approaches the disk posteriolaterally with an 18-gauge probe and advances it to the center of the nucleus pulposus. A 14-gauge dilating cannula is slipped over the probe until its tip touches the annulus fibrosus.

At this point in the standard procedure, a trephine would be inserted to excise the annulus and gain access to the nucleus. By contrast, during the laser procedure, a 17-gauge "introducer," which contains a stylet, is placed in the cannula and advanced through the annulus to the center of the nucleus. The stylet is removed and replaced by a 600-mm optical fiber that carries a KTP laser beam. The laser vaporizes nucleus material and opens up a cavity that extends distally from the tip of the optic fiber.

The introducer is removed and another is inserted in the cannula. The optic fiber in this introducer exits the tip at a 15-degree angle. This allows the nucleus cavity to be significantly enlarged as the tip is rotated during lasing. When the instruments are removed, the reduced pressure effected by the laser-created cavity allows the extruded nucleus material to return to the center of the disc. This relieves pressure on the root nerve and alleviates pain.

Opening a cavity with a laser takes less than 10 minutes, and the entry wound can be covered with a simple bandage.

The procedure was cleared by the FDA early this year [1990]. Candidates should meet the protocols established for standard diskectomy: positive x-ray evidence of lumbar disk herniation consistent with clinical findings, such as 1) no significant pain relief following 6 months of conservative treatment, 2) significant unilateral leg pain greater than back pain, 3) demonstrated specific paresthetic complaints, 4) demonstrated indications from a physical examination, and 5) demonstration of neurologic findings indicating a herniated disk.

Suggested Reading

Ascher PW, Choy DS, Yuri H. Percutaneous nucleus pulposus denaturation and vaporization of protruded discs. American Society for Laser Medicine and Surgery, annual meeting, 1989.

Davis GW, Onik G. Clinical experience with automated percutaneous discectomy. *Clin Orthop* 1989:238;98-103.

Kapandji IA. The trunk and vertebral column. In: *The physiology of joints*. New York: Churchill Livingstone, 1987.

—by Robert H. Overmyer

Robert H. Overmyer is *Modern Medicine*'s medical science writer.

Chapter 23

Back Surgery

Nobody ever really wants to have back surgery.

It's a major operation, it's expensive and it may not work.

But then there's the reality of back pain—relentless, excruciating, all-encompassing. The kind of pain that takes your breath away and knocks you to the floor and ruins your life.

Beverly Sweeney didn't want a spinal fusion operation, but she felt it was the only way to relieve the pain. She was 32 years old and in nursing school. She suffered from a condition called spondylolisthesis in which one vertebra overlaps another and squeezes the nerve.

"I had no choice, stand or lie down the rest of my life or go for surgery," she recalled. "I gave in to the surgeon thinking that would take care of the pain. Now I know better."

Thirteen years later Sweeney, who works for a home health agency in Cherry Hill, N.J., is still in daily pain. She can sit only for limited periods in a special pressure-reducing chair. The pain hits her in the lower back and sometimes travels down her leg. She takes anti-depressant medication and ibuprofen, "otherwise I couldn't function," she said.

"I can remember the doctor telling me: 'You have a 70 percent chance of being better,'" she said.

"It was a risk I had to take. I wouldn't take it again unless I couldn't walk. I would try all noninvasive things and for a great length of time too."

The U.S. Public Health Service agrees with Sweeney's conclusions. In this country, surgeons perform more than 250,000 lower back operations annually—at an average hospital cost of $11,000, excluding surgeon's fees—and health officials think that much of the surgery is unnecessary. In a recent report on acute lower back problems in adults by the federal Agency for Health Care Policy and Research (AHCPR), the message was clear: In most cases you're just as well off toughing out the pain for six weeks before even considering an operation. With conservative treatment—brief bed rest, painkillers and a mild exercise program—90 percent of back patients will get better within six weeks without surgery. The latest thinking is to get patients up and around as soon as possible. Only about 5 percent will develop chronic pain syndromes persisting beyond three months.

But how to predict who will get better? Among the unlucky 5 percent with persistent pain, the chronic sufferers, who will benefit from surgery and who will go through an operation for nothing?

There are situations where surgery can provide a cure just short of miraculous. That's what happened to Lyonne Withers, a swimming pool contractor in Southern Maryland.

"It's like having a new life again," said Withers, 38, after surgery to remove part of a ruptured disc in his lower back. He was felled by paralyzing back pain after a season of heavy lifting. "There were times my back would get a severe pain bad enough I would just collapse and wouldn't be able to move. The pain felt like it encompassed my lower back and my butt, and in a split second it'd run all the way down my right leg." Doctors told him it was the classic pain called sciatica, and gradually he was losing use of the leg.

Withers lived with the pain for two months and then sought out a spinal surgeon, Neil Kahanovitz, former chief of back surgery at the Hospital for Joint Diseases in New York and now in private practice in Virginia. Less than a year after surgery, Withers said, he was able to go hunting, hiking 10 to 12 miles per day "with a backpack and no pain. Incredible."

Cautious Approach

Low back pain is like the common cold of orthopedics—except that it hangs on for weeks on end. According to the Department of Health and Human Services, 80 percent of Americans will experience an episode of back pain during their lifetime. In any one year, 50 percent of all working adults have low back pain.

The condition is rarely life-threatening. The first step for physicians is to make sure there is no infection, tumor or inflammatory process that is underlying the patient's pain. When these are ruled out, doctors look for the mechanical problem that is causing the pain to see if they can treat it.

In the process, many back sufferers enter the gray zone of whether to operate or not. Back surgery ranks only behind Caesarean section and tubal ligation as a cause of hospitalization for surgery. Rates have been rising steadily since 1980—along with the supply of orthopedic and neurosurgeons.

The general consensus among surgeons is that it's not so much operating technique but rather selection of the right patients that is the real high wire act of the profession.

"I think that the vast majority of patients with acute back problems and with chronic problems are best treated with nonoperative measures," said Edward Hanley, chairman of the spine committee for the American Academy of Orthopedic Surgeons. At the same time, he pointed out the crux of the surgeon's dilemma. As he put it:

"I do believe there is a subset of patients with chronic back pain that can be helped with surgery. However, I do not know how to properly select them, and I don't know anybody who does."

Many factors come into play. Psychological pressures, for example, on the physician as well as the patient can influence the decision to operate. "The patient's and doctor's frustration that the pain is not improving is not an indication for back surgery," said Virginia surgeon Kahanovitz. "For people who have had all sorts of treatment and still have pain, it's very difficult to look them in the face and say 'The last thing you need is an operation that's not going to make you better and could make you worse.'"

Exploratory surgery to search for the cause of a patient's pain is also useless, he said. "Unless you can put your finger on [the cause of pain] clinically and diagnostically before surgery, you can be assured [the operation] is going to fail."

The profession's leaders agree on the obvious: You don't operate on a chronic patient unless the pain is intolerable, unless you know for sure that the pain is generated by a specific malfunction in the back and that surgery has been shown to correct this particular problem.

But these rules of thumb are not always followed. Some surgeons may think it pointless or even cruel to delay surgery for many weeks in the name of conservative care and they chafe at the federal guidelines. One is Arthur White, medical director of the San Francisco Spine Institute and a past president of the North American Spine Society.

"I feel strongly that those guidelines are very limiting to the sub specialist who is trying to get patients better faster and off the starting block," White said. "Why not do a surgery that has a 90 percent success rate when it is a slam-shut case? ... Strike while the iron is hot! That is not saying operate prematurely or on everyone who has back pain."

Treating the Image

One area in which surgeons may go wrong is in relying too heavily on the findings of imaging technology to make a diagnosis, instead of verifying that the problem on the screen correlates with the symptoms they find when examining the patient.

A report last year in the *New England Journal of Medicine* advised caution in using one of the most high-tech diagnostic devices, magnetic resonance imaging, to justify spinal surgery. The researchers did MRIs on the lower backs of a group of people who had no complaints of back pain—and found nonetheless that more than half of them had "abnormal" MRI readings, showing bulging discs. The researchers warned that a bulging disc on an MRI may be purely coincidental and not the cause of the patient's pain.

"If you operate on just what you see, you are going to make some major errors," said Sam Wiesel, chairman of the department of orthopedics at Georgetown University Medical Center. "You can never base your surgery on the pure diagnostic test."

"I think the criticism of spine surgery is that the criteria are not met all the time," said surgeon David Selby, of the University of Texas Health Center and a past president of the North American Spine Society. "It's the doctor's job to be able to absolutely prove where the pain is coming from."

There are three mechanical emergencies where there is little argument about the need for prompt surgery: when trauma causes an instability in the spine, such as a fracture or dislocation; when a patient has acute symptoms of cauda equina syndrome, damage to the tailbone area (symptoms include loss of bladder control); and when there is severe, disabling pain in the limbs and paralysis.

In addition to these emergency situations, there are several malfunctions of the spine that, when pinpointed accurately, can be alleviated by surgery.

Spinal stenosis, for example, is an arthritic condition that usually affects people over age 60. The primary symptoms of severe spinal stenosis are leg pain when walking or standing, relieved by sitting or flexing the spine, and occasionally weakness of the legs.

In reviewing the scientific literature on surgery for spinal stenosis, the federal panel on low back pain found that for patients with severe and persistent symptoms, an operation called decompressive laminectomy was likely to lessen leg pain and make walking more tolerable. The panel cautioned in its report that "there is some indication that these results tend to deteriorate over time."

Laminectomy may also help to relieve the pain of spondylolisthesis, where one vertebra slips forward on the one below and may compress the nerve.

"Relieving spinal stenosis is really fun and [so is] spondylolisthesis," said Selby. "People normally get a lot of leg pain. Neither of these conditions responds well to conservative treatment." The fun comes, he said, in the immediate and dramatic effect of the surgery. People who enter the hospital immobilized by pain often can leave shortly after the operation able to walk again.

Most common—and most challenging from a diagnostic point of view—is a ruptured or herniated disc. The pressure on the spinal nerve can feel like a burning pain centered in the back or it can travel down the nerve path into the limbs. This is called radicular pain. When pressured by a ruptured disc, the sciatic nerve can relay pain down through the buttocks, down the back of the thigh and the back of the leg to the foot, causing numbness and tingling or even difficulty moving the foot. If the pain is only in the buttocks or doesn't really travel past the knee, it probably isn't true sciatica.

The complete or partial removal of a herniated disc that is pressing on a nerve—called a diskectomy—is the most frequently performed back operation. Before attempting diskectomy, some surgeons like to try chemical treatment methods for shrinking discs. Called chemonucleolysis, it involves the injection of chymopapain or other enzymes to dissolve the disc's jelly-like center. Chymopapain, approved by the FDA in 1982, is derived from the papaya and is ordinarily used as a meat tenderizer. Common in Europe, chemical methods have recently lost popularity here. Surgeons argue about chymopapain's effectiveness, but the federal panel said chemical treatments like chymopapain "are less efficacious than standard or microdiskectomy and have rare but serious complications." Even if a surgeon gets the checklist right before doing a disc operation—the MRI shows a ruptured disc, the patient has more leg pain than back pain, there is a corresponding nerve problem (such as numbness) and

247

the patient has already tried conservative care—still, the patient might not need an operation.

The federal panel's report states that even among patients for whom the case for disc surgery is obvious it may be unnecessary: "With or without an operation, more than 80 percent of patients with obvious surgical indications eventually recover. Surgery seems to be a luxury for speeding recovery of patients with obvious surgical indications but benefits fewer than 40 percent of patients with questionable physiological findings. Moreover, surgery increases the chance of future procedures with higher complication rates. Overall, the incidence of first-time disc surgery complications, including infection and bleeding is less than 1 percent. The figure increases dramatically with older patients or repeated procedures."

Even more contentious is the decision to operate on patients who have back pain but no sciatica, said Richard Deyo, a member of the federal panel on low back pain. A general internist and professor at the University of Washington School of Medicine, Deyo has published widely on the outcomes of surgery for back pain patients. As he put it: "Many people, myself included, believe surgery is not indicated in that circumstance."

Spinal Fusion Under Fire

In 1975, Michelle Cutrow's car was rear-ended on a Los Angeles freeway. Thus began her back surgery saga.

"I tried acupuncture, biofeedback, medication, bed rest," she said. "Surgery was truly a last resort for me." A neurosurgeon performed a laminectomy and presto. "It took care of the problem. I was fine for 10 years."

Then suddenly, and for no apparent reason, in 1987 Cutrow started feeling "shooting pains" down her back and leg. "The right side of my back felt like someone was taking a poker and drilling into it," she said. "I was in the hospital seven times over that year.... I had nerve blocks, CAT scans, discograms, you name it.

"I was in my thirties; I had two young kids. I didn't feel I wanted to live the rest of my life that way."

She agreed to have exploratory surgery. When the surgeons discovered that one of her lower vertebrae "was wobbling like spaghetti," they fused her back on the left side. "I still had pain, the same kind of pain ...

"I tried to get on with my life. It wasn't easy. I lived on pain medication."

So Cutrow underwent a third operation. The orthopedic surgeon fused the other side of her back. Recovery has been slow. The site of the bone graft didn't heal properly and a portion of her back is hypersensitive to touch.

"I'm in pain all the time," she said.

The idea behind this controversial operation is to make the joint rigid so it will not impinge on the spinal nerve.

"Fusion surgery is a major operation, a big deal," said Deyo, "and the complication rate is higher than ordinary disc surgery, and the success rate is less." He also noted that the rates of fusion surgery vary among geographic regions and among specialties. Neurosurgeons, for example, are far less likely to perform fusion surgery than orthopedic surgeons, even when patients appear to be similar. These variations suggest that there is no consensus on the appropriate use of this procedure.

San Francisco's White, who defends the aggressive use of back surgery when warranted, is also cautious. "Fusion, it has a great danger of being severely abused," he said. "Surgeons being surgeons, they think that they can fix everything: If a part is broken, fuse it and use it. But if you haven't covered the psychological basis, the conditioning basis and the diagnostic basis, you're going to be making mistakes 40 percent of the time. I make my living cleaning up the messes of other surgeons who have operated prematurely with inadequate diagnosis and inadequate training."

At the same time, Selby of the University of Texas defends the usefulness of spinal fusion in certain circumstances. "There should be a specific reason to fuse a spine, such as an instability," he said. "There's overwhelming evidence if you decompress [remove some bone to relieve the nerve] and don't fuse, patients will continue to have pain."

Yet the federal panel wrote, "Although the usual reasons stated for doing spinal fusion for degenerative problems are instability of the spine and disc disease, there is lack of scientific agreement on how to define spinal instability." There are no studies that compare the long-term success or failure rates of different back operations.

"The real issue is the efficacy of fusion in general," said Deyo, who is principal investigator for the federal panel's Patient Outcome Research Team. "Our group has called attention to the fact that the complication rate appears to be higher. Whatever else it does, it doesn't seem to make future surgery less likely. You can't tell from the literature whether or when this type of surgery works. The advocates say, 'We know it works.' The skeptics are saying this procedure has complications; it's unclear how effective it is for some indications, and we need to slow down."

The Psychology of Back Pain

Who is likely to get back problems? In a study published in 1991 of blue-collar workers at Boeing Corp., Stanley Bigos and fellow University of Washington researchers found that among those who initially had no back pain symptoms, the best predictor of whether they eventually reported back problems at work was job dissatisfaction and emotional distress. Physical factors were not important.

It was not that workers were intentionally shirking, the researchers reported. But "symbolically, back pain may be the proverbial 'last straw' that breaks the back of the worker already burdened by job dissatisfaction or distress. Removing back pain alone may not spring the individual back to their feet, to work or to their normal place in life."

Physicians, chiropractors and physical therapists all note the importance of a person's emotional state in dealing with back pain. The recent federal report on back pain cited several studies that "have detected a strong correlation between the outcomes of ... spine surgery and the preoperative psychological status of the patient."

Consequently, surgeons like Neil Kahanovitz in Virginia and Arthur White in San Francisco send their patients to see a psychiatrist before performing an operation. "It's to see if there's something in their background that might keep them from getting better," said White, "such as child abuse or alcoholic parents, something that's driving their pain, that has to be treated."

The psychiatrist can also confirm that the patient has realistic expectations for the operation, he said, and has made a firm decision to go through this major operation.

Louis Sportelli, in chiropractic practice for 33 years and a spokesman for the American Chiropractic Association, agrees that a person's attitude can tip the scales on whether an operation is necessary—or will be successful. He has seen a change in attitude among many back pain patients toward taking more responsibility for their recovery. "They are not in the mindset of dropping their bodies at the office and picking them up the next day, fixed," he said. "They're doing lifestyle changes, exercise in homes. The ones that are diligent and interested are doing a great job."

"Conditioning is a major piece of the puzzle," added White, the San Francisco spine surgeon. "A patient who is not willing to take responsibility, to exercise, train and learn—you can't solve his problem. Any good you do, he'll undo."

Chapter 24

Pedicle Screws

Medical Apparatus Tangled in Dispute

Glen Steinkopff says a medical device known as the pedicle screw all but saved his life. A 1990 skiing accident crushed a vertebra in his lower back and ruptured two disks. Now 25, he's back at work with the ski patrol at a Tahoe City, Calif., resort. The framework of screws and rods that holds three of his surgically fused vertebrae left Steinkopff with only occasional soreness in his back and enviable flexibility. "I can touch my toes," he says, "though I can't put my palms on the ground."

Gloria Perdue says the same device ruined her life. The apparatus loosened in its moorings after her 1992 operation, and "I could feel the screws in my back going 'clank clank clank,'" she said. After three additional surgeries, Perdue, 39, depends on a combination of prescribed narcotics, muscle relaxers and antidepressants to get through the day. Perdue, who lives near Roanoke, says, "My pain is so bad that if I weren't a Christian, I'd have blown my brains out."

At least 300,000 patients in the United States have received some combination of pedicle screws, rods and plates, many to repair serious problems such as crushed vertebrae but sometimes for lesser ailments. Like Steinkopff, most appear to be pleased with their operations,

"Medical Apparatus Tangled in Dispute" *Washington Post*, March 29, 1996, copyright 1996 *The Washington Post*. Reprinted with permission; FDA fact sheet "Update on Pedicle Screws," December 20, 1994; and excerpts from *Federal Register*, Wednesday, October 4, 1995.

which generally cost between $8,000 and $10,000. But some 7,000 patients have sued manufacturers, alleging injury from the devices, which surgeons fasten to the bony struts, or "pedicles," that connect the front and back of the vertebrae along the spine.

That could be the story of any medical invention sold in this country. No device or operation is free of risk. But the pedicle screw's path from drawing board to operating room has implications even for people who have never felt a twinge of back pain. Behind this simple piece of hardware is a tangled regulatory history that both patients and manufacturers cite—for opposite reasons—as proof that the federal Food and Drug Administration needs to change the way it regulates medical devices and drugs.

For patients who say the device caused them injury, the pedicle screw is a case study of how companies can exploit loopholes in the rules that the FDA has made to protect the public from dangerous devices. For the manufacturers, however, it is a prime example of their contention that companies have to scale needless FDA roadblocks to bring promising new treatments to market.

The pedicle screw also has become a key prop in the raging debate in Congress over the FDA. The Republican majority is pushing legislation, now in committee, that would speed up the FDA's approval process. Opponents of the legislation, including consumer advocacy groups, contend that the agency's safety net already has too many holes in it.

Fifteen years ago, the pedicle screw was merely an idea in the head of a Cleveland orthopedic surgeon named Arthur Steffee. Today, it is the foundation of a $100 million industry and a popular treatment that many spine surgeons regard as a true advance in orthopedic medicine. Last October, after years of opposition, the FDA recommended that the industry be allowed to market the screws for spinal surgery.

How the screws became so widely used, and whether the FDA intended that to happen, are matters of dispute. Twice in the mid-1980s, the FDA rejected applications from Steffee's company, AcroMed Corp., to market the device for spinal operations; the second time, the agency cited the risk that the screws could cause nerve damage and bone fractures.

The pedicle screw had not been proven safe or effective for spinal surgery, and it had not received formal FDA approval for use in the spine. But the company was able to make its pedicle screw device available anyway through what AcroMed's co-founder, Edward

Wagner, once called a regulatory sleight-of-hand done with the FDA's blessing.

Instead of asking for permission to "label" the device for lower back surgery, AcroMed filed a new application in 1985 to sell the device for general bone surgery—such as in arms and legs, where bone plates and bone screws already were being used. FDA gave the go-ahead.

Once the product was labeled for general use, physicians were free to try it for other surgeries. FDA permits such "off-label" uses—indeed, it has become common to experiment with off-label drugs in treating cancer—as long as companies and doctors don't advertise or promote the product for these unapproved purposes. FDA officials deny that AcroMed had the agency's approval to pursue this backdoor strategy.

Whether AcroMed and a half-dozen competitors violated the FDA's rules is an issue in the bitter legal battle being fought in federal and state courts. The patients' lawyers, who stand to make millions of dollars in contingency fees if they win, have a nine-member committee to manage the mounting number of cases being heard in courtrooms throughout the country.

As the federal courts have done in other large product liability cases, one judge has been assigned to supervise pretrial discovery. The lawsuits, which allege that pedicle screws are defective in design and pose unreasonable dangers to patients, are coordinated in Philadelphia under a single name: *In Re: Orthopedic Bone Screw Products Liability Litigation.*

The patients' lawyers, in pushing their lawsuits, have unleashed a broad attack on the manufacturers. They allege that the industry subverted FDA's rules by using physicians as a kind of sales force. According to the lawyers, the companies recruited doctors to serve as advisers and consultants, bought the loyalty of some physicians with financial incentives and sent them to teach their colleagues how to use the device in the spine.

The lawyers also allege that patients became human guinea pigs. They contend that companies and surgeons tried out their products on thousands of patients instead of testing them through rigorous clinical trials that involve a limited number of patients who give their informed consent.

The industry and the surgeons vigorously deny these charges. The companies say they are victims of a vague and ever-changing FDA process that provides them with little guidance on the difference between education and promotion. The surgeons say they have found the device to be a necessary and vital option, and that's the only reason they choose to use it.

"I think it's 'state of the art' for certain indications," said Neil Kahanovitz, an Arlington orthopedic surgeon. Kahanovitz, who said he has received no industry money for pedicle screw research, has implanted pedicle screws and plates in about 75 to 100 patients who had fractures, instability of their spines or tumors that required removal of bone. "When those indications present themselves in my office, I have no hesitation about doing that operation," he said.

But some doctors say the pedicle screw has been used too often for general lower back pain of unspecified origin—a condition about which there has long been debate about whether surgery is effective.

The FDA, before making a final decision on pedicle screws, is required by law to seek public comment. On March 1, the committee of plaintiffs' attorneys weighed in with a 231-page response. They took this unusual step, the lawyers said, to forestall the FDA action, which they said manufacturers could exploit as support for their position that pedicle screws are safe for spinal surgery. "You fight the war on all fronts," said John Coale, one plaintiff lawyer.

Drawing on industry documents recently unsealed in Philadelphia, the attorneys accused the FDA of basing its recommendation on sloppy science, much of which they said came from doctors with financial ties to the industry. The devices came into widespread use "not because they were a good medical idea but because they were a good business idea," wrote attorneys John Cummings III of New Orleans and Arnold Levin of Philadelphia on behalf of the plaintiffs' committee.

In 19 volumes of supporting material filed with the FDA, the lawyers included an electronic mail message that they said shows the industry mentality. In the May 1994 message, a salesman at Synthes (U.S.A.), a Paoli, Pa., device maker, reported to his colleagues after observing a medical team as they implanted the device. "Well I did my first case the other day and the patient died on the table" for reasons unrelated to the screws, he wrote. "Second case went better, patient lived."

The representative included a p.s. to another sales rep with a good track record for selling the devices: "It sounds to me like you're on a 'gravy train!'"

Industry officials reject the notion that this message symbolizes anything other than one man's colorful language. AcroMed's Wagner said no medical company can survive by putting profits before patients' safety. "I didn't want to build an airplane that wasn't going to fly," he said. "You don't build a company making bad products."

Getting to the Marketplace

Before the pedicle screw could turn the first penny of profit, it had to get to the marketplace. Steffee, an orthopedic surgeon with an entrepreneurial bent, formed AcroMed with Wagner in the early 1980s to sell a "spinal fixation" system Steffee had developed. The device acts as an internal splint, holding the vertebrae in place until the bones' own healing mechanism can bring about fusion. Surgeons consider Steffee's approach an improvement over existing spinal stabilization techniques that depended on hooks and wires.

In a mid-1980s demonstration video, Steffee described his trial-and-error development of the device. "The early design," he says on the video, "proved to exhibit a number of imperfections." In some 160 early procedures, 21 screws broke, and he had to redesign the system, he said.

In 1984 and 1985, AcroMed twice asked the FDA to clear the device, saying the implant was substantially equivalent to bone plates and bone screws already in use. The FDA turned down both requests, saying the device was not equivalent. The agency's second rejection cited "potential risks," including nerve damage and fractures.

Steffee, who declined to be interviewed for this story, met with FDA officials on Dec. 12, 1985, and was "very aggravated," one agency official later wrote in a memo. Steffee "badgered the FDA staff at length demanding the right to immediately sell" the device, the memo said.

AcroMed and FDA officials do not agree on what happened next. During the meeting, AcroMed officials say, an FDA representative suggested the company change its vocabulary: AcroMed should apply again and should call the devices "bone plates" and "bone screws" and ask permission to use them for general bone surgery. A few weeks later, the company filed a third application using this approach.

The FDA says it never coached the company on how to bend the rules. Wagner, who retired in 1991, retorted in an interview: "They knew. They've known from day one. There was nothing secretive. We weren't meeting in tunnels in Chicago in the dark."

The contemporaneous record reflects some evidence for AcroMed's version. On Jan. 16, 1986, Wagner wrote to a surgeon on the company's advisory board that "we have acceded to FDA's position that we refer to the plates as 'bone plates' and the screws as 'bone screws,' a labeling slight-of-hand [sic] that satisfies the agency's regulations but in no way changes the intended use of the plates and screws."

The FDA then gave the green light. Soon after, it also approved a separate AcroMed request to conduct clinical trials that would determine whether the device was safe and effective.

Now the company could distribute the device to a surgeon who wanted to employ it off-label—in this case, in the spine. But the rules prohibit companies from promoting off-label uses, limiting them to presenting scientific papers and demonstrating the device.

The plaintiffs' lawyers have alleged, and some FDA officials believe, that the company crossed the line by turning education into a form of promotion. The lawyers assert that AcroMed formed an advisory panel of physicians, sponsored training sessions for hundreds of spine surgeons and offered videos, catalogues and brochures.

At least five other pedicle screw manufacturers adopted the same strategy, the lawyers allege. The industry developed financial ties with about 200 spine surgeons and these doctors provided services that ranged from consulting work to spreading the word about the pedicle device's utility, the lawyers allege. According to their FDA comment, surgeons made more than 1,000 appearances at some 230 professional meetings where pedicle screw devices were demonstrated.

All told, the lawyers allege, the industry paid out more than $29 million in cash and gave out stock or stock options. The firms also donated $5 million to medical institutions where these doctors worked, their FDA comment asserts.

In the early 1990s, the FDA warned the industry that its sales and training practices were a form of illegal promotion and told manufacturers they faced administrative sanctions if they did not stop, FDA documents show. The FDA investigated AcroMed and referred the case to the Justice Department for prosecution. But the case went nowhere; one internal FDA memo suggested a jury might decide that the agency had full knowledge of the company's tactics, and therefore shared any blame. AcroMed officials say the case was dropped because there was no merit to the allegation.

Former AcroMed executive Wagner said his company followed FDA rules—at least so far as company officials could understand them—and didn't improperly advertise or promote the device for spinal use. The FDA never drew a bright line for the company describing where training ended and promotion began, Wagner said. FDA officials seemed reluctant to give straight answers, according to Wagner. "Everybody ducked and bobbed and weaved and avoided," he said.

The surgeons also dispute that what they did could be called marketing and say their loyalty could not be bought. "I see what appears to me to be a very useful procedure, and then those doctors want to learn how to do that useful procedure. Is that promoting or is that science?" said Steven Garfin, a spine surgeon at the University of

California at San Diego who has acted as a consultant for three pedicle screw companies. "I'm instructing; at least that's what I see my role as."

AcroMed and other companies say their consulting doctors always gave honest information to their colleagues. "They are out there talking about the risks and benefits," AcroMed lawyer Richard Werder said. "A number of the doctors AcroMed was associated with did nothing but talk about complications."

In their FDA comment, the plaintiffs' attorneys also criticize the industry's clinical trials, saying the data were flawed. The FDA also has questioned the data. In 1990, the agency withdrew its approval for one AcroMed study. AcroMed defended the study, saying it generated valid, useful information.

The plaintiffs' attorneys also attacked the body of scientific literature about pedicle screw devices, alleging conflicts of interest. Of 206 journal articles the FDA reviewed, about 90 were by authors with financial relationships to pedicle screw companies and fewer than a dozen disclosed those ties, the lawyers alleged.

In one case, AcroMed advised Marc Asher, a University of Kansas orthopedic surgeon, that be did not need to disclose his company ties in an article he had written for the *Journal of Bone and Joint Surgery*, even though he had been receiving royalties from AcroMed for his work in developing a pedicle device. The company told Asher that because his article dealt with a different AcroMed device, he could state on the medical journal's conflict of interest form that he had received "no benefits in any form" from "a commercial party related directly or indirectly to the subject of this article."

Asher decided to disclose his ties anyway, Werder, the AcroMed lawyer, said the company still believes Asher's disclosure was unnecessary.

Spine surgeon Garfin, who helped supervise an industry-sponsored study requested by the FDA said the industry's support has not tainted the research. "That's where the money came from. I can't hide it," he said. "But they didn't influence anything. I'd like to think I'm above that."

'A Uniquely Valuable Device'

In early 1993, representatives of the American Academy of Orthopedic Surgeons met with FDA officials to discuss the growing use of the device—and the increasing numbers of lawsuits and the much-criticized clinical trials. Some surgeons argued that the pedicle screw "is a uniquely valuable device for certain diagnoses, but probably not for the general usage it now enjoys!" according to notes of the meeting included in the plaintiffs' FDA comment.

The FDA asked orthopedic professional societies to conduct a new study, funded by the industry, to gather data about past pedicle screw operations. In July 1994, an FDA advisory panel, citing that study and other evidence, voted unanimously to recommend that the pedicle screw be reclassified as a less risky device that did not require premarket studies. It said the devices had become the standard of care for certain spinal operations in the lower back and merited approval.

The plaintiffs' lawyers fault the FDA's reliance on the study, asserting that its methodology was weak and that it was overseen by doctors with conflicts of interest. The industry and the doctors contend the study was a thorough, un-tainted review based on the records of 314 surgeons in operating on some 3,500 patients.

FDA spokesman Jim O'Hara said the agency is reviewing the plaintiffs' allegations as it weighs a final decision. "Is this a case of bad science being sold to the agency?" O'Hara said. "A lot of charges are being made on both sides of this issue. The agency is committed to getting answers to all of the questions."

— by Benjamin Weiser and John Schwartz

Benjamin Weiser and John Schwartz are *Washington Post* staff writers.

Update on Pedicle Screws

FDA has recently received a number of inquiries about certain screws used in surgery to stabilize the spine. We hope the following information helps to answer these questions.

How are the screws used?

Screws are used to stabilize the spine after spinal injury, or to correct severe spinal curvatures and other abnormalities. A pair of the screws is placed horizontally into the rear of the bony bridges, called pedicles, that are connected to each vertebra, one on each side. (Thus they are called "pedicle screws" when used for this purpose.) Vertical rods (or plates) are attached to the screws. The rods are connected to the pedicles of a second vertebra by means of another set of pedicle screws, straightening or strengthening the spine.

How widespread is this use?

Pedicle screws have largely replaced other methods of spine stabilization such as wires, rods and hooks in the 30-70,000 spine stabilization procedures performed annually in the U.S. About 300,000 people have been implanted with the screws.

Why is FDA concerned about the screws?

Because, despite their widespread use, not enough is known about the possible short-term adverse effects of the screws when they are used in the pedicles of the spine, nor about their long-term effectiveness. Under the law, before orthopedic screws can be marketed as pedicle screws, their manufacturers must submit scientific data to FDA establishing that these devices are safe and effective for this purpose. Limited studies of pedicle screws have been ongoing for a number of years, and FDA has approved using the screws in these studies. But the studies are still not complete, and the manufacturers have not yet accumulated enough data to show, one way or the other, whether the screws are safe and effective.

Are there any spinal screws approved by FDA?

Yes. Those that are inserted into the front of the spine rather than the rear have been approved. Screws used in certain portions of the lower spine (the sacrum) are also approved. But no screws have been approved for use in the pedicles of the spine.

If pedicle screws aren't approved how can they be used so widely?

In practice, surgeons often use orthopedic screws that FDA has cleared for other purposes, such as repairing long bones in the arms and legs, as pedicle screws. Such use of approved medical devices for non-approved purposes is called "off-label use," and has traditionally been regulated by the hospitals in which physicians practice and by their state medical boards, not by FDA.

However, FDA has taken two actions to be sure that all parties are adequately informed that using screws in the pedicles of the spine is considered an "off-label" use. First, to be sure physicians understand the regulatory status of the screws, FDA requires that manufacturers include in the labeling for the screws a statement that they are not approved for use in the spine. And second, FDA has advised physicians that they have an obligation to discuss any "off-label" use of these screws with the patient, explaining the benefits, drawbacks and limitations of knowledge about the procedure, and making it clear to the patient that this particular use of the screws has not been approved by FDA.

Widespread use of screws in the pedicles of the spine was encouraged in the past by some of the screw manufacturers, who promoted this practice to surgeons through training courses given during professional meetings. As a result of FDA warnings, this type of illegal promotion has largely ceased.

Does the lack of FDA approval mean the screws are unsafe?

Not necessarily. There simply isn't enough scientific information at this point to say for sure whether the screws are safe for use in the pedicles of the spine or not. There is some evidence that the screws might be beneficial in treating certain specific conditions, such as spinal fractures, degenerative spondylolisthesis (slippage of the spine), tumors and scoliosis (spinal curvature). In light of this evidence, an FDA advisory panel of outside experts recommended in July 1994 that FDA re-classify those pedicle screw device systems intended for two specific uses—treating spinal fractures and spinal slippage—into a less stringent regulatory category. FDA is now considering whether to take this action.

But the effectiveness of the screws—or any other surgical procedure—in treating low back pain or simple disc problems is far more uncertain. Despite this, many of the 30-70,000 spine stabilization procedures performed annually in the U.S. are to treat these conditions.

What about the problem of screws breaking inside the body?

Although some news stories have implied that the screws break very commonly, the actual breakage rate is not known. Limited information suggests that the screws now being used break less frequently than those used in the mid-1980s, because of improvements in product design and testing. More information is needed about breakage rates before FDA can decide whether the screws are safe and effective for use in the spine.

Is progress being made in getting scientific information on the effectiveness of the screws?

Yes. FDA is working with surgeons and manufacturers to design sound clinical studies and get them underway. These studies will provide the needed information about which spinal conditions, if any, can be successfully treated with the screws, the kinds of adverse effects that can be expected, and how often they occur.

In the meantime, what about people contemplating back surgery?

Patients considering back surgery in which pedicle screws might be used to stabilize the spine should keep in mind that these devices have not been approved for this purpose, and that FDA cannot assure that they are safe and effective. They should also remember that there is little evidence that the screws are effective in treating low back pain or simple disc problems. Patients should ask their doctors to explain beforehand both the potential benefits and risks of the screws, as well as alternative treatments, including nonsurgical ones. Patients should also keep in mind that, as with any surgery, it is important to choose a surgeon who is skilled and experienced in performing the procedure.

What are the surgical alternatives to the screws?

The goal in these procedures is to stabilize the spine temporarily until two or more adjacent vertebrae permanently fuse together. This can be done with the use of hooks or wires, which are approved by FDA, rather than the screws. Surgery can also be done using implants attached from the front of the spine rather than the rear. And fusion can be accomplished surgically without the use of implants by inserting bone grafts between the vertebrae, followed by the prolonged use of braces or casts.

How about people who already have the screws?

Some news stories have implied that a large proportion of pedicle screws fail in use. Although the actual failure rate is still unknown, the medical literature indicates that the screws probably fail only a small percentage of the time. This means that most patients with the screws are not likely to have serious problems with them. However, patients who are experiencing problems or concerns that relate to their surgery should consult with their doctors.

Proposed Rule Regarding Pedicle Screws

In October 1995, the FDA published a proposed rule regarding pedicle screws. The final regulation had not yet been announced at the time this volume went to press. For updated information concerning the status of the rule regulating pedicle screws, contact:

Mark N. Melkerson
Center for Devices and Radiological Health (HFZ-410)
Food and Drug Administration
9200 Corporate Blvd.
Rockville, MD 20850
(301) 594-2036

The following section discussing the proposed rule is excerpted from the *Federal Register*, Vol. 60, No. 192, Wednesday, October 4, 1995:

Highlights of the Proposal

FDA is issuing for public comment several recommendations of the Panel [Orthopedic and Rehabilitation Devices Panel] concerning the classification of pedicle screw spinal systems. The Panel recommended that FDA classify into class II the unclassified preamendments pedicle screw spinal system intended for the treatment of severe spondylolisthesis (grades 3 and 4) of the fifth lumbar vertebra in patients receiving fusion by autogenous bone graft having implants attached to the lumbar and sacral spine with removal of the implant after the attainment of a solid fusion. The Panel also recommended that FDA reclassify the postamendments pedicle screw spinal system intended for degenerative spondylolisthesis and spinal trauma from class III to class II. For all other indications, pedicle screw spinal systems are considered postamendments class III devices for which premarket approval is required. The Panel made its recommendations after reviewing information presented at two public meetings on August 20, 1993 and July 23, 1994, and after reviewing information which was solicited in response to an April 3, 1995, letter. FDA is also issuing for public comments its tentative findings on the Panel's recommendations. FDA is proposing to expand the intended uses of the device identified by the Panel to include pedicle screw spinal systems intended to provide immobilization and stabilization of spinal segments as an adjunct to fusion in the treatment of acute and chronic instabilities and deformities, including spondylolisthesis, fractures and dislocations, scoliosis, kyphosis, and spinal tumors. Finally, FDA is proposing to codify the classification of both the preamendments and the postamendments device in one regulation. Comments received in response to this proposed rule, along with other relevant information that the agency may obtain, will be relied upon by the agency in formulating a final position on each of the foregoing issues and provide the basis for a final agency regulation.

FDA's Tentative Findings

FDA agrees with the Orthopedic and Rehabilitation Devices Panel's recommendation and is proposing that the pedicle screw spinal system intended for the treatment of degenerative spondylolisthesis, severe spondylolisthesis, and spinal trauma be classified into class II. FDA believes that there exists sufficient information to develop special controls which will provide reasonable reassurance of the safety and effectiveness of these devices. FDA believes that appropriate special controls should include mechanical testing standards of performance, special labeling requirements, and postmarket surveillance. FDA also believes that premarket approval is not necessary to provide reasonable assurance of the safety and effectiveness of the device.

The data demonstrate the use of pedicle screw-based instrumentation in the treatment of degenerative spondylolisthesis and fractures results in significantly higher fusion raters, improved clinical outcomes, and comparable complication rates when compared with treatment with no instrumentation or with currently available preamendments class II spinal devices.

The data also demonstrate that the use of pedicle screw-based instrumentation in the treatment of severe spondylolisthesis results in equivalent or higher fusion rates, similar clinical outcomes, and comparable complication rates when compared with treatment with no instrumentation or with currently available preamendments class II spinal devices.

Chapter 25

Electrical Bone-Growth Stimulation and Spinal Fusion

Since 1911, fusion of the spine by a variety of techniques has been used to restore stability in a number of congenital, acquired, and degenerative spinal disorders. The failure to obtain spinal fusion has persisted over the years as a relatively common problem. The documented failure of solid fusion 1 year after surgery is referred to as pseudoarthrosis. Pseudoarthrosis has been attributed to inadequate surgical technique, failure to neutralize excessive motion or shear stresses at the segment to be fused, or underlying metabolic abnormalities in the patient.[1] Some have even suggested that the responsibility for the occurrence of pseudoarthrosis may be entirely within the hands of the surgeon.[2]

Estimates of the incidence of pseudoarthrosis in lumbar spinal fusion procedures range from 0 to greater than 30%, depending on the type of procedure. Cameron and Bridges[3] reviewed the results published from 1948 to 1979 and estimated the incidence of pseudoarthrosis according to the type of procedure (Figure 25.1).

Steinmann and Herkowitz[1] noted the incidence of pseudoarthrosis reported in some of the same studies and other more recent reports as follows: 4%-68% for anterior interbody fusion, 3%-25.5% for intertransverse fusion, and 6%-27% for posterior interbody fusion. They pointed out that, short of surgical exploration, the detection of pseudoarthrosis before the occurrence of late signs of fusion failure (such as pain or recurrence of spinal instability) often necessitated

Agency for Health Care Policy and Research (AHCPR) Pub. No. 94-0014, January 1994.

Spinal fusion procedure	Rate	Percent	Range (percent)
Posterior	350/2032	17.2	7.7 - 33.3
Anterior	88/453	19.4	14.5 - 29.6
Intertransverse	68/593	11.5	0 - 28.6
Posterior interbody	128/575	22.3	nr

nr = not reported
Source: Cameron and Bridges.[3]

Figure 25.1. *Posterior spinal fusion: Incidence of pseudoarthrosis according to type of procedure.*

the use of more than one of the following procedures: conventional roentgenograms, tomography, discography, bone scintigraphy, computed tomography, or magnetic resonance imaging. They considered the following criteria as being most useful for establishing the presence of pseudoarthrosis: (1) lack of trabecular bone continuity, (2) collapse of the graft height, (3) shift in position of the graft, (4) loss of fixation, and (5) unexplained pain in the area of fusion.

The clinical significance of pseudoarthrosis is, however, questionable. For example, DePalma and Rothman[2] found that 39 (9%) of their 448 patients who had lumbar intertransverse spinal fusion had evidence of pseudoarthrosis. The 39 patients with pseudoarthrosis demonstrated the ability to return to work and resumed a level of activity similar to that of a group of 39 age-matched patients with solid fusion. Relief from back pain and sciatica was only slightly and insignificantly better in the patients with solid fusion. Other studies have also noted that approximately 40%-50% of patients with pseudoarthrosis are asymptomatic.[4,5]

Direct electrical current has been demonstrated to have stimulatory effects on bone formation in *in vitro* biologic models and animal models. In humans, constant, direct-current stimulation has been accepted as a standard for treating long-bone nonunion and as an adjunct in the treatment of congenital pseudoarthrosis of the tibia.[6]

The results of two studies done in animals suggest that direct-current application may have stimulatory effects on spinal fusion. Kahanovitz and Arnoczky[7] studied the effect of a direct-current electrical stimulator on the fusion of the posterior lumbar facets in dogs. They noted little or no roentgenographic or histologic differences between the control and stimulated fusion at 2, 4, and 6 weeks, but found that all of the stimulated facet joints showed solid bony fusion at 12 weeks while none of the eight control facet joints showed any osseous bridging of the fusion site. Nerubay et al.[8] found evidence at 2 months, but not at 1 month, that the constant-current stimulator enhanced the fusion of the lower lumbar spine in 1-month-old pigs.

The suggestion that a substantial number of pseudoarthroses may be the result of inadequate surgical technique may be of concern as the data on the possible effects of direct-current therapy on enhancing spinal fusion are examined. For example, Steinmann and Herkowitz[1] cited a number of studies that suggest that identification of the factors that lead to nonunion, and adjustment for these factors before repair was attempted, resulted in significantly improved outcomes. For example, Brodsky et al.[9] found that 95% of their patients with failed anterior cervical fusion had successful fusion after a subsequent posterior procedure, in contrast to a 47% success rate in similar patients who underwent a second anterior procedure. Edwards and Weigel[10] treated 51 low lumbar nonunions in 28 patients with reexploration, regrafting, and internal fixation with compression rods that resulted in 84% of the repairs proceeding to solid fusion.

The earliest demonstration that direct current may stimulate lumbosacral fusion was described in 1974 by Dwyer and Wickham of Australia.[11] They reported that direct-current stimulation resulted in successful fusion in 11 (91.7%) of 12 patients. In a later study, published in 1975, Dwyer[12] reported that fusion was documented radiographically in 40 (85.1%) of 47 patients, 27 of whom were at high risk for fusion failure because of the need for multiple-level fusion and previous fusion failures.

After these demonstrations by Dwyer,[11,12] a multicenter clinical trial was initiated in the United States in 1978 to study the role of implantable bone-growth stimulators in spinal fusion surgery. Although the data did not formally appear in the literature, Kane[13] briefly reviewed the data that were available in 1981 on 84 stimulated patients from the study and on 159 historical control patients. The 84 patients were from 23 orthopaedic surgeons in 18 clinical centers in 12 States, and 82 of these patients were available for followup. The 159 historical control patients were from the University of South Carolina and Northwestern University, Chicago. The two groups were comparable in age and sex, but the incidence of previous surgery and that of pseudoarthrosis were 2-4 times higher in the stimulated group (80% and 55% vs. 28% and 20%, respectively). This difference in patient characteristics might have led to a bias against finding successful fusion in the stimulated group. Fusion was successful, however, in 75

(91%) of 82 patients in the stimulated group compared with 128 (81%) of 159 in the control group (p=.02). In a subgroup of 46 patients who had pseudoarthrosis and were included in the stimulated group, 42 (91%) achieved successful fusion. Kane noted that the results of the control group were comparable to the overall success rate of 74% that was derived from 31 papers on lumbosacral fusions in 3,383 patients, which were reviewed in a presentation "at the International Society for the Study of the Lumbar Spine in 1981," but not published, by Evans of England.

Kane[13] then directed a randomized, prospective, controlled trial that showed that the rate of radiographically successful spinal fusion was higher when the direct-current implantable stimulator was used as an adjunct to the conventional spinal fusion procedure than when the surgery was performed alone. This multi-investigator trial included only patients who were classified as "difficult" spinal fusion patients with (1) one or more previous failed spinal fusions, (2) grade II or worse spondylolisthesis, (3) extensive bone grafting necessary for multiple-level fusion, or (4) other high-risk factors for failure of fusion, including gross obesity. Randomization was in blocks of four patients per investigator, with two patients implanted with the stimulator and two without. To maintain randomization validity, investigators were required to enter at least four patients. Measurement of success was based on radiographic assessments for fusion.

Of 99 patients entered into the trial, 63 were from investigators meeting the criterion of submitting at least four patients. Of the 63 patients, 59 from seven investigators were available for followup. Thirty-one patients received stimulation therapy and 28 control patients had the usual surgical procedures. The randomization procedure succeeded in the assignment of subjects with comparable characteristics, such as age and other entry criteria, into the

Criteria	Successful fusions			
	Control group		Treatment group	
Failed fusion	4/10	40.0%	9/11	81.8%
Spondylolisthesis	5/6	83.3%	2/2	100.0%
Extensive grafting	6/12	50.0%	11/15	73.3%
Risk	6/8	75.0%	8/9	88.9%

Source: Kane[13]

Figure 25.2. Random study results by entry criteria.

treatment and control groups. Eighteen months after surgery, successful fusion was achieved in 25 (81%) of 31 treated patients compared with 15 (54%) of 28 in the control group (p=.026). Kane presented a table on the rate of successful fusions obtained in the control and treatment groups to illustrate that "higher success rates were seen in the treatment groups for all entry criteria" (Figure 25.2).

The data show that, among patients who had had failed fusion or extensive grafting (two or more levels of fusion), successful fusion occurred in more patients in the stimulated group than in the control group; however, for patients meeting the other two entry criteria, the rate of successful fusion was essentially the same in the stimulated and control groups.

Kane also reported that 13 (81%) of 16 electrically stimulated patients who were not included in the former analysis had successful fusion; this rate was comparable with that in the randomized treated group described above. Similar data on the remaining 20 of 36 excluded patients were not given.

The Food and Drug Administration's (FDA) summary of data on the safety and effectiveness of the implantable bone-growth stimulator[14] contained the data on all of the patients in Kane's randomized trial. The FDA report noted that, of the original 99 patients, 8 were lost to followup, 4 did not complete the treatment, and 2 did not meet the entry criteria. Of the 36 patients who were not included in the randomized group, 26 were available for analysis (10 controls and 16 treated patients). As Kane had noted, 13 of the 16 treated patients had successful fusions. However, 10 (100%) of the 10 untreated control patients also had successful fusions.

Kane[13] also reported briefly on a nonrandom study that took place at the same time as his randomized study described above. The number of surgeons contributing data for this study was not stated. Kane reported that 108 (93%) of 116 patients treated with the implantable stimulator achieved successful fusion. The poorest result, 26 (87%) of 30, was seen in the subgroup of patients who had the highest risk of fusion failure according to the criteria for patients selected for the randomized trial.

Cameron and Bridges[3] reported qualitative radiologic evidence for an increased rate of bone graft incorporation in 41 scoliosis patients who received electrical bone-growth stimulation. An intertransverse fusion procedure with the lowest known failure rate of 11.5% was accomplished with bone grafted on both sides of the spine. The cathode from an implantable stimulator was applied to one side, with the other side serving as "control." Radiologic examinations were done at 3 months, 6 months, and 1 year and then at 6-month intervals until fusion occurred and the battery was removed. Only 1 patient (2.5%) failed to achieve fusion, although the theoretically expected rate of failure was 16%. Visually significant differences between the two sides were said to have been evident in 80% of the patients at the 3- and 6-month followup examinations. The differences became less apparent with time, and "fusion" in 40 of the 41 patients was reported by the hospital radiologist 12 months after surgery.

It appears clear that direct electrical current stimulates bone formation, and it has been used as a standard of care in the treatment of long-bone fractures that have failed to fuse. Direct-current stimulation may play a similar role in spinal fusion, especially in patients who have had fusion failures or are at high risk for fusion failure. Although many of the spinal fusion failures may be the result of less-than-optimal surgical technique, the available data appear to indicate that direct-current stimulation increases the chances for obtaining solid fusion in these patients. This seemed apparent from results with high-risk patients reported by Dwyer[12] and by Kane.[13] However, the highly varied rate of unsuccessful spinal fusion that had been reported (ranging from 0 to 30% following initial surgery) makes it difficult to assess the effects, if any, of direct-current stimulation on initial spinal fusion attempts. For example, the uncontrolled study by Nerubay and Katznelson[15] that showed that a solid fusion was obtained in all five children with spondylolisthesis cannot be readily interpreted as a demonstration of the influence of the implanted electrical stimulator. Perhaps a study of electrical stimulation in smokers might yield definitive information regarding the possible benefit of electrostimulation as an adjunct for spinal fusion in high-risk patients such as smokers, who have been shown to have a five-fold increased risk for fusion failure compared with nonsmokers in a retrospective study of patients who had had spinal surgery during 1977 and 1978.[16]

Although the published data on the effects of direct-current stimulators in lumbar spinal fusion are old and involve a relatively small number of patients, they indicate that the use of a direct-current stimulator as an adjunct to spine surgery may result in a better chance for solid fusion, especially in patients at high risk for fusion failure. Most studies purporting to demonstrate the beneficial effect of direct-current stimulation on lumbar spinal fusion have indicated that they included some high-risk patients, but they did not report the fusion results separately for these patients. The only controlled study that gave data on patients identified with specific high-risk criteria[13] showed that direct-current stimulation appeared to influence spinal fusion only in patients with two of the four entry criteria for high risk.

Direct-current application has been shown to stimulate osteogenesis in spinal fusion studies with animal models[7,8] and appears to increase the rate of bone graft incorporation in humans.[3] Although these studies and reports of better fusion success rates in uncontrolled studies[11-13] imply that direct-current electrical stimulation may increase the success rate of spinal fusion, other studies that were cited by Steinmann and Herkowitz[1] indicate that improved surgical technique may obviate the need for using electrical stimulators. On the other hand, direct-current stimulation may optimize the chances for solid fusion in patients who are considered to be at high risk for fusion failure.

The available data appear to suggest that an implantable bone-growth stimulator may be a useful adjunct that could enhance the probability of fusion success in patients who have had previous fusion failure or need extensive bone grafting for multiple-level fusion. Although direct-current stimulation might also increase the likelihood for successful spinal fusion in other high-risk patients such as those who have severe spondylolisthesis, are obese, or are smokers, there are insufficient data available at the present time to include these latter patients among those who may benefit from electrical stimulation.

References

1. Steinmann JC, Herkowitz HN. Pseudoarthrosis of the spine. *Clin Orthop* 1992;284:80-90.

2. DePalma AF, Rothman RH. The nature of pseudoarthrosis. *Clin Orthop* 1968;59:113-118.

3. Cameron HU, Bridges A. Pseudoarthrosis in lumbar spine fusion. *Prog Clin Biol Res* 1985;187:479-484.

4. Watkins MB, Bragg C. Lumbosacral fusion: Results with early ambulation. *Surg Gynecol Obstet* 1956;102:604-606.

5. Hannon KM, Wetta WJ. Failure of technetium bone scanning to detect pseudoarthroses in spinal fusion scoliosis. *Clin Orthop* 1977;123:42-44.

6. Connolly JF. Selection, evaluation and indications for electrical stimulation of ununited fractures. *Clin Orthop* 1981;101: 39-53.

7. Kahanovitz N, Arnoczky SP. The efficacy of direct current electrical stimulation to enhance canine spinal fusions. *Clin Orthop* 1990;251:295-299.

8. Nerubay J, Mrganit B, Bubis JJ, et al. Stimulation of bone formation by electrical current on spinal fusion. *Spine* 1986;11: 167-169.

9. Brodsky AE, Khalil MA, Neuman BP. Comparison of posterior vs anterior repair of pseudoarthrosis of anterior interbody fusions of the cervical spine. *Orthop Trans* 1988;12:47.

10. Edwards CC, Weigel MC. A prospective study of 51 low lumbar nonunions. *Orthop Trans* 1988;12:608.

11. Dwyer AF, Wickham GG. Direct current stimulation in spinal fusion. *Med J Aust* 1974;1:73-74.

12. Dwyer AF. The use of electrical current stimulation in spinal fusion. *Orthop Clin North Am* 1975;6:265-273.

13. Kane WJ. Direct current electrical bone growth stimulation for spinal fusion. *Spine* 1988;13:363-365.

14. Food and Drug Administration. Summary of safety and effectiveness data: Implantable electrical bone growth stimulator (unpublished report). 1987.

15. Nerubay J, Katznelson A. Clinical evaluation of an electrical current stimulator in spinal fusions. *Int Orthop* 1984:7:239-242.

16. Brown CW, Orme TJ, Richardson HD. The rate of pseudoarthrosis (surgical nonunion) in patients who are smokers and patients who are nonsmokers: A comparison study. *Spine* 1986;11:942-943.

—by S. Steven Hotta, M.D., Ph.D.

Chapter 26

What to Do about a
Pain in the Neck

Good Posture and Certain Exercises Can Help

You've been to the doctor and there's nothing seriously wrong. No slipped disk, no arthritis, no injuries, no tumors or other worrisome findings. But your neck still hurts.

That's not unusual. Most neck pain is caused not by some identifiable underlying ailment but by the extra strains and stresses you put on your neck. Better posture and a few neck exercises may ease your pain.

Keep Your Head on Straight

Your neck bears the weight of your head more easily when the head is centered above the spine, with only a slight forward curve at the back of the neck. Holding the head too far forward puts extra strain on the muscles, ligaments, and vertebrae in the neck, causing discomfort and leaving the neck vulnerable to injury. To decrease the strain, pay attention to your posture, especially when you're sitting for long periods or lying down.

Sitting. As you sit, your muscles relax and your back tends to curve forward, along with your shoulders and head. To discourage that tendency, fill the hollow between your chair and the small of your back with a small pillow or a rolled-up towel. Or you can buy a "lumbar (low-back) roll" made for the purpose, available at medical supply stores. To minimize bending forward when working at a desk, prop up books or papers, and align your computer screen at eye level. When you must sit with your head forward, be sure to change your position frequently.

Lying down. Lying on your stomach forces you to turn your neck too far to one side or the other. Sleep on your side or back instead. Use only one pillow that supports your neck and cradles your head. It shouldn't lift your head when you're on your back, or tilt it too far up or down when you're on your side. The pillow should be filled with feathers or some other material that you can contour to the shape of your head and neck. If the pillow alone doesn't provide enough neck support, you can slip a 3-inch foam roll into the pillowcase.

When You're in Pain

Neck exercises can help relieve pain that's not caused by any serious disorder. Before trying exercise, see a physician to be sure there's no such problem (see below).

Your physician may refer you to a physical therapist or suggest a self-care exercise program designed to relieve pain and restore your neck's full range of motion. One such exercise program comes from the book *Treat Your Own Neck*, by Robin McKenzie, director of The McKenzie Institute International, which trains health-care professionals to teach exercises to patients. All of these exercises are usually performed while seated, and all (except neck flexions) are repeated 10 times.

The following exercises, which should be approved by your physician, are designed to relieve pain and stiffness:

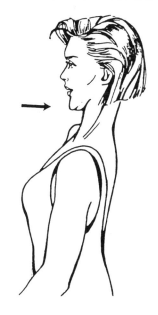

Figure 26.1.

Head retraction. Relax and let your head move forward slightly. Keep looking straight ahead. Now slowly retract your head—that is, move it backward as far as possible, without raising your chin (Figure 26.1). After a few seconds, relax and let your head move forward. (If the exercise is too painful or makes you dizzy, try it lying on your back, pressing your head down into the mattress.)

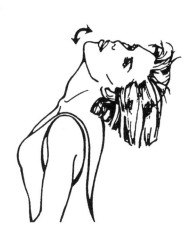

Figure 26.2

Neck extension. (This basic exercise may not be advisable for some people. Check with your physician first.) Do neck extensions after each set of head retractions. With your head retracted, lift your chin so that your head drops all the way back. Tilt your head slightly to the left and then the right, about a half-inch each way (Figure 26.2). After completing about half a dozen arcs, return to the retracted position.

Extensions and retractions should be done after each of the exercises described below.

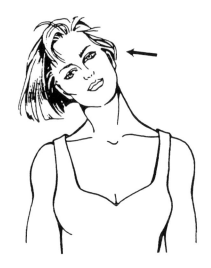

Sidebend. If your neck hurts more on one side than the other, try this: First do a few head retractions. With your head still retracted, tilt it toward the more painful side (Figure 26.3). After a few seconds, return to the retracted position.

Figure 26.3.

As Pain Lets Up

Although there may be some additional discomfort during your first session, the pain should be better, not worse, when the session's over. After pain begins to let up, other exercises can offer additional relief and begin to get your neck back into shape:

Neck rotation. This is especially helpful if it still hurts for you to turn your head to the side. Again, do a few retractions. Keeping your head retracted, turn it all the way to the left, then to the right (Figure 26.4). Hold the position for a few seconds on each side.

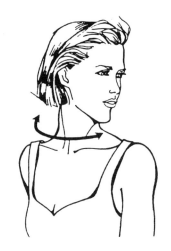

Figure 26.4.

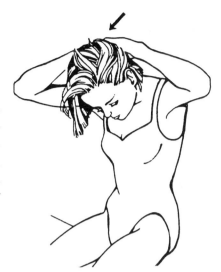

Neck flexion. If bending forward is still painful, or if headaches accompany the pain, a set of two or three flexions can help. Lower your head as far as possible, then let the weight of your arms push your chin farther down (Figure 26.5). After a few seconds return to the starting position.

Figure 26.5.

Once pain and stiffness are gone, keep them from returning by doing rotations, retractions, and extensions twice a day.

You should begin to feel less pain and have a greater range of motion within a few days. If you don't, check with your physician or physical therapist for further instruction or treatment.

See a Doctor First

Don't do neck exercises before you've seen your physician to check for underlying disorders, such as arthritis or a herniated ("slipped") disk. Here are some signs of trouble:

- Severe pain lasts more than two days.
- Pain follows a recent accident, especially if you also have difficulty moving your arms or legs.
- Pain shoots down your shoulders and arms, especially when you move your neck.
- Pain or numbness strikes your wrist, hand, or fingers.
- You experience drowsiness, nausea, sensitivity to bright light, severe headache, or vomiting.

Your physician may use X-rays, computerized tomography (CT) scans, magnetic resonance imaging, or other tests to assess your problem. If there's no specific diagnosis, your physician is likely to attribute the pain to stresses and strains.

Isometric Exercises (Non-moving exercises)

In each instance keep your head in the neutral position. Attempt to move each direction. Resist with your hand(s). Hold four seconds. Relax. Do each exercise five times.

Forward

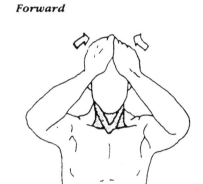

Backward

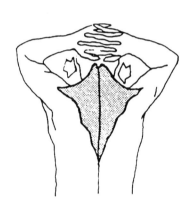

Left then Right

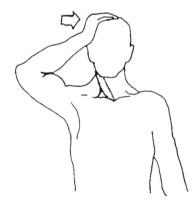

Figure 26.6.

Part Four

Chiropractic Care

Chapter 27

Basic Facts about Chiropractic

- Chiropractic is the fastest growing and second-largest primary health care profession. There are approximately 50,000 doctors of chiropractic (DCs) in active practice in the United States. More than 10,000 students are currently enrolled in chiropractic educational programs accredited by a federally-recognized body (CCE).

- Chiropractic services are in high demand. In 1993, more than 30 million consumers made chiropractic part of their health care regimen.

- Doctors of chiropractic receive extensive, demanding professional education on par with medical doctors (MDs) and osteopaths (DOs). To receive the doctor of chiropractic degree, candidates must complete extensive undergraduate prerequisites and four years of graduate-level instruction and internship. Comprehensive knowledge of all systems of the body and diagnostic procedures enable the DC to thoroughly evaluate a patient, address disorders relating to the spine and determine the need for referral to another health care provider.

- Doctors of Chiropractic are primary health care providers. According to the Center for Studies in Health Policy, "The DC can

The International Chiropractors Association, nd; reprinted with permission.

283

provide all three levels of primary care interventions and therefore is a primary care provider, as are MDs and DOs."

- Doctors of chiropractic are licensed in all 50 states. DCs have
  been licensed and recognized for many decades in all states, the
  District of Columbia and Puerto Rico.

- Chiropractic is recognized by governmental health care programs. Chiropractic is included in Medicare, Medicaid, Federal
  Employees Health Care Benefits Programs, Federal Workers'
  Compensation and all state workers' compensation programs.
  Chiropractic students are qualified to receive federal student
  loan assistance and DCs are authorized to be commissioned as
  health care officers in the U.S. Armed Forces.

- The practice of chiropractic is based on sound scientific principles. The existence of the nervous system as the primary control mechanism of the body is an undisputed scientific fact. Its
  relationship with the spine is the focus of the practice of chiropractic. When the vertebrae of the spine become misaligned
  through trauma or repetitive injury, two major consequences
  will result: (1) range of motion becomes limited and (2) spinal
  nerves emerging from the spinal cord are compromised. DCs
  use the term "subluxation" to describe such disruptions. Interruption of nerve flow can lead to pain, disability, and an overall
  decrease in quality of life. Conversely, removal of that interference has been shown to have significant, lasting health benefits.
  Through the adjustment of the subluxation, the DC endeavors
  to restore normal nerve expression. The body is then able to respond appropriately to any imbalance in the system, thus relieving symptoms and restoring health.

- Doctors of chiropractic provide effective, low-cost health care for
  a wide range of conditions. Studies conducted according to the
  highest scientific standards and published by organizations not
  affiliated in any way with chiropractic institutions or associations continue to show the clinical appropriateness and effectiveness of chiropractic care. One of the most recent, funded by
  the Ontario Ministry of Health, stated emphatically that:

"On the evidence, particularly the most scientifically valid
clinical studies, spinal manipulation applied by chiropractors is

shown to be more effective than alterative treatments for low back pain.... There would be highly significant cost savings if more management of low back pain was transferred from physician to chiropractors."

- The doctor of chiropractic is an effective source of preventative and wellness care. The anatomical focus of the DC on the human spine has created the perception of the DC as just a "back doctor." Although this perception is not entirely incorrect, it is very much incomplete. Doctors of chiropractic are a highly appropriate resource in matters of work-place safety, stress management, ergonomics, injury prevention, postural correction and nutritional counseling.

- The process of chiropractic adjustment is a safe, efficient procedure which is performed nearly one million times every working day in the United States. There is a singular lack of actuarial data that would justify concluding that chiropractic care is in any way harmful or dangerous. Chiropractic care is non-invasive, therefore, the body's response to chiropractic care is far more predictable than its reactions to drug treatments or surgical procedures. Of the nearly one million adjustments given every day in this country, complications are exceedingly rare. Perhaps the best summary statement on the subject of safety was published in 1979 by the Government of New Zealand which established a special commission to study chiropractic. They found:

  "The conspicuous lack of evidence that chiropractors cause harm or allow harm to occur through neglect of medical referral can be taken to mean only one thing: that chiropractors have on the whole an impressive safety record."

- Chiropractic offers a significant alternative to traditional medicine. A recent *New England Journal of Medicine* article affirmed that Americans made more visits to non-M.D. [including DCs] providers (425 million visits) than to M.D.s (388 million visits).

- Compare malpractice statistics. As testament to the safety and effectiveness of chiropractic care, consider that according to the AMA, the average medical doctor paid $14,900 for malpractice coverage in 1991. Doctors of chiropractic paid one fourth or less of that figure. This is true despite the fact that DCs see more patients per day than most MDs.

• A victory for chiropractic. The shifts in consumer behavior pose a significant threat to health care competitors who have vested interests in maintaining the status quo. Negative "disinformation" campaigns have routinely been employed to frighten patients and influence public policy decision makers about chiropractic. In 1987, chiropractic won an important lawsuit wherein the American Medical Association (AMA) was found guilty of attempting to "contain and eliminate" chiropractic. Chiropractic was awarded a permanent injunction order against the AMA. (*Chester A. Wilk v. AMA*)

For more information contact:
The International Chiropractors Association
1110 N. Glebe Road, Suite 1000
Arlington, Virginia 22201
1-800 423-4690

Chapter 28

What Is Manipulation

What is manipulation?

Manipulation is treatment using the doctor's hands to apply body leverage and a physical thrust to one joint or a group of related joints to restore joint and related tissue function. Through the use of manipulation, the doctor seeks to provide relief from symptoms, improve joint and muscle function, and speed recovery. Spinal manipulation is the most common form of manipulation. Manipulation should not be confused with other forms of manual therapy such as mobilization and massage.

Is manipulation effective?

Yes! As more of the benefits and safety of manipulation are made public, it is becoming more universally recognized as a safe and effective choice for the care of back problems.

The most recent evidence of manipulation's effectiveness comes from a landmark study[1] conducted by the Agency for Health Care Policy and Research, a federal government research organization. In

Source: http://www.cais.net/aca/man-qa.htm. Adapted from ACA's booklet, *What is Manipulation & How Can it Help Me?* The booklet, available from ACA Press, includes additional questions and answers, and extensive references. For ordering information, call ACA's Department of Marketing at 1-800-986-INFO. © 1995 American Chiropractic Association. Reprinted with permission.

this study, a panel of health care experts analyzed the scientific evidence available on all methods of examination and treatment used for acute adult low back problems and formed conclusions regarding their appropriateness and effectiveness. Among their most significant conclusions, they confirmed that spinal manipulation is a safe and effective initial form of treatment for this problem. This panel also strongly recommended that both doctors and patients consider using the most conservative treatment approach first for this common problem. Spinal manipulation is a drugless, nonsurgical (conservative) approach to the treatment of back pain and its related disorders.

Is manipulation safe?

Yes! When administered by a qualified doctor who is well trained and experienced in the use of manipulation, it is one of the safest drugless, nonsurgical procedures available.

Clinical surveys show that complications from manipulation are rare. So low, in fact, that doctors who perform manipulation have the lowest malpractice insurance costs of all practicing doctors. And within the group of doctors who use manipulation, chiropractic costs are lowest[2]. This means that when manipulation is performed by a Doctor of Chiropractic, the potential risk of complications from manipulation is at its lowest.

A word of caution. Manipulation is as much an art as it is a clinical science. It should not be used by unskilled persons. As more people become aware of manipulation's effectiveness, unlicensed or untrained persons might believe they too can use it safely and effectively. For your own safety, when selecting a doctor to provide manipulation for your back problem, be sure you choose a doctor who is well trained and experienced in this form of care.

Which doctors are most skilled at manipulation?

Doctors of Chiropractic (DCs) are the public's first choice of doctors for treatment using manipulation. A Summer, 1994 study by the respected health care research organization Louis Harris & Associates confirms this as a fact. This nation-wide survey reveals that nearly one-half of the general public and six in ten of those who sought professional care for a back problem in the recent past regard DCs as most skilled in the use of spinal manipulation. And the majority of those who visited other doctors for a back problem also consider

DCs more skilled in the use of manipulation than their medical or osteopathic doctor.

The DC's clinical expertise is derived from his/her training and the clinical experience gained from spending over 85% of his/her daily practice in the differential diagnosis of the patient's complaint and the management of neuromusculoskeletal (NMS) disorders. The DC's training and experience enable him/her to identify those health problems that are most likely to be responsive to chiropractic management and to administer the appropriate treatment personally, safely and effectively.

What if chiropractic manipulation is not covered in my insurance plan?

Ask your insurance plan administrator to add full, direct access chiropractic services coverage to your plan for both you and your dependents. And be sure to specify that you want these chiropractic services to be provided only by a Doctor of Chiropractic.

References

1. In December 1994 the Agency for Health Care Policy and Research (AHCPR), an agency of the United States Public Health Service, made public its findings from a two-year study of acute low back problems. A panel of twenty-three health care experts from different disciplines carefully examined the available research for all forms of evaluation and treatment for low back problems, debated the issues involved, and formed conclusions based on both the controlled clinical trial evidence available in the research literature and their collective expertise in these forms of treatment.

   Within the nonsurgical category of treatment, the panel concluded that only spinal manipulation, and certain over-the-counter and prescription drugs provided sufficiently effective relief from low back discomfort to be recommended as the safest and most effective initial form of drugless professional treatment for these low back problems.

Bigos S, Bowyer O, Braen G, et al. *Acute Low Back Problems in Adults. Clinical Practice Guideline No. 14.* AHCPR Publication No. 95-0642.

Rockville, MD: Agency for Health Care Policy and Research, Public Health Service, U.S. Department of Health and Human Services, December 1994.

2. Malpractice insurance costs reflect the rate of treatment complications that have occurred within different provider groups. In 1991, Medicare reported the average malpractice insurance costs for all health care providers in the Medicare system. The five provider groups practicing manipulation have the following mean liability expenses, as reported by their respective national associations: Chiropractic 1.8%; Physical Medicine and Rehabilitation 3.0% Manipulative Therapy 4.8% and Physical Therapy 4.8%.

Medical Program: Fee Schedule for Physicians' Services, Federal Register, Part II: Department of Health and Human Services, 42 CFR Parts 405, 413, and 415. Monday, November 25, 1991.

For More Information on Chiropractic Care, Please Call: The American Chiropractic Association 1-800-986-INFO

Chapter 29

Advice from the International Chiropractors Association on Whiplash and Arm and Shoulder Pain

Whiplash

What is whiplash?

Whiplash is more than just a pain in the neck. It can cause injury to the bones (cervical vertebrae) and connective tissues of the neck. The injury may be mild—causing only stiffness or soreness in the neck—or it can be severe—resulting in pain, tingling, numbness in the neck, shoulders, arms and hands as well as headaches, blurred vision, and nausea. Whiplash injuries can be severe and result in permanent damage.

What can cause whiplash?

Whiplash (known as hyperextension/hyperflexion injury) is usually the result of a backward-and-forward or sideways motion of the head and neck, both of which are often caused by a forceful impact from behind or the side. While whiplash occurs in the neck area most frequently, it may also strike in other areas of the spine, such as in the low-back or lumbar spine.

A whiplash injury can happen to anyone. A bad fall, a car accident, a sudden blow in a football game—all have the potential for causing whiplash.

"Whiplash," and "Arm and Shoulder Pain," International Chiropractors Association, nd; reprinted with permission.

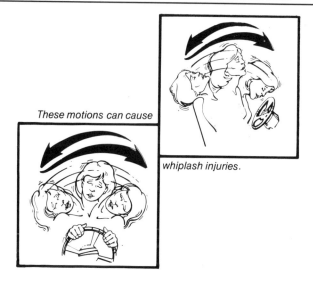

These motions can cause whiplash injuries.

Figure 29.1. *These motions can cause whiplash injuries.*

How can I tell if I have a whiplash?

Many mild whiplash injuries cannot be felt immediately. Sometimes hours, weeks or even months go by before any symptoms surface. In other cases of mild whiplash, the pain and other symptoms appear immediately after the injury and then lessen with the passage of time. Much later, however, severe reactions may reappear, caused by the long term effects of the injury.

A more severe whiplash can usually be detected immediately after the injury. It may result in many of the same symptoms as mild whiplash, as well as severe headaches, neck and shoulder pain, dizziness, blurred vision and general disorientation.

Should I be concerned about whiplash?

Yes! Even with mild whiplash—called a strain injury—a stretching or possible tearing of the neck muscles or other tissue can occur. When the head is "whipped" by an impact, the tendons, ligaments, and muscles which protect and cushion the spine are damaged. When these tissues are stretched or torn, depending on the severity, your spine may be significantly less stable.

Whiplash injuries may result in one or more vertebral subluxations—biomechanical alterations of the spinal vertebrae—which may cause nerve and blood-vascular interference. Prolonged instability of the spine can result not only in symptoms directly related to the whiplash, but in other symptoms resulting from a general deterioration in the involved area. Symptoms may arise that are far removed from those thought to be normally associated with a whiplash—low-back pain; knee, ankle and leg pain; diminished hand-to-eye coordination; irregular gait, and lethargy.

In the most traumatic, but rare, cases of whiplash, the vertebrae can actually fracture and damage the spinal cord itself, often resulting in tragic, debilitating, permanent injury.

What can I do to ease the pain?

If you experience whiplash, immediately stabilize and protect the head so that it cannot be exposed to further injury. Movement of the head may cause additional trauma to damaged tissue.

Apply ice packs to the area to help reduce inflammation and swelling and thereby decrease the pain. Use the ice packs for periods of 20 to 30 minutes with at least a 30-minute interval between each application.

A word of caution: these are temporary remedies and not a substitute for seeking immediate professional care. If you have been involved in an automobile accident or have other reason to suspect that you have sustained a whiplash, do not wait, consult your doctor of chiropractic as soon as possible.

What can the Doctor of Chiropractic do to help?

Mild whiplash often responds well to chiropractic care and usually heals rather quickly. Severe whiplash usually requires more healing time because of the extensive injury to the cervical spine and its supportive muscles, tendons and ligaments. Whatever the degree of injury, most whiplash cases will respond more readily under normal conditions if immediate chiropractic care is initiated.

Doctors of Chiropractic are educated and trained in the care of the spinal column. Your chiropractor will make a thorough examination. If no conditions exist which would call for referral to another specialist, he or she will determine what type of chiropractic care is appropriate in your case and recommend a course of treatment.

While every case is different, in most instances chiropractic care will help relieve the pain from the initial whiplash, as well as help allow your body to return to normal more quickly.

What can I do to prevent whiplash?

Since whiplash occurs frequently in automobile mishaps, you can help protect yourself by observing common sense driving practices:

- Drive defensively—always anticipate the actions of other drivers.
- Wear your seatbelts at all times—don't drive off without them fastened.
- Make sure your headrest is positioned properly.
- Avoid making sudden and unexpected starts and stops—be especially cautious when driving in heavy traffic.
- Don't tailgate—maintain an adequate stopping distance between you and the cars ahead and behind you.
- Be sure your tail lights and directional signals work properly.
- Concentrate on your responsibility if you are driving—don't let distractions inside or outside of the car divert your attention.
- Courtesy while driving is contagious—and can save your life.

Arm and Shoulder Pain

What can cause arm and shoulder pain?

Pain and other symptoms in the arm and shoulder may be due to injury of the neck or cervical spine. The seven cervical vertebrae (spinal bones) in the neck have highly mobile joints so that you can bend and tilt your neck. Since the neck is exceptionally flexible, it is susceptible to injury and pain which can be referred to the shoulder and the arm. (It should be noted, however, that pain in the arm and shoulder may be due to other conditions not related to the cervical spine such as frozen shoulder, strain/sprain syndromes, osteomas, etc.)

The vertebrae are separated by discs, which are stiff jelly-like pads that act as elastic cushions between the spinal bones. Neck, shoulder and arm pain may be caused by an abnormal bulging or protrusion of a disc in the cervical spine. The disc may impinge on the spinal nerve roots or irritate the spinal cord itself. This is also known as a herniated or slipped disc.

Cervical disc lesions that can cause arm and shoulder pain can be acute or chronic. For example, sudden and severe pain (acute torticollis) can result from lying too still for too long, on a pillow too thick or too thin, or in a position that keeps the neck in a sideways position for a long period.

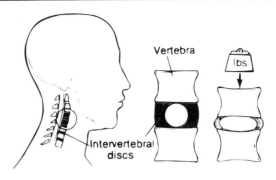

Figure 29.2.

Another way of developing acute torticollis is a whiplash injury or by simply stretching. Severe neck stiffness can result, sometimes with discomfort in both arms, and pins and needles in the fingers.

Pain in the shoulder blade (the scapula) may also be due to cervical disc trouble. It is also a common site for referred pain secondary to gall stones or a transverse humeral ligament tear or rupture. This scapular pain may radiate from the shoulder blade up to the base of the skull. Pressure on the nerve that innervates the arm area (the brachial nerve) from cervical disc injury can also cause pain in the shoulder, arm and chest.

Still other causes of shoulder and arm pain may include referred pain, such as from a heart attack, as well as regional disorders of the shoulder, elbow, wrist and hand. These conditions may include osteoporosis, tumors or cancerous growths, bursitis, neuritis and damage to the nerves and spinal cord.

What can I do to ease the pain temporarily?

- Apply an ice pack(s) to the area to reduce inflammation and swelling and thereby decrease the pain. Use the ice pack(s) for periods of 20 to 30 minutes with at least a 30-minute interval between each application.

- If you have insidious, recurring pain, apply moist heat to the back of the neck, arm and shoulders. Use the heat for periods of 20 minutes with at least a 30 minute interval between each application. A word of caution: these are temporary remedies and not a substitute for seeking immediate professional evaluation and care.

What can the Doctor of Chiropractic do to help?

Doctors of chiropractic are educated and trained in the detection and care of problems related to the spine. Your first visit to the chiropractor will include a complete chiropractic examination. X-rays may be ordered to screen for possible underlying pathologies and to reveal extreme distortions of the spine.

If your doctor of chiropractic feels that chiropractic care is appropriate in your case, he/she may give you an adjustment to help reduce the misalignments and ease the pressure on the spinal nerve roots. In addition your chiropractor may advise you on therapeutic exercises, job safety, work-related posture and dietary information.

What can I do to prevent arm and shoulder pain?

Your doctor of chiropractic cannot correct pain in the arm and shoulder without your help. These steps can help:

- Don't sleep on a stack of pillows, or even one thick pillow. By doing so you can put stress on the upper back and neck.

- Don't read or watch television while lying down. This can contort the neck. Always sit upright.

- Don't carry heavy purses or bags with a shoulder strap. The weight can pull on the neck and shoulder causing further pain.

- When doing work that requires you to bend your neck downward or face the same direction for long periods take frequent breaks.

- Be strict in following good postural habits when standing, sitting and walking.

- Follow a regular schedule of appropriate exercises to help strengthen your back and neck. Your chiropractor can recommend the best exercise program for you.

Chapter 30

Chiropractic Offers Long-Term Headache Relief

Chronic tension headache sufferers should consider chiropractic treatment as a long-term solution to their ailment without the side effects of drugs, according to a study funded by the Foundation for Chiropractic Education and Research (FCER). The study found that when six weeks of spinal manipulative treatment by chiropractors was compared to six weeks of medical treatment with amitriptyline, an antidepressant used to control severe headache pain, the chiropractic patients experienced fewer side effects, and the positive effects of chiropractic proved to be longer term, with patients reporting continued relief after the study was completed.

While anecdotal evidence has supported chiropractic treatment of tension headaches for years, until now, there have been no clinical trials that corroborate this reported success. The study that brings scientific support to these claims, "Chiropractic Spinal Manipulative Therapy vs. Amitriptyline for the Treatment of Chronic Tension-type Headaches: A Randomized Comparative Clinical Trial," was conducted by Dr. Patrick D. Boline (principal investigator) at Northwestern College of Chiropractic and published in the March/April issue of the Journal of Manipulative and Physiological Therapeutics.

For the study, a total of 126 patients between the ages of 18 and 70 were divided into two groups that were screened and randomly assigned to receive either chiropractic spinal manipulation or pharmaceutical treatment consisting of amitriptyline, a tricyclic antidepressant

Source: http://www.cais.net/aca/ha-study.htm. ACA Online; reprinted with permission.

commonly known by the brand name Elavil. The spinal manipulation group received short-lever, low-amplitude, high-velocity thrust techniques with moist heat and light massage of the cervicothoracic musculature prior to manipulation. Patients were palpated to determine the cervical, thoracic, or lumbar spinal segment to be manipulated with special attention to the upper three cervical segments. The patients in the amitriptyline therapy group received 10 mg daily for the first week, 20 mg daily for the second week, and 30 mg daily thereafter. This dosage was decreased if adverse side effected weren't tolerated by the patient.

During the six weeks that both groups received treatment, both reported similar improvements; however, four weeks after the end of the clinical trial, the superiority of chiropractic treatment was evident. The group receiving spinal manipulation showed a reduction of 32 percent in headache intensity, 42 percent in headache frequency, 30 percent in over-the-counter medication usage, and a 16 percent improvement in functional health status. The group receiving amitriptyline reverted to the levels recorded at the beginning of the study. The groups also differed greatly in their reporting of side effects. While 82.1 percent of the patients who received medical treatment suffered from drowsiness, dry mouth and weight gain, only 4.3 percent of the spinal manipulation group reported side effects consisting of neck soreness and stiffness.

"At last, with the results of this study, the claims of thousands of chiropractic patients who have enjoyed relief from pain without drugs will have to be taken seriously by the medical community," said Stephen R. Seater, CAE, Executive Director of FCER. "At last, chiropractic will be recognized as a viable and scientific alternative for relief of common tension headaches."

Chapter 31

Studies Regarding the Effectiveness of Chiropractic Care

In recent years, numerous independent researchers and various government agencies have conducted studies which focus on the efficacy, appropriateness and cost-effectiveness of chiropractic treatment. Several of these important studies are listed below.

U.S. Government Agency Report

A 1994 study published by the U.S. Agency for Health Care Policy and Research (AHCPR) and the U.S. Department of Health and Human Services endorses spinal manipulation for acute low back pain in adults in its Clinical Practice Guideline #14. An independent multidisciplinary panel of private-sector clinicians and other experts convened and developed specific statements on appropriate health care of acute low back problems in adults. One statement cited, relief of discomfort (low back pain) can be accomplished most safely with spinal manipulation, and/or nonprescription medication.

The Manga Report

A major study to assess the most appropriate use of available health care resources was reported in 1993. This was an outcomes

Information in this chapter was prepared in 1995 by the National Board of Chiropractic Examiners, 901 54th Avenue, Greeley, CO 80634; (970) 356-9100; reprinted with permission.

study funded by the Ontario Ministry of Health and conducted in hopes of sharing information about ways to reduce the incidence of work-related injuries and to address cost-effective ways to rehabilitate disabled and injured workers. The study was conducted by three health economists led by University of Ottawa Professor Pran Manga, Ph.D. The report of the study is commonly called the Manga Report. The Manga Report overwhelmingly supported the efficacy, safety, scientific validity, and cost-effectiveness of chiropractic for low-back pain. Additionally, it found that higher patient satisfaction levels were associated with chiropractic care than with medical treatment alternatives.

"Evidence from Canada and other countries suggests potential savings of hundreds of millions annually," the Manga Report states. "The literature clearly and consistently shows that the major savings from chiropractic management come from fewer and lower costs of auxiliary services, fewer hospitalizations, and a highly significant reduction in chronic problems, as well as in levels and duration of disability."

RAND *Study on Low-Back Pain*

A four-phase study conducted in the early 1990s by RAND, one of America's most prestigious centers for research in public policy, science and technology, explored many indications of low-back pain.

In the RAND studies, an expert panel of researchers, including medical doctors and doctors of chiropractic, found that:

- chiropractors deliver a substantial amount of health care to the U.S. population.

- spinal manipulation is of benefit to some patients with acute low-back pain.

The RAND reports marked the first time that representatives of the medical community went on record stating that spinal manipulation is an appropriate treatment for certain low-back pain conditions.

The New Zealand Commission Report

A particularly significant study of chiropractic was conducted between 1978-1980 by the New Zealand Commission of Inquiry. In its 377-page report to the House of Representatives, the Commission called its study "probably the most comprehensive and detailed independent examination of chiropractic ever undertaken in any country." The Commission entered the inquiry with "the general impression ... shared by many in the community: that chiropractic was an unscientific cult, not to be compared with orthodox medical or paramedical services."

By the end of the inquiry, the commission reported itself "irresistibly and with complete unanimity drawn to the conclusion that modern chiropractic is a soundly-based and valuable branch of health care in a specialized area..." Conclusions of the Commission's report, based on investigations in New Zealand, the U.S., Canada, the United Kingdom, and Australia, stated:

- Spinal manual therapy in the hands of a registered chiropractor is safe.

- Spinal manual therapy can be effective in relieving musculoskeletal symptoms such as back pain, and other symptoms known to respond to such therapy, such as migraine.

- Chiropractors are the only health practitioners who are necessarily equipped by their education and training to carry out spinal manual therapy.

- In the public interest and in the interests of patients, there must be no impediment to full professional cooperation between chiropractors and medical practitioners.

Florida Workers' Compensation Study

A 1988 study of 10,652 Florida workers' compensation cases was conducted by Steve Wolk, Ph.D., and reported by the Foundation for Chiropractic Education and Research. It was concluded that "a claimant with a back-related injury, when initially treated by a chiropractor versus a medical doctor, is less likely to become temporarily disabled, or if disabled, remains disabled for a shorter period of time; and claimants treated by medical doctors were hospitalized at a much higher rate than claimants treated by chiropractors."

Washington HMO Study

In 1989, a survey administered by Daniel C. Cherkin, Ph.D., and Frederick A. MacCornack, Ph.D., concluded that patients receiving care from health maintenance organizations (HMOs) within the state of Washington were three times as likely to report satisfaction with care from chiropractors as they were with care from other physicians. The patients were also more likely to believe that their chiropractor was concerned about them.

Utah Workers' Compensation Study

A workers' compensation study conducted in Utah by Kelly B. Jarvis, D.C., Reed B. Phillips, D.C., Ph.D., and Elliot K. Morris, JD, MBA, compared the cost of chiropractic care to the costs of medical care for conditions with identical diagnostic codes. Results were reported in the August 1991 *Journal of Occupational Medicine.*

The study indicated that costs were significantly higher for medical claims than for chiropractic claims; in addition, the number of work days lost was nearly ten times higher for those who received medical care instead of chiropractic care.

Patient Disability Comparison

A 1992 article in the *Journal of Family Practice* reported a study by D.C. Cherkin, Ph.D., which compared patients of family physicians and of chiropractors. The article stated "the number of days of disability for patients seen by family physicians was significantly higher (mean 39.7) than for patients managed by chiropractors (mean 10.8)." A related editorial in the same issue referred to risks of complications from lumbar manipulation as being "very low."

Oregon Workers' Compensation Study

A 1991 report on a workers' compensation study conducted in Oregon by Joanne Nyiendo, Ph.D., concluded that the median time loss days (per case) for comparable injuries was 9.0 for patients receiving treatment by a doctor of chiropractic and 11.5 for treatment by a medical doctor.

Stano Cost Comparison Study

A study by Miron Stano, Ph.D., reported in the June 1993 *Journal of Manipulative and Physiological Therapeutics* involved 395,641 patients with neuromusculoskeletal conditions. Results over a two-year period showed that patients who received chiropractic care incurred significantly lower health care costs than did patients treated solely by medical or osteopathic physicians.

Saskatchewan Clinical Research

Following a 1993 study, researchers J. David Cassidy, D.C., Haymo Thiel, D.C., M.S., and W. Kirkaldy-Willis, M.D., of the Back Pain Clinic at the Royal University Hospital in Saskatchewan concluded that "the treatment of lumbar intervertebral disk herniation by side posture manipulation is both safe and effective."

Wight Study on Recurring Headaches

A 1978 study conducted by J.S. Wight, D.C., and reported in the *ACA Journal of Chiropractic*, indicated that 74.6% of patients with recurring headaches, including migraines, were either cured or experienced reduced headache symptomatology after receiving chiropractic manipulation.

1991 Gallup Poll

A 1991 demographic poll conducted by the Gallup Organization revealed that 90% of chiropractic patients felt their treatment was effective; more than 80% were satisfied with that treatment; and nearly 75% felt most of their expectations had been met during their chiropractic visits.

1990 British Medical Journal Report

A study conducted by T.W. Meade, a medical doctor, and reported in the June 2, 1990, *British Medical Journal* concluded after two years of patient monitoring, "for patients with low-back pain in whom manipulation is not contraindicated, chiropractic almost certainly confers worthwhile, long-term benefit in comparison with hospital outpatient management."

Virginia Comparative Study

A 1992 study conducted by L.G. Schifrin, Ph.D., provided an economic assessment of mandated health insurance coverage for chiropractic treatment within the Commonwealth of Virginia. As reported by the College of William and Mary, and the Medical College of Virginia, the study indicated that chiropractic provides therapeutic benefits at economical costs. The report also recommended that chiropractic be a widely available form of health care.

1992 America Health Policy *Report*

A 1992 review of data from over 2,000,000 users of chiropractic care in the U.S., reported in the *Journal of American Health Policy*, stated that "chiropractic users tend to have substantially lower total health care costs," and "chiropractic care reduces the use of both physician and hospital care."

1985 University of Saskatchewan Study

In 1985 the University of Saskatchewan conducted a study of 283 patients "who had not responded to previous conservative or operative treatment" and who were initially classified as totally disabled. The study revealed that "81% ... became symptom free or achieved a state of mild intermittent pain with no work restrictions" after daily spinal manipulations were administered.

Chapter 32

Glossary of Chiropractic Terms

Adjustment. A form of manipulation, where the thrust or application of force is of a high velocity-low amplitude magnitude. This type of manipulation can be likened to quickly pulling an apple off of a branch to obtain the specific apple, as opposed to pulling the apple slowly and obtaining multiple apples.

Arthritis. A general term referring to a condition of the joints. Literally it refers to an inflammation of the joints. There are many types of arthritides. The form which will inflict most people with age is known as osteoarthritis. Other types include rheumatoid and psoriatic arthritis.

Brain. This is the portion of the central nervous system where higher mental and body functions occur. It is protected by the skull at the top of the head, and makes a smooth transition into the spinal cord at its base.

Cervical. When discussing the spinal column, this refers to the region of the neck.

Chiropractor. Doctor trained in the science, art and philosophy of manipulation (adjustment) of the human body. Chiropractic procedure is directed at evaluating causative factors in the bio-mechanical and

Source: http://www.panix.com/~tonto1/pat_ed.html. Chiropractic OnLine Today, Todd Eglow, editor; reprinted with permission.

structural derangements of the spine which could affect the nervous system and the body's natural defense mechanism.

Chiropractic Subluxation Complex. An extension of joint dysfunction. At this point, symptoms arise which are no longer simply musculoskeletal. Now, through faulty transmission of information through the nervous system, various organs (heart, liver, stomach, etc) may malfunction.

Degeneration. A wear and tear phenomena. When the joints of the body wear out, it is referred to as osteoarthritis, also known as degenerative joint disease.

Herniation. Condition of the intervertebral disc, whereby some of the material which makes up the disc shifts to a position which irritates the nearby nerve for that spinal area.

Intervertebral disc. This is the soft tissue found between the bones of the spinal column, the vertebrae. They help cushion the spine from everyday stress (i.e., running, walking, jumping, etc.). Through improper posture (i.e., bending forward at the waist and twisting), discs can wear out (degenerate). When this occurs a condition known as spondylolysis occurs. This can lead to the condition known commonly by the laymen, as a "slipped disc," or a disc herniation.

Joint. The area between two bones where movement occurs. If movement is abnormal, pain and degeneration may occur.

Joint dysfunction. A condition, whereby the joints of a particular area are not moving properly. Any sort of physical, chemical or mental trauma may bring this about.

Lumbar. When discussing the spinal column, this refers to the region of the low back.

Manipulation. This is a form of manual therapy where an application of forces to structures such as muscles, joints and bones, with the goal is the restoration of normal spinal motion and the elimination of pain secondary to disturbed biomechanics (Manip #1 p. 280). Grieve mentions Korr's definition of manipulation as follows: "the application of an accurately determined and specifically directed manual force to the body, in order to improve mobility in areas that are restricted; in joints, in connective tissues or in skeletal muscles" (Manip #2 p. 857).

Manual Therapy. To work with one's hands.

Massage. This is the application, usually by hand, of systematic stroking or manipulation to the soft tissues of the body for therapeutic purposes, i.e., to alleviate pain and discomfort. The most well known massage movements are those that involve stroking and gliding (effleurage), kneading (petrissage), and percussion (tapotement) to soft tissues of the body (Manip #1 p. 286-289).

Nervous System. The telephone communication center of the body. All information from outside the body and from the inside the body must pass through this system. The two parts of the nervous system include the central and peripheral nervous systems.

Nerves. The extensions of the brain and spinal cord which carry information to all parts of the body.

Osteoarthritis. Also known as degenerative joint disease. A form of arthritis in which a wear and tear phenomena occur at the joint. A common form of arthritis, especially in older people.

Range-Of-Motion. This is a description for the movement which occurs at a particular joint. In the spinal column, there are six (6) different movements which may occur. These include flexion (bending forward), extension (bending backward), rotation (twisting right and left) and lateral flexion (bending to each side, right and left).

Spinal Column. The bones of the back. The spinal column protects the spinal cord and allows for movement of the body. There are 24, movable bones (also known as vertebrae), plus a sacrum and a coccyx at the bottom of this column.

Spinal Cord. The extension of the brain. Coming off of the spinal cord are 31 pairs of spinal nerves which communicate with the body as a whole. The spinal cord is protected by the spinal column.

Spondylolysis. A degeneration of the intervertebral disc.

Symptom. The feeling, perceived by a patient that something is not right.

Thoracic. When discussing the spinal column, this refers to the region of the back between the neck and the pelvis.

Vertebrae. The bones of the spinal column. There are three (3) areas of vertebrae; a cervical, thoracic and lumbar area.

References to Glossary

Manip #1. Rehabilitation Medicine-Principles and Practice 2nd Ed. Joel A. DeLisa. Lippincott (1988).

Manip #2. Modern Manual Therapy. Gregory P. Grieve. Churchill Livingstone (1986).

Part Five

Information for Spinal Cord Injury Patients

Chapter 33

Spinal Cord Injuries: Causes and Statistics

What is spinal cord injury?

Spinal Cord Injury (SCI) is damage to the spinal cord that results in a loss of function such as mobility or feeling. Frequent causes of damage are trauma (car accident, gunshot, falls, etc.) or disease (polio, spina bifida, Friedreich's Ataxia, etc.). The spinal cord does not have to be severed in order for a loss of functioning to occur. In fact, in most people with SCI, the spinal cord is intact, but the damage to it results in loss of functioning. SCI is very different from back injuries such as ruptured disks, spinal stenosis or pinched nerves.

A person can "break their back or neck" yet not sustain a spinal cord injury if only the bones around the spinal cord (the vertebrae) are damaged, but the spinal cord is not affected. In these situations, the individual may not experience paralysis after the bones are stabilized.

What is the spinal cord and the vertebra?

The spinal cord is the major bundle of nerves that carry nerve impulses to and from the brain to the rest of the body. The brain and

"Common Questions About Spinal Cord Injury." National Spinal Cord Injury Association (545 Concord Avenue, Suite 29, Cambridge, MA 02138) March 1996; and "Spinal Cord Injury: Facts and Figures at a Glance," The National SCI Statistical Center (1717 6th Avenue South, Room 544, Birmingham, AL 35233-7330) May 1996.

the spinal cord constitute the *Central Nervous System*. Motor and sensory nerves outside the central nervous system constitute the *Peripheral Nervous System*, and another diffuse system of nerves that control involuntary functions such as blood pressure and temperature regulation are the *Sympathetic and Parasympathetic Nervous Systems*.

The spinal cord is surrounded by rings of bone called vertebra. These bones constitute the spinal column (back bones). In general, the higher in the spinal column the injury occurs, the more dysfunction a person will experience. The vertebra are named according to their location. The eight vertebra in the neck are called the *Cervical Vertebra*. The top vertebra is called C-1, the next is C-2, etc. Cervical SCIs usually cause loss of function in the arms and legs, resulting in *quadriplegia*. The twelve vertebra in the chest are called the *Thoracic Vertebra*. The first thoracic vertebra, T-1, is the vertebra where the top rib attaches. Injuries in the thoracic region usually affect the chest and the legs and result in *paraplegia*.

The vertebra in the lower back—between the thoracic vertebra, where the ribs attach, and the pelvis (hip bone), are the *Lumbar Vertebra*. The *sacral* vertebra run from the pelvis to the end of the spinal column. Injuries to the five Lumbar vertebra (L-1 thru L-5) and similarly to the five *Sacral Vertebra* (S-1 thru S-5) generally result in some loss of functioning in the hips and legs.

What are the effects of SCI?

The effects of SCI depend on the type of injury and the level of the injury. SCI can be divided into two types of injury—complete and incomplete. A *complete injury* means that there is no function below the level of the injury; no sensation and no voluntary movement. Both sides of the body are equally affected. An *incomplete injury* means that there is some functioning below the primary level of the injury. A person with an incomplete injury may be able to move one limb more than another, may be able to feel parts of the body that cannot be moved, or may have more functioning on one side of the body than the other. With the advances in acute treatment of SCI, incomplete injuries are becoming more common.

The level of injury is very helpful in predicting what parts of the body might be affected by paralysis and loss of function. Remember that in incomplete injuries there will be some variation in these prognoses. Cervical (neck) injuries usually result in quadriplegia. Injuries above the C-4 level may require a ventilator for the person to breathe.

C-5 injuries often result in shoulder and biceps control, but no control at the wrist or hand. C-6 injuries generally yield wrist control, but no hand function. Individuals with C-7 and T-1 injuries can straighten their arms but still may have dexterity problems with the hand and fingers.

Injuries at the thoracic level and below result in paraplegia, with the hands not affected. At T-1 to T-8 there is most often control of the hands, but poor trunk control as the result of lack of abdominal muscle control. Lower T-injuries (T-9 to T-12) allow good trunk control and good abdominal muscle control. Sitting balance is very good. Lumbar and Sacral injuries yield decreasing control of the hip flexors and legs.

Besides a loss of sensation or motor functioning, individuals with SCI also experience other changes. For example, they may experience dysfunction of the bowel and bladder. Sexual functioning is frequently affected: men with SCI may have their fertility affected, while women's fertility is generally not affected. Very high injuries (C-1, C-2) can result in a loss of many involuntary functions including the ability to breathe, necessitating breathing aids such as mechanical ventilators or diaphragmatic pacemakers. Other effects of SCI may include low blood pressure, inability to regulate blood pressure effectively, reduced control of body temperature, inability to sweat below the level of injury, and chronic pain.

How many people have SCI? Who are they?

Approximately 450,000 people live with SCI in the U.S. There are about 8,000 new SCIs every year; the majority of them (82%) involve males between the ages of 16-30. These injuries result from motor vehicle accidents (42%), violence (24%), or falls (22%). Quadriplegia is slightly more common than paraplegia.

Is there a cure for SCI?

Currently there is no cure for SCI. There are many researchers attacking this problem, and there have been many advances in the lab. Many of the most exciting advances have resulted in a decrease in damage at the time of the injury. Steroid drugs such as methylprednisolone reduce swelling, which is a common cause of secondary damage at the time of injury. The experimental drug Sygen® appears to reduce loss of function, although the mechanism is not completely understood.

Do people with SCI ever get better?

When a SCI occurs, there is usually swelling of the spinal cord. This may cause changes in virtually every system in the body. After days or weeks, the swelling begins to go down and people may regain some functioning. With many injuries, especially incomplete injuries, the individual may recover some functioning as late as 18 months after the injury. In very rare cases, people with SCI will regain some functioning years after the injury. However, only a very small fraction of individuals sustaining SCIs recover all functioning.

Does everyone who sustains SCI use a wheelchair?

No. Wheelchairs are a tool for mobility. High C-level injuries usually require that the individual use a power wheelchair. Low C-level injuries and below usually allow the person to use a manual chair. Advantages of manual chairs are that they cost less, weigh less, disassemble into smaller pieces and are more agile. However, for the person who needs a powerchair, the independence afforded by them is worth the limitations. Some people are able to use braces and crutches for ambulation. These methods of mobility do not mean that the person will never use a wheelchair. Many people who use braces still find wheelchairs more useful for longer distances. However, the therapeutic and activity levels allowed by standing or walking briefly may make braces a reasonable alternative for some people.

Of course, people who use wheelchairs aren't always in them. They drive, swim, fly planes, ski, and do many activities out of their chair. If you hang around people who use wheelchairs long enough, you may see them sitting in the grass pulling weeds, sitting on your couch, or playing on the floor with children or pets. And of course, people who use wheelchairs don't sleep in them, they sleep in a bed. No one is "wheelchair bound."

Do people with SCI die sooner?

Yes. Before World War II, most people who sustained SCI died within weeks of their injury due to urinary dysfunction, respiratory infection or bedsores. With the advent of modern antibiotics, modern materials such as plastics and latex, and better procedures for dealing with the everyday issues of living with SCI, many people approach the lifespan of non-disabled individuals. Interestingly, other than level of injury, the type of rehab facility used is the greatest indicator of long-term survival. This illustrates the importance of and the difference made by going to a facility that specializes in SCI. People who use vents are at some increased danger of dying from pneumonia or respiratory infection, but modern technology is improving in that area as well. Pressure sores are another common cause of hospitalization, and if not treated—death.

Do people with SCI have jobs?

People with SCI have the same desires as other people. That includes a desire to work and be productive. The *Americans with Disabilities Act* (ADA) promotes the inclusion of people with SCI to mainstream in day-to-day society. Of course, people with disabilities may need some changes to make their workplace more accessible, but surveys indicate that the cost of making accommodations to the workplace in 70% of cases is $500 or less.

Can people with SCI have sex, children?

SCI frequently affects sexual functioning. However, there are many therapies that allow people with SCI to have an active and satisfying sex life. Fertility is also frequently affected in men with SCI. Methods similar to those used for non-disabled men with fertility problems have allowed many men with SCI to father their own children. Of course, adoption is another option. The fertility of women with SCI may be affected in the first months after injury. However, most women regain the ability to become pregnant after SCI. Many women with SCI are able to carry babies to full term. However, it is important that she consult a physician experienced in SCI.

What do I say when I meet a person with SCI?

"Hi."
A person with a SCI is no different from a non-disabled individual except in a few ways. People with SCI have the same hopes, interests and desires as other people. People with SCI are interested in sports—or not (just like non-disabled people). Although disabled individuals do some things differently than non-disabled individuals, the result is the same. It's important to remember that although SCI changes a person, they are still people, so treat them that way.

315

The most important thing to remember is: *Life does not end with spinal cord injury.*

This Factsheet is offered as an information service and is not intended to cover all treatments or research in the field, nor is it an endorsement of the methods mentioned herein. The National Spinal Cord Injury Resource Center (NSCIRC) provides information and referral on many subjects related to spinal cord injury. Contact the resource center at 1-800 962-9629.

Facts and Figures At a Glance

Incidence. It is estimated that the annual incidence of spinal cord injury (SCI), not including those who die at the scene of the accident, is between 30 and 40 cases per million population in the U.S. Based on the 1992 census population of 254 million, these rates correspond to between 7,600 and 10,000 new cases each year. Since there have not been any overall incidence studies of SCI in the U.S. since the 1970's it is not known if incidence has changed in recent years.

Prevalence. The number of people in the United States who are alive today and who have SCI has been estimated to be between 721 and 906 per million population. This corresponds to between 183,000 and 203,000 persons. (Note) Incidence and prevalence statistics are not derived form the National SCI Database.

The National Spinal Cord Injury Database. The National Spinal Cord Injury Database has been in existence since 1973 and captures data from an estimated 15% of new SCI cases in the U.S. Since its inception, 24 federally funded Model SCI Care Systems have contributed data to the National SCI Database. As of September 1995 the database contained information on more than 16,799 persons who sustained traumatic spinal cord injuries. All the remaining statistics on this sheet are derived from this database or from collaborative studies conducted by the Model Systems.

Detailed discussions of all topics on this sheet may be found in the latest Model Systems' book, *Spinal Cord Injury: Clinical Outcomes from the Model Systems* (Aspen Publishers, order #20697).

Age at injury. SCI primarily affects young adults. Fifty-seven percent of SCIs occur among persons in the 16 to 30 year age group,

316

and the average age at injury is 31.1 years. Since 1973 there has been an increase in the mean age at time of injury. Those who were injured before 1979 had a mean age of 28.6 while those injured after 1990 had a mean age of 33.8 years. Another trend is an increase in the proportion of those who were at least 61 years of age at injury. In the 1970's persons older than 60 years of age at injury comprised 4.7% of the database. Since 1990 this has increased to 9%. This trend is not surprising since the median age of the general population has increased from 27.9 years to 33.1 years during the same time period.

Gender. Overall, 82.1% of all persons in the national database are male. This grater than four-to-one male to female ratio has varied little throughout the 22 years of Model Systems data collection.

Ethnic groups. A significant trend over time has been observed in the racial distribution of persons in the Model System database. Among persons injured between 1973 and 1978, 77.5% of persons in the database were Caucasian, 13.6% were African-American, 6% were Hispanic, 2% were American Indian and 0.8% were Asian. However among those injured since 1990 only 55.2% were Caucasian, while 29% were African-American, 12.8% were Hispanic, 0.5% were American Indian and 1.9% were Asian.

Etiology. Since 1991, motor vehicle crashes account for 35.9% of the SCI cases reported. The next largest contributor is acts of violence (primarily gunshot wounds), followed by falls and recreational sporting activities. Interesting trends in the database show the proportions of injuries due to motor vehicle crashes and sporting activities have declined while the proportion of injuries from acts of violence has increased steadily since 1973.

Etiology of SCI Since 1991

- Vehicular Crashes: 35.9%
- Violence: 29.5%
- Falls: 20.3%
- Sports: 7.3%
- Other: 7.1%

Neurologic level and extent of lesion. Persons with tetraplegia (52%) have sustained injuries to one of the eight cervical segments of the spinal cord; those with paraplegia (46.7%) have lesions in the thoracic, lumbar, or sacral regions of the spinal cord.

Since 1991 the most frequent neurologic category is complete paraplegia (29.1%), followed by incomplete tetraplegia (27.6%), incomplete paraplegia (22.6%), and complete tetraplegia (18.7%). Trends over time indicate an increasing proportion of persons with incomplete paraplegia and a decreasing proportion of persons with complete tetraplegia.

Occupational status. More than half (61%) of those persons with SCI admitted to a Model System reported being employed at the time of their injury. The post-injury employment picture is better among persons with paraplegia than among their tetraplegic counterparts. By post-injury year 8, 36.2% of persons with paraplegia are employed during the same year.

Residence. Historically, many persons with SCI were forced to live out the remainder of their lives in institutional settings such as nursing homes. Today however, 89.2% of all persons with SCI who are discharged alive from the system are sent to a private, noninstitutional residence (in most cases their homes before injury.) Only 4% are discharged to nursing homes. The remaining are discharged to hospitals, group living situations or other destinations.

Marital status. Considering the youthful age of most persons with SCI, it is not surprising that most (53.7%) are single when injured. Among those who were married at the time of injury, as well as those who marry after injury, the likelihood of their marriage remaining intact is slightly lower when compared to the uninjured population. The likelihood of getting married after injury is also reduced.

Length of stay. Overall, average days hospitalized for acute care and rehabilitation for those who enter a Model System immediately following injury has declined from 137 days in 1974 to 63 days in 1994. Similar downward trends are noted for those with paraplegia (from 122 to 53 days) and persons with tetraplegia (from 150 to 75 days).

Lifetime costs. Average yearly health care and living expenses (in 1992 dollars) that are directly attributable to SCI vary greatly according to severity of injury. (See Figure 33.1.)

Severity of Injury	First Year	Each Subsequent Year
High Tetraplegia (C1-C4)	$417,067	$74,707
Low Tetraplegia (C5-C8)	$269,324	$30,602
Paraplegia	$152,396	$15,507
Incomplete Motor Functional at Any Level	$122,914	$8,614
All Groups	$198,335	$24,154

Figure 33.1.

Estimated lifetime costs discounted at 4% depend on severity of injury and age at injury. (See Figure 33.2.)

Severity of Injury	Age At Injury	
	25 years old	50 years old
High Tetraplegia (C1-C4)	$1,349,029	$876,287
Low Tetraplegia (C5-C8)	$748,234	$528,021
Paraplegia	$427,733	$326,272
Incomplete Motor Functional at Any Level	$287,001	$231,018

Figure 33.2.

These figures do not include any indirect costs such as losses in wages, fringe benefits and productivity which could average almost $38,000 but vary substantially based on education, severity of injury and pre-injury employment history.

Life expectancy. Life expectancy is the average remaining years of life for an individual. Life expectancies for persons with SCI continue to increase, but are still somewhat below normal. (See Figure 33.3.)

Mortality rates are significantly higher during the first year after injury than during subsequent years, particularly for severely injured persons.

Cause of Death. In years past, the leading cause of death among persons with SCI was renal failure. Today, however, significant advances

Current Age	Normal	Ventilator Dependent at Any Level	High Tetra (C1-C4)	Low Tetra (C5-C8)	Para	Motor Functional at Any Level
20	56.3	19.9	32.8	38.6	44.8	49.0
30	46.9	15.9	26.8	30.7	36.7	40.5
40	37.6	12.4	20.9	23.6	28.8	31.7
50	28.6	9.3	15.5	17.0	21.2	23.4
60	20.5	6.6	11.0	11.2	13.8	15.9

Figure 33.3. Life expectancy for those who survive the first year post-injury by severity of injury and age at injury

in urologic management have resulted in dramatic shifts in the leading causes of death. Person enrolled in the National SCI Database since its inception in 1973 have now been followed for 22 years after injury. During that time the causes of death that appear to have the greatest impact on reduced life expectancy for this population are pneumonia, pulmonary emboli and septicemia.

The Model Regional Spinal Cord Injury Care System

The Model Regional Spinal Cord Injury Care System program was established in the early 1970s. Presently there are 18 systems sponsored by the National Institute on Disability and Rehabilitation Research, U.S. Department of Education:

University of Alabama at Birmingham
Birmingham, AL
(205) 934-3330

Regional SCI Care System of Southern California
Downey, CA
(310) 401-7161

Northern California SCI System
San Jose, CA
(408) 295-9896

Rocky Mountain Regional SCI System
Englewood, CO
(303) 789-8203

Georgia Regional SCI System
Atlanta, GA
(404) 350-7580

Midwest Regional SCI Care System
Chicago, IL
(312) 908-3425

Boston University Medical Center Hospital
Boston, MA
(617) 638-7300

University of Michigan Model SCI System
Ann Arbor, MI
(313) 763-0971

Southeast Michigan Regional SCI System
Detroit, MI
(313) 745-9876

University of Missouri
Columbia, MO
(314) 882-6271

Northern New Jersey SCI System
West Orange, NJ
(201) 243-6805

Mt. Sinai SCI Model System
New York, NY
(212) 241-6593

MetroHealth Medical Center
Cleveland, OH
(216) 778-8781

Regional SCI System of Delaware Valley
Philadelphia, PA
(215) 955-6579

Texas Regional SCI System
Houston, TX
(713) 797-5910

Medical College of Virginia
Richmond, VA
(804) 828-9328

Northwest Regional SCI System
Seattle, WA
(206) 543-8171

Medical College of Wisconsin
Milwaukee, WI
(414) 259-3657

Chapter 34

General Spinal Cord Injury Anatomy and Physiology

Even though the brain controls the majority of the activities of your body, it only extends down as far as the top of your neck. Beyond that, the *spinal cord* takes over and acts like telegraph wires for messages coming and going between the brain and all the other parts of your body. Your face has a direct connection to the brain stem, so it is independent of your spinal cord.

To look at it, the spinal cord is a long, rope-like cord about the width of your little finger. It runs from the base of your brain down to the lower part of your back and is fairly fragile. Damage to your spinal cord can affect your ability to move or feel. It can also affect the workings of some internal organs. If you are injured at a given level of your spinal cord, parts of your body will be affected at and below that level.

To avoid damage, the spinal cord is protected by bone—specifically, by your *back bones*. The back bones are 29 small bones stacked one on top of the other. These bones are called *vertebrae (VERT-i-bray)*. Because of all the jarring and bending your back must do, each *vertebra (VERT-i-brah)* is cushioned from the next by disks. Disks are made of spongy material that act on your back like shock absorbers do on your car. Ligaments hold the vertebrae together and allow your neck and back to twist and bend.

Excerpted from *Yes, You Can: A Guide to Self-Care for Persons with Spinal Cord Injury*, copyright 1989, Paralyzed Veterans of America (PVA); reprinted with permission. For information on how to obtain a complete copy of this manual or receive a list of other available resources contact the PVA at 1-800-424-8200.

Each vertebra has a hole in it, so when stacked together with other vertebrae, they provide a hard, boney tunnel through which the spinal cord passes. This is called the *spinal column*. In this way, the cord is protected from the possibility of damage. (See Figure 34.1)

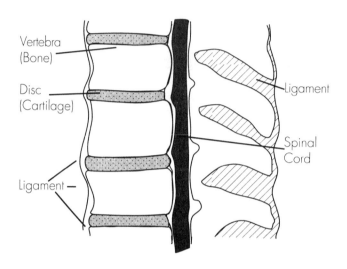

Figure 34.1. The spinal column.

There are four sections of your spine. The top is the *cervical (SURR-vick-ull)* section, which makes up your neck. The next down is the *thoracic (thor-ASS-ick)* section, which runs to just about the level of your waist. The *lumbar (LUMM-bar)* level comes next and coincides with your lower back. And last but not least is the *sacral (SAY-crull)* part, down around your seat and tailbone. (See Figure 34.2)

There are eight pairs of nerves and seven vertebrae in the cervical section of your spine. In this case, the nerves numbered C1 through C7 are above the corresponding numbered vertebrae. C8 then slips through between the C7 and T1 bones.

For the thoracic and lumbar sections, each of the numbered nerves lies below the corresponding numbered vertebra. There are 12 thoracic vertebrae and 5 lumbar vertebrae.

At the lower end of your spinal cord (below the second lumbar vertebra), the nerves coming out do not match up exactly with the bones in your back. This is because the spinal cord itself ends much higher than where your tailbone marks the lower end of your backbone.

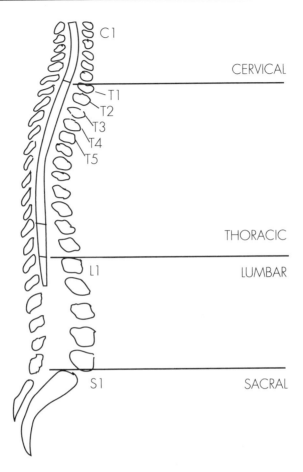

Figure 34.2. *The spinal cord.*

This makes the lower lumbar and sacral nerves look like a horse's tail inside the spinal column. It is known as the *cauda equina (CODD-ah eh-QUINE-ah)*, which means "horse's tail" in Latin.

Your sacral section is really only one piece of bone with five nerve pairs coming out through holes in it.

What the Spinal Cord Does

The spinal cord is the communicating link between the *spinal nerves* and the brain. The nerves that lie only within the spinal cord itself are called *upper motor neurons (UMNs)*. These run only between

325

the brain and the spinal nerves. The spinal nerves branch out from the spinal cord into the tissues of your body. Spinal nerves are also called *lower motor neurons (LMNs)*. (See Figure 34.3)

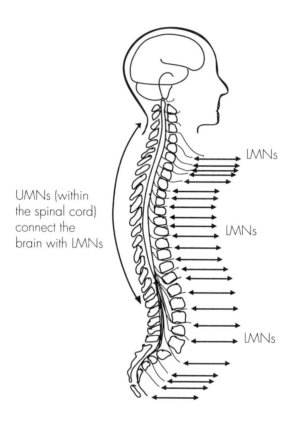

Figure 34.3. *LMNs connect the spinal cord (UMNs) with muscles, blood vessels, glands, organs, etc.*

In movement, the brain sends messages through the spinal cord (UMNs) to the spinal nerves (LMNs). The LMNs then carry these messages to the muscles to coordinate complicated movements such as walking. In this way, the brain can influence movement.

In sensation, information is collected by the LMNs and sent up the spinal cord to the brain. This allows conscious awareness of feelings such as heat or cold.

You may wonder how the spinal cord keeps these messages from getting confused, what with all the running back and forth between

brain and body. The LMNs and the UMNs carry messages in different nerve fibers.

Within the cord itself, the UMN nerve fibers are combined into
spinal tracts. Each tract carries messages one way, either up or down.
They are similar to the lanes on a freeway. (See Figure 34.4)

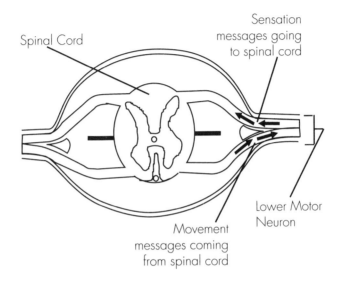

Spinal Cord

Sensation
messages going
to spinal cord

Lower Motor
Neuron

Movement
messages coming
from spinal cord

Figure 34.4.

What Is an LMN and What Does It Do?

Each LMN, or spinal nerve, has two main parts: One part carries
information related to movement from the spinal cord to the muscles.
It is called the *motor* portion of the nerve. Each motor portion of a
spinal nerve connects to a specific muscle group. Each level of the
spinal cord causes movement in a corresponding group of muscles.

The other part of the LMN carries messages of feeling, such as heat
and cold, from the body to the spinal cord. It is called the sensory
portion of the nerve.

Different types of sensation or feeling are carried up the spinal cord
to the brain. These include pain, touch, heat, cold, vibration, pressure,
and knowing where a body part is located in space without looking
at it.

Each sensory portion of the spinal nerve collects information about feelings from a given area of skin. Each area is called a *dermatome (DER-muh-tome)* and matches a specific spinal cord level. See the map of dermatomes (Figure 34.5).

You might want to make your own map of dermatome sensation using the blank map (Figure 34.6). Color in the sections where you have feeling. See if the map can tell you your level of injury.

Spinal Cord Injury (SCI)

A spinal cord injury is often caused by the movement of vertebrae. When bones in your back and neck are broken or when ligaments are torn, the spinal cord can get caught between two vertebrae. Sometimes stab wounds or gunshot wounds can damage the cord without breaking bones.

Damage to your spinal cord can cause changes in your movement, feeling, bladder control, or other bodily functions. How many changes there are depends on where your spinal cord was injured. The main problem is that the connection between your brain and the parts of your body below the injury is impaired.

A numbering system is used to name levels of injury. It is the same as the system used to name bone and nerve levels in your back. A spinal cord injury is named for the lowest level of the spinal cord that still functions the way it did before your injury. It becomes very important to your rehabilitation that you know your level of injury and, more importantly, how it affects your body.

The Difference Between Complete and Incomplete Injuries

When there is no voluntary movement (spasms don't count—they are involuntary) or feeling below your spinal cord injury level, you have a *complete injury*.

If you do have some feeling or voluntary movement below your injury, you have an *incomplete injury*. This happens when there is only partial damage to your spinal cord.

Upper Motor Neuron (UMN) and Lower Motor Neuron (LMN) Injuries

Earlier in this chapter, we discussed the difference between upper motor neurons (UMNs) and lower motor neurons (LMNs). This section will tell you why it is important that you know this.

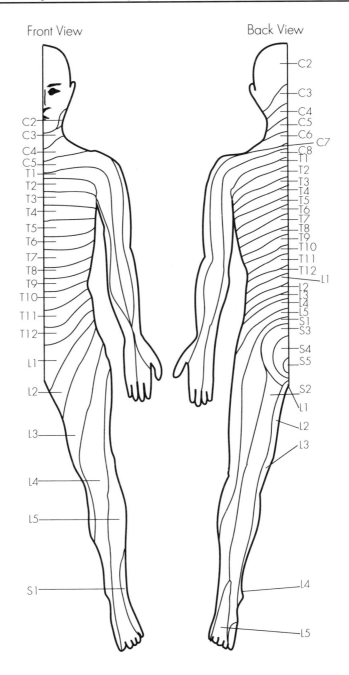

Front View

Back View

Figure 34.5.

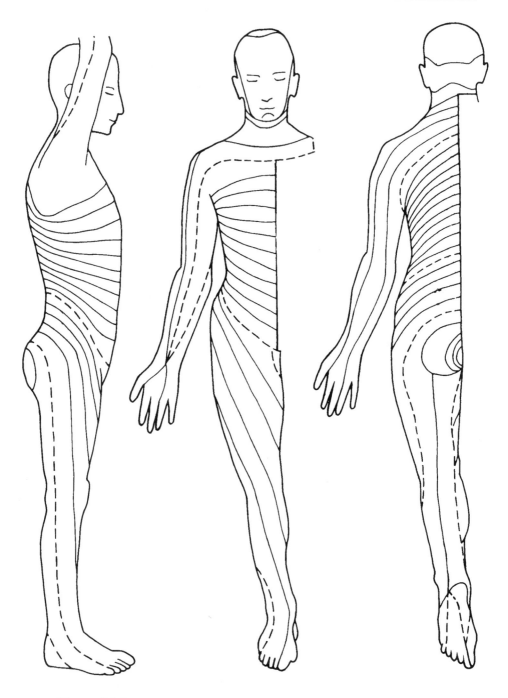

Figure 34.6.

Most spinal injuries damage UMNs and LMNs. A complete injury cuts right across all the UMNs running up and down the spinal cord. This disrupts the connection between the brain and the parts of the body below the injury. On the other hand, only the LMNs *right at the level* of injury are damaged. Because they are in charge of reflex actions, only a small portion of those reflexes (governed by the LMNs at the level of injury) are lost. All other reflexes, above and below the level of injury, are still in working order. This is a *UMN injury*. (See Figure 34.7)

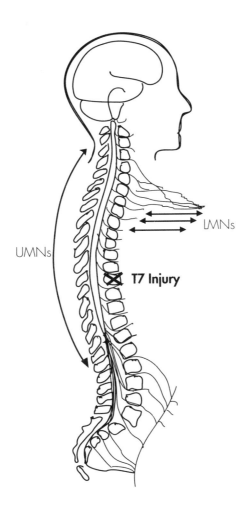

Figure 34.7. *Upper motor neuron injury.*

The reflex action that the LMNs carry out below the level of injury may still work, but there is one problem. In reflexes, the brain keeps control on how much your nerves react. In an UMN injury, control by the brain no longer exists because messages from the brain can't get through the point of injury. The LMNs act by themselves, causing reflexes without limit. One example is *spasticity (spa-STI-si-ti)*. *Spasticity* is the uncontrolled movement of your arms or legs.

LMN injuries are a different story. This kind of injury is found for the most part at the lower tip of the spinal cord, or the cauda equina. Damage to the cauda equina impairs reflex actions. This is because the cauda equina is made up entirely of LMNs. Other LMNs above the injury are still in good shape. (See Figure 34.8)

Spasticity is not found in LMN injuries as it is in UMN injuries, because muscles governed by these LMNs tend to shrink or *atrophy (AT-row-fee)*. This is because they do not have any direct nerve contact to stimulate them.

Stated simply, a *UMN injury* is one where the UMN pathway is broken and the only LMNs that get damaged are at the site of injury. An *LMN injury*, usually at the cauda equina, breaks the connection of the LMNs to the spinal cord. It will be very important for you to know which type of injury you have, because how your spinal cord injury is managed will differ depending on that fact.

Recovery

Right after your injury occurs, your spinal cord stops doing its job during a period of time called "spinal shock." All the reflexes below your level of injury are absent during this period of several weeks or months. Usually, the return of reflexes below the level of injury marks the end of spinal shock. At this time, your doctor can determine if you have a complete or an incomplete injury.

If you have an incomplete injury, some feelings and movement may come back. *Will this happen to you?* No one can say. If you do regain some feeling and movement, it will likely start in the first few weeks after your injury.

Rehabilitation begins immediately. You will be instructed in strengthening exercises, new styles of movement, and the use of special equipment to work with what you have. If you do get additional recovery of feeling or movement, your rehabilitation team will develop new goals with you.

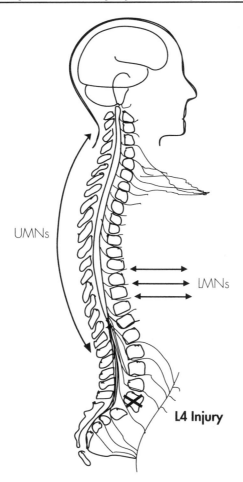

UMNs

LMNs

L4 Injury

Figure 34.8. *Lower motor neuron injury.*

Educational Materials Available

The goal of the Paralyzed Veterans of Americans Spinal Cord Injury Education and Training Foundation (ETF) is to enhance the quality of life for people with spinal cord injury and/or disease. To that end, the following items have been produced.

Inform Yourself: Alcohol, Drugs, and Spinal Cord Injury

This resource guide will help individuals with a spinal cord injury, their families and caregivers to understand the health consequences and safety issues associated with alcohol and drug use. The guide offers up-to-date, pertinent research and resource information to assist in identifying, assessing and seeking help.

Available From:
Novation, Inc.
2165 Bunker Hill Drive
San Mateo, CA 94402
(415) 578-8047

Audience: Consumers, families, caregivers, health-care professionals
Price: $10.00

National Database of Educational Resources on Spinal Cord Injury

This comprehensive database serves as a central information resource and retrieval center for disseminating information on such topics as, but not limited to, rehabilitation management, psychosocial-vocational management, sexuality, equipment and recreation. You can write or call to receive a free list of materials available on the topic you're interested in.

Available From:
The Institute for Rehabilitation and Research
1333 Moursund
Houston, TX 77030-3405
(713) 797-5945

Audience: Consumers, families, health-care professionals
Price: Free

The Economic Consequences of Traumatic Spinal Cord Injury

This 200-page book provides an understanding of the demographics and economics of living with SCI. The book is the first comprehensive analysis of who becomes spinal cord injured and of occupational data before and after SCI, including its impact on lifestyles and career goals.

Available From:
Demos Publications
386 Park Avenue South
Suite 201
New York, NY 10016
(212) 683-0072

Audience: Consumers, professionals, policy-makers
Price: $59.95

Reducing Risks to Secondary Conditions

The booklets in this series address prevention and management of secondary conditions affecting individuals with spinal cord injury and other sensory/motor disabilities. The booklets offer references and suggest prevention or treatment techniques in an easy-to-read format. Available in English or Spanish. The topics are:

- Urinary Tract Infections
- Pressure Sores
- Chronic Pain Management
- Chronic Fatigue
- Joint Pain
- SCI and Aging
- Spasticity

Available From:
The Research and Training Center on Independent Living
University of Kansas, Life Span Institute
4089 Dole
Lawrence, KS 66034-2930
(913) 864-4095

Audience: Consumers, caregivers, health-care professionals
Price: $2.50 (each)

Sexuality Reborn

This 48-minute video is intended to supplement discussions and educational sessions about sexuality after spinal cord injury. Designed to illustrate sexuality issues in SCI through a discussion of social, psychological and emotional concerns.

Available From:
Sexuality Reborn
Kessler Institute for Rehabilitation
Education Department
1199 Pleasant Valley Way
West Orange, NJ 07052
(800) 435-8866

Audience: Consumers, families, health-care professionals
Price: $39.95
Shipping/Handling: $8.00

Handbook on Sexuality for People with SCI

This handbook is to insure that all men and women with spinal cord injury have available, up-to-date information on sexuality, fertility and parenting. Designed to be easily understood by consumers, the book will serve as an authoritative reference on sexuality and spinal cord injury.

Available—Spring 1996
Audience: Consumers, families, health-care professionals

Yes, You Can! A Guide to Self-Care for Persons with Spinal Cord Injury 2nd Edition

This 161-page manual provides comprehensive and easy-to-read practical knowledge on a large number of medical, psychological, social and vocational issues for people with spinal cord injury or disease. Available in English or Spanish.

Available From: PVA
Audience: Consumers, families, health-care professionals
Price: $9.50
Shipping/Handling: $2.50

Resource Guide on Functional Electrical Stimulation (FES)

This comprehensive guide will provide a list of FES programs and providers and illustrate the state of the art in electrotherapy and FES for people with spinal cord injury or multiple sclerosis.

Available From:
University Bookstore
Case Western Reserve University
10900 Euclid Ave.
Cleveland, OH 44106
(216) 368-1656
(800) 666-2353

Audience: Consumers, families, health-care professionals
Price: $13.35
Shipping/Handling: $2.00

Conditioning with Physical Disabilities

This book provides easy and safe exercises for people with all levels
and classifications of physical disabilities. It contains step-by-step
descriptions and more than 250 illustrations/pictures.

Available From:
Rehabilitation Institute of Chicago
Education and Training Dissemination
345 East Superior Street
Chicago, IL 60611
(312) 908-6000

Audience: Consumers, families, health-care professionals
Price: $22.95
Shipping/Handling: $3.00

A Guide to Wheelchair Selection: How to Use the ANSI/ RESNA Wheelchair Standards to Buy a Wheelchair

This book provides an incredible amount of useful information on wheelchair standards and test procedure in a well-organized, consumer-
friendly format. By explaining how to use the information disclosed
by wheelchair test procedures, the book can help wheelchair users be
more involved when selecting their next wheelchair.

Available From: PVA
Audience: Consumers, families, health-care providers.
Price: $12.00

Rebecca Finds a New Way—intended for children under 10 years old

Follow Your Dreams—intended for children 11-13 years old

The two books are designed for and about children with a spinal cord injury or disease. These books help children foster their own coping devices by understanding the variety of reactions they might receive due to their injuries. In addition, it assists with personal relationships and integration into the community, which will enable them to learn, play and live productively with a spinal cord injury.

Available From:
National Spinal Cord Injury Association
545 Concord Avenue
Suite 29
Cambridge, MA 02138
(800) 962-9629

Audience: Young consumers, families
Price: Free
Shipping/Handling: $3.00

The Challenges of Working with the Spinal Cord Injured

This manual includes 16 teaching modules (including slides) and is designed to provide health-care professionals with a basic knowledge of spinal cord injury management. The modules include teaching objectives, methodologies, presentation formats and evaluation instruments.

2nd Edition Available Spring 1996

Take Control—A Multimedia Guide to Self-Care for Persons with SCI

This is an innovative, self-paced, interactive computer module that mixes video, animation, graphics, photographs and sound to teach people with SCI, their families and health-care providers about SCI. The program will be available on multiple computer operating systems. People with a wide range of impairments will be able to independently use the program.

338

Available Summer 1996
Audience: Consumers, families, care-givers, health care professionals

An Introduction to Spinal Cord Injury: Understanding the Changes

This booklet provides basic information about spinal cord injury, suggests reading materials and has a glossary. Available in English or Spanish.

Available From: PVA
Audience: Consumers, families, health-care professionals
Price: First copy free. additional copies $1.50

The Quest for Cure: Restoring Function After Spinal Cord Injury

This unique 200-page book explains the complexity of spinal cord injury and the scientific theories that may lead to treatments to help restore function. *The Quest for Cure* gives readers a comprehensive understanding of the neuroscience involved in spinal cord research in clear and understandable language.

Available From: PVA
Audience: Consumers, families, health-care professionals
Price: $22.45

Ordering Information

Call or write directly to the organization the item you want is available from. **To order those items available from PVA only**—send your request and a check made payable to "Paralyzed Veterans of America" to:

Paralyzed Veterans of America
Office Services
801 Eighteenth Street, NW
Washington, DC 20006

For quantity rates, please call (800) 424-8200 ext. 609

Chapter 35

Psychosocial Adjustment to a Spinal Cord Injury

The first section of this chapter is primarily directed toward the newly injured individual. It discusses various reactions to disability and provides insights into adjustment. However, the "not-so-new" spinal cord injured person may enjoy reading this section too. You may find yourself reflecting on the early days after your own injury and re-examining the way you relate to spinal cord injury. In addition, this section provides useful information about assertiveness training, stress management, relaxation training, time management, and setting priorities in your life. These are areas *everyone* can benefit from whether they have spinal cord injuries or not.

Having a disability, such as a spinal cord injury, produces lots of questions about who you are; who you want to be; how other persons, including your family, will interact with you; and how you live your life as a person with a disability. This chapter will offer some ideas and suggestions on ways to think about these personal questions. Unlike questions about your physical needs, personal and social questions have no exact answers or procedures to follow. What you decide to do with your personal and social life is up to you. Since some of these issues are difficult, this chapter will try to offer you some help.

Excerpted from *Yes, You Can: A Guide to Self-Care for Persons with Spinal Cord Injury*, copyright 1989, Paralyzed Veterans of America (PVA); reprinted with permission. For information on how to obtain a complete copy of this manual or receive a list of other available resources contact the PVA at 1-800-424-8200.

In addition, this chapter includes information about independent living and your legal rights as a person with a disability. General self-improvement and civil rights books have made lots of nondisabled authors very rich, so you know these must be important topics! If questions regarding personal or family concerns come to mind, remember that you can talk to your social worker, psychologist, or other team member.

You Are Still the Same Person

Becoming spinal cord injured was probably the worst thing that has ever happened to YOU. YOU cannot change what has happened, leave it behind, or ignore it. One way or another, YOU have to deal with it. It's not easy.

To make a very important point, we've purposely emphasized the word YOU in the above paragraph. Many people each year are involved in accidents that result in spinal cord injury. Everyone is unique, and this does not change after injury.

There are many life experiences all rolled together that make you who you are and that is not going to change just because you may have to use a wheelchair now instead of legs for getting around. To put it another way, there is no reason to assume that your personality, intelligence, style of interacting with other people, and other personal traits will change as a result of injury. If you were smart, friendly, obnoxious, hard-to-get-along-with, finicky, argumentative, bossy, or goal-oriented before your injury, chances are very good that you will be the same way after injury.

Don't be surprised, however, if you experience feelings such as intense sadness, frustration, and anger. These are normal human reactions that can occur in response to unfortunate things that happen to you. This is very common after injury and will lessen with time and new learning experiences. Tips on how to deal with these and other feelings and reactions are provided next.

Examining Your Feelings Toward Disabilities

It's often said that one of the hardest things about coping with abrupt onset of disability is that you're suddenly thrust into it with all your able-bodied beliefs, attitudes, and misconceptions.

Do you know any people with disabilities? Are any friends or family members disabled? How about fellow employees or fellow students?

If you have known someone well, you have probably discovered that the disability gradually seemed less important as the relationship grew. First impressions or initial attitudes are not always accurate, and they may change over time.

Many people have varying attitudes and impressions that show how they feel about people with disabilities. You may discover that you possess some of these beliefs as well, especially if your association with people with disabilities has been very limited or nonexistent. What are some common attitudes toward or first impressions about people with *obvious* physical disabilities? Here are some examples:

- Pity or sympathy for the individual, which often results in a condescending or patronizing attitude.

- Personal discomfort, anxiety, or fear of being around the individual with a disability. Therefore, such a person is actively avoided.

- Assumed cognitive/mental impairment because of physical disability.

- Assumed dependency because of physical disability.

- Assumed "second class" citizen status. Therefore, people with disabilities may not be included in many activities or functions of their communities, or they may not be treated with equal respect by others.

- Unearned praise of the individuals because they are "so brave" or "have coped so well."

However, your attitudes about yourself and the attitudes of others (family, friends, and even strangers) can change. But beliefs do not change overnight. This is a gradual process that occurs with new learning and behaving. You may find that you are a "student" in the rehabilitation facility and a "teacher" on the outside who helps others to reassess their attitudes about physical disability.

The Art of Living

Each individual has a unique way of responding to major changes in lifestyle. How you respond to having a spinal cord injury is very personal and involves a wide variety of thoughts and feelings. Not everyone has the same experiences, but sometimes it helps to know that there are some problems that others have had to face. Others have found useful ways to cope with those problems, and these are available to you.

As mentioned earlier in this manual, it is important to consider "who you are." Some people prefer to ignore personal problems, others like to talk all the time, and others may want to call their favorite talk-show host or write to "Dear Abby" for advice. There are many ways to respond to personal needs and concerns. Most important, whether you read a book, talk with a friend, go to an educational group, or seek professional counseling, it is essential to choose what is best for YOU.

Why Me?

Almost all patients go through a "why me?" phase when they are first injured. They ask themselves questions like, "Why did this happen to me?" "I always treated everyone fairly and did what I thought was right! So, why have I been singled out for this unfortunate thing to happen?" Or you may be saying, "I am being punished for all the wrongs I have done before my injury." Some patients bargain: "I promise to lead a good life from now on, if only I can be allowed to walk again." A very good book by Harold S. Kushner, *When Bad Things Happen to Good People*, describes these feelings in more depth.

Regardless of what conclusions you come to about why you were injured, you must reach some sort of conclusion and psychologically put the issue aside and look toward the future.

Different people accept change at different speeds. The process of accepting change is often called the "adjustment period." It is very difficult to estimate how long it will take you to adjust to your new lifestyle after being injured. What is important to you right after injury may not be as important later on in your life. The following example may help describe this process.

Imagine yourself learning to fly an airplane. Early on, you must learn a great deal of technical information and how to operate new, unfamiliar equipment. When you first sit in the cockpit, your attention is focused on the dials, levers, gadgets, and switches on the panels in front of you. After some basic training and practice, you will progress to the point at which you can fly to a given destination and not focus all your attention on gadgets or equipment. These things move to the background, and your attention is focused on the open sky beyond.

A similar process occurs after spinal cord injury. You first learn technical information about how your body works and how to operate new equipment like braces, wheelchairs, catheters, etc. After training and practice, you begin to focus your attention on other parts of your life.

The speed of your adjustment is greatly influenced by your philosophical attitude toward life. Some people's attitudes toward living are very flexible. They take each day as it comes. Others, though, are more rigid and have their lives planned for years to come. Their plans do not, of course, include a spinal injury. A good clue as to the progress of your adjustment is when you start thinking and verbalizing such statements as, "I wonder what the future holds for me?" or "I would like to know what kind of work I could be trained to do with the amount of function I still have?" or "In what direction am I headed now?"

Believe it or not, there is a positive side. Patients who have been injured for some years have said: "Life is richer for me now than it was before I became injured because I have slowed down. I have done much soul-searching in adjusting to my injury, and as a result, I have become a more mature and appreciative person. I am able to appreciate and admire things and qualities that in the past I would have missed." No one chooses to have a spinal cord injury, but as with most things in life, there is another side of the coin.

"Normal" Feelings

It is important to keep in mind that the personal and psychological issues you face will, over time, be less focused on your injury and have more to do with everyday life. The following discussion of feelings applies to emotions of crisis (right after your injury) as well as emotions that may come and go throughout your life. It is normal for people to experience a wide range of feelings after a major crisis. *Anger, sadness, frustration, irritation, confusion, and isolation* are common. How *you* feel is probably different from how others may feel. However, some people like to know that others have similar feelings. This section will discuss what you can do to help yourself in dealing with the emotional reactions you experience. Not all those emotions are going to be uncomfortable ones! The process of rehabilitation also involves *humor, pride, hope, and a sense of accomplishment.*

Anger

If you find yourself snapping at others, yelling when things go wrong or "boiling over" most of the time, know that many people experience anger. However, it may become difficult for you to work with others if that anger carries over into everything you do. A good test is to ask yourself: "Would I like to be treated the way I treat others?" If the answer is "No," ask yourself: "*Who or what is getting in my way? Why am I angry?*"

This kind of self-talk can help you step back from a problem, cool off, and develop a positive plan of action. Also, ask others to help you stay calm by talking about problems openly, rather than letting something build up to the boiling point and exploding in anger.

Humor

When was the last time you had a good, long, belly shaking laugh? It seems that this type of "therapy" is often overlooked or discounted, especially when you are in the hospital. Recent medical writers have discussed the positive effect that laughing has upon both mental and physical health. Norman Cousins, author of *Anatomy of an Illness*, discusses how he has used joke books, funny movies, and other forms of humor to help improve his ability to combat illness. Certainly, laughing is no "cure," but it can help you deal with difficult problems, and it usually sets up a positive mood.

Some suggestions to help you find humor are:

- Spend more time with friends who make you laugh.
- Go to a bookstore and look at joke books or humorous notecards.
- Read newspaper comics or comic books.
- Rent a video recorder (with some friends) and watch a funny movie.
- Start a joke contest.

Sadness

It is very common for someone to feel intense sadness after a major loss or significant change in health. This is similar to the grief you might feel when someone close to you has died. Some people express this sadness with tears, withdrawal, avoidance of the "usual routine," or talking about the sad feelings with a close friend. These are normal, common reactions. However, when these feelings seem to be overwhelming, persistent, or hopeless, you should consider getting help in dealing with your sadness. The main differences between *grief* and *significant depression* are that depression is often accompanied by hopelessness, a sense of "giving up," physical exhaustion, trouble sleeping, and a change in appetite. Try talking to someone close, thinking about something positive in your future, or maybe setting out to do something enjoyable (like listening to a concert, having a special dessert, or reading a good book). If you feel like "it's not worth trying," then talk with a member of your rehab team about those feelings. You can get some help.

Pride

How you feel about yourself is very important, especially in a rehabilitation setting. It influences how you look, talk, and act. Think of someone you know who is very proud and confident (not false pride). How do they look and act? When you feel good about yourself, other people will know because you care enough to groom well and present yourself nicely to others. This feeling starts when you tell yourself: "I am worthwhile as a person." Sure, you have faults, but you have some unique qualities as a person. You can learn to feel good about those qualities and that will begin to help you improve your sense of pride. A recent book called *A New Guide to Rational Living* by Albert Ellis and Robert Harper describes specific ways of improving and maintaining a positive sense of self-esteem and pride.

Frustration/Confusion

Having to try new ways of doing things can be both frustrating and confusing. First, try to identify the source of frustration. If you can identify a person, talk with that person about the problem as openly as you can. *Clear communication helps!* If talking about things makes you more upset, ask for a "third party" to help out or try to use some relaxation activities (mentioned later in this section) before you talk. *Being calm and relaxed can help!*

Sometimes you can identify why you are frustrated, but you can't figure out how to improve or change it. *Ask for help!* Another person can help you "brainstorm," which may lead to a solution, or you may find a way to stay relaxed in the face of some very frustrating situations.

Learn to Let Others Know What You Need Without Being Rude

Many times, people feel upset, angry, and frustrated when they miss out on something they want. This section focuses on learning how to achieve certain things without hurting or stomping on others. This involves being assertive, *without being nasty or aggressive.*

There will be times when you need to ask for assistance with something you cannot accomplish on your own, or you may need to let someone else know they are doing something that *really* bothers you. Also, recent research has shown that people with spinal cord injuries often need to take the extra step in making some able-bodied persons feel comfortable when talking to someone in a wheelchair. This often helps to set the stage for positive communication.

The following discussion will focus on three basic communication styles: *assertion, aggression, and passivity.*

The general style will be described, followed by descriptions of specific *behaviors* that are typical of each style. Notice that these are *behaviors*, not words. It is how you say something (body language, tone of voice, etc.) that is important, not necessarily the *words* you use.

Assertion

Assertion involves standing up for your own personal rights. Express your ideas and feelings directly and honestly, but take into account other people's feelings, too. This involves respect—respect for yourself *and* respect for other people. To do this requires that you communicate clearly *and* that you ask what others might think and feel. In other words, cooperation and fair play are essential to being assertive.

In assertive behavior, your body actions are consistent with the verbal messages and add support, strength, and emphasis to what is being said verbally. The voice is appropriately loud to the situation; eye contact is firm, but not a stare-down; body gestures that denote strength are used; and the speech pattern is fluent—without awkward pauses—expressive, clear, and with emphasis on key words.

Aggression

Aggression involves standing up for your personal rights, but in a way that ignores others' rights. This is not an honest way to communicate.

348

It is almost always inappropriate and may create strong, negative feelings, such as anger or disgust.

The usual goal of aggression is domination and winning, forcing the other person to lose. Winning is insured by humiliating, degrading, belittling, or overpowering other people so that they become weaker and less able to express and defend their needs and rights. The basic message is: This is what I think—you're wrong for believing differently. This is what I want—what you want isn't important. This is what I feel—your feelings don't count.

In aggressive behavior, the nonverbal behaviors are ones that dominate or demean the other person. These include eye contact that tries to stare down and dominate the other person, a forceful voice that does not fit the situation, sarcastic or condescending tone of voice, and parental body gestures such as excessive finger pointing.

Passivity

Passivity involves violating your own rights by failing to express honest feelings, thoughts, and beliefs. Expressing your thoughts and feelings in such an apologetic, self-defeating style may allow others to easily disregard you. The total message communicated is: I don't count—you can take advantage of me. My feelings don't matter—only yours do. My thoughts aren't important—yours are the only ones worth listening to. I'm nothing—you are superior.

Passivity is nonassertion and shows a lack of respect for your own needs. It also shows a subtle lack of respect for another person's ability to take disappointments or to shoulder some responsibility. The goal of nonassertion is to appease others and to avoid conflict at any cost.

In nonassertive behavior, the nonverbal behaviors include avoiding eye contact, hand wringing, clutching the other person, stepping back from the other person as an assertive remark is made, hunching the shoulders, covering the mouth with a hand, nervous gestures that distract the listener from what the speaker is saying, and wooden body posture. The voice tone may be singsong or overly soft. The speech pattern is hesitant and filled with pauses, and the throat may be cleared frequently. Facial gestures may include raising of the eyebrows, laughs, and winks when expressing anger.

In general, the nonassertive gestures are ones that convey weakness, anxiety, pleading, or a self "put-down." They reduce the impact of what is being said verbally, which is precisely why people who are scared of acting assertively use them. Their goal is to "soften" what they're saying so that the other person will not be offended.

Relaxing in This Stressful World

Frequently, it seems there are too many things going on around you and no way to deal with all the daily hassles. Although no one can eliminate stress from your life, there are some ways of reducing the impact stress can have on your health. A great many health problems are directly linked to the strains of muscle tension, increased blood pressure, and increased heart rate that usually come along with stressful activities. Many people with spinal cord injuries say they find that the *initial* demands of rehabilitation are stressful. But even most able-bodied people you talk to will say that their days are often busy and stressful. This section offers two specific methods of dealing with stress: relaxation techniques and time management skills.

Progressive Relaxation

You cannot have the feeling of warm well-being in your body and at the same time experience psychological stress. Progressive relaxation of your muscles reduces pulse rate and blood pressure as well as decreasing perspiration and breathing rates. Deep muscle relaxation, when successfully mastered, can be used as an "anti-anxiety" pill.

Most people do not realize which of their muscles are chronically tense. Progressive relaxation provides a way of identifying particular muscles and muscle groups and learning the difference between tension and relaxation.

The following is a procedure for achieving deep muscle relaxation quickly. Whole muscle groups are simultaneously tensed and then relaxed. You may not be able to complete all the muscle movements, but do what you can. Repeat each procedure at least once, tensing each muscle group from five to seven seconds and then relaxing from 20 to 30 seconds. Remember to notice the contrast between the sensations of tension and relaxation. Try these exercises in a comfortable position (such as in a sitting position with your head supported), and practice at least twice a day until you have mastered these exercises.

1. Curl both fists, tightening biceps and forearms, pulling your fist toward your shoulder. Relax. Allow your arms to rest at your side.

2. Wrinkle up your forehead. At the same time, press your head as far back as possible, roll it clockwise in a complete circle, then reverse. Now wrinkle up the muscles of your face like a walnut: frowning, eyes squinted, lips pursed, tongue pressing the roof of the mouth, and shoulders hunched. Relax.

3. Straighten your back as you take a deep breath into the chest. Hold. Relax. Take a deep breath, pressing out the stomach. Hold. Relax.

Special Considerations

1. Since some of the actions require neck and back movement, you need to get clearance from your doctor.

2. You may want to make a cassette tape of the basic procedure to improve your relaxation program. Remember to space each procedure so that time is allowed to experience the tension and relaxation before going on to the next muscle or muscle group.

3. Most people have somewhat limited success when they begin deep muscle relaxation, but it is only a matter of practice. Although 20 minutes of work might initially bring only partial relaxation, it will eventually be possible to relax your whole body in a few moments.

4. In the beginning, it may seem to you as though relaxation is complete. But although the muscle or muscle group may well be partially relaxed, a certain number of muscle fibers will still be contracted. Relaxing these additional fibers will bring about the emotional effects you want. It is helpful to say to yourself during the relaxation phase, "Let go more and more." Also, focus on deep breathing when you relax.

Time Management

This is another important way to deal with stress. When you leave the hospital after a recent injury, you will no longer have a staff member to help schedule your activities. For those of you working or returning to work for the first time after your injury, it is essential to develop skills in planning your daily routine. Parts of the following discussion were taken from *The Relaxation & Stress Reduction Workbook*, by Martha Davis, Elizabeth Eshelman, and Mathew McCay.

Time can be thought of as an endless series of decisions, small and large, that gradually change the shape of your life. Inappropriate decisions produce frustration, lowered self-esteem, and stress. They result in the six symptoms of poor time management:

1. Rushing.
2. Always being caught in the middle of unpleasant alternatives.
3. Fatigue or listlessness with many slack hours of nonproductive activity.
4. Constantly missed deadlines.
5. Insufficient time for rest or personal relationships.
6. The sense of being overwhelmed by demands and detail and having to do what you do not want to do most of the time.

Time management techniques for relieving these symptoms have been developed by management consultants and efficiency experts who teach busy people to streamline their lives. Alan Lakein, who wrote *How to Get Control of Your Time and Your Life*, sees himself as a "time planning and life goals consultant." Many therapists, such as Harold Greenwald (author of *Direct Decision Therapy*), have also contributed to time management theory by developing techniques for facing and clarifying decision-making.

All methods of time management can be reduced to three steps:

1. You can establish priorities that highlight your most important goals and that allow you to base your decisions on what is important and what is not.

2. You can create time by realistic scheduling and the elimination of low-priority tasks.

3. You can learn to make basic decisions.

Before examining the three steps to effective time management, it will be useful to explore how you really spend your time. An easy way to do this is to divide up your day into three segments:

1. From waking through lunch.
2. From the end of lunch through dinner, and
3. From the end of dinner until going to sleep.

Carry a small notebook with you, and at the end of each segment (after lunch, after dinner, in bed just before sleep), write down every activity you engaged in. Note the amount of time each one took. The total amount of time for all activities should be fairly close to the total number of hours you were awake.

Unless you are particularly interested in improving time utilization at work, simply describe work activity as socializing, routine tasks, low-priority work, productive work, meetings, and telephone calls.

Keep this time inventory for three days. At the end of three days, note the total amount of time spent in each of the categories. If you wish, you can divide by three to get the average daily time for each activity. You can also order the categories from the most- to the least-time consuming to get a rough picture of your current obligations.

You should modify or add categories to suit yourself. You might wish to distinguish between conversation at home with intimates and talk at social gatherings or between shopping for pleasure and shopping for necessities. You may want to have specific categories for your daily self-care activities or just a general "hygiene" category. You might want to break down household chores into several categories. The important thing is to separate and examine categories of time use, and then determine if you want to spend more or less time engaged in each of these activities.

Setting Priorities

Having made your own time inventory, you can begin to compare your current use of time to important goals.

What did you want to accomplish in your life, what are you most proud of, and what might you most regret? Limber up your imagination and put anything down that comes to mind. Don't think about it or analyze it—if something occurs to you, write it down. Distill what you have written into your long-range goals.

Second, make a list of your one-year goals that stand a reasonable chance of being accomplished. Finally, put down all your goals for the coming month, including work priorities, improvement schemes, recreational activities, etc.

You have created three lists of goals: long-, medium-, and short-range. Each list can be prioritized by deciding which are the top-, middle-, and bottom-drawer items:

1. Top drawer: those items ranked most essential, most desired.

2. Middle drawer: those items that could be put off for a while but that are still important.

3. Bottom drawer: those items that could easily be put off indefinitely with no harm done.

Breaking Priorities Down into Manageable Steps

Now it is time to break down the top-drawer items into manageable steps that can be easily accomplished.

You have goals to work on. They are your top priorities. Give them a month. Next month you will make a new list. Some goals will remain top drawer, others will drop off. The goals will always be accompanied by a list of specific steps. Set aside a certain time period each day to work on your top-drawer goals. Emphasize results rather than activity. Try to accomplish one step toward your goal each day, no matter how small that step may be.

If you are a very busy person or one who finds it hard to keep focused on top-drawer items, you will need a daily "to-do" list. The to-do list includes everything you would like to accomplish that day. Each item is rated top, middle, or bottom. If you find yourself doing a bottom-drawer item when some of the tops are not yet finished, you can be almost certain that you are wasting your time. Work your way down. When the top items are completed, get to the middle-drawer tasks. Only when everything else is done should you permit your time to go to the bottom drawer.

You will find that it is often possible to just ignore the bottom items. They may never be missed. In making and following your to-do list, it is useful to be aware of the 80-20 rule. Eighty percent of the value will come from only 20 percent of the items.

It is easy sometimes to let top-drawer goals slip to the back of your mind and say, "Not today. I'll get to it after I get the house cleaned up." One solution to this tendency is to make signs describing your current top-drawer goals and post them conspicuously around the house or office. Every time you look at them you'll be reminded of your priorities.

Making Time

There are four "must" rules and nine optional rules for making time. The four must rules are as follows:

1. *Learn to say "no."* Unless it's your boss who asks, keep away from commitments that force you to spend time on bottom-drawer items. Be prepared to say, "I don't have the time." If you have trouble saying no, see the section in this chapter on assertiveness training.

2. *Banish bottom-drawer items* unless you have completed all higher priority items for the day. Bottom-drawer items can wait.

3. *Build time into your schedule for interruptions,* unforeseen problems, unscheduled events, etc. You can avoid rushing by making reasonable time estimates for activities and then adding on a little extra time for the inevitable problems.

4. *Set aside several periods each day for quiet time.* Arrange it so that you will only be interrupted in an emergency. Focus on deep relaxation, using the techniques presented in this chapter.

Listed below are the nine "optional" rules for making time. Check three of them that would be most helpful to you. Begin the habit of following the rules you have marked right now.

1. Keep a list of short five-minute tasks that you can do any time you are waiting or are "between things."

2. Learn to do two things at once. Organize an important letter in your mind while driving to work, plan dinner while vacuuming.

3. Delegate bottom-drawer tasks. Give them to your children, your secretary, your housecleaner, your mother-in-law.

4. Get up a half hour or an hour earlier.

5. Watch less television.

6. When you have a top-drawer item to do, block off your escape routes:

   - Schedule daydreaming for a later time.
   - Stop socializing.

- Put away the books.
- Put away tiny, unimportant tasks.
- Don't run out for ice cream or other sudden indulgences.
- Forget the errands you could probably do more efficiently later.

7. Cut off nonproductive activities as soon as possible (e.g., socializing on the phone when top-drawer items are begging to be done).

8. Throw away all the mail you possibly can. Scan it once and toss it.

9. Stop perfectionism. Just get it done. Everyone makes mistakes.

Independent Living: Is There Life Beyond the Hospital Walls?

Yes, there is a life beyond the hospital walls, and independent living is a way to approach your day-to-day life in society. Independent living means being in charge of your life and taking responsibility for your actions. Independent living is *how* you live your life, not *where* you live. For example, some people think that being alone in an apartment is independent living. It is independent living only if the person freely chooses that lifestyle based on his or her individual physical, social, and financial needs and on the available resources. For other people, independent living means choosing to reside in a nursing home. In the following paragraph, July Gulliom explains her choice to live in a nursing home.

> "A lot of people seem to feel that if they end up in a nursing home, that's the end of life and they will never see daylight or any of their friends again. One of the facts about a nursing home is that it's one of the most efficient mechanisms for getting an unwieldy body attended to... I have a full-time job and heavy volunteer activities. If I had to devote a lot of time to administering a mini-institution on my own behalf, I wouldn't be able to do what I want to do. I don't choose to spend my time that way....
>
> "The nursing home has a lot of space and a lot of staff, and the economies of scale make a lot of difference when they mean that you're able to come and go as you please. If I arrive at two

*o'clock in the morning, there are people waiting to put me to bed.
I really could not afford to hire someone to sit in my own house
and do that for me."*

How you make decisions about your equipment needs is another
good example of independent living. Some persons prefer to use equipment for assistance with tasks ("high-gadget tolerance"). Other people
like the physical and mental challenge of doing difficult tasks, or they
may prefer to limit their equipment ("low-gadget tolerance") and use
"people" power when they need some help.

Remember: Free choice means making a decision based upon:

- Your needs.
- What you would like to happen.
- The resources available to you.

Social Survival Tactics

A person with a spinal cord injury needs social survival tactics
because:

- You are a member of a minority group in our society.
- You will run into negative stereotypes that people have about
  wheelchair or crutch users.
- You will be noticed by the general public.
- You will be dealing with agencies and bureaucracies more than
  the average American!

Social survival tactics are the tools you use to get the services,
emotional support, and physical help you need. Some tools, such as
the social skills of time management and assertiveness, have already
been discussed. Other tools for survival and independent living include how you think through the social decisions that you face most
frequently. This section will present some ways to solve basic social
questions.

Social Decisions

These decisions are crucial to your physical future. There are no
right answers to these questions. It all depends on personal goals, and
these goals can change throughout your life. Remember that these

decisions are the foundation for your social and emotional survival. Listed below are two important questions.

- Where will I live?
- Will I live alone or with someone?

You Will Need New or Different Social Skills to Get What You Want and Need

Meeting new people after your spinal cord injury is really no different from before your injury. Be yourself, make eye contact, and talk sports, weather, or whatever you used to do.

Once you become aware of the particular social challenges that your disability may create, you will learn how to handle them. There are two major approaches to meeting these challenges. First, decide if you have the necessary basic social and communication skills that everyone needs! Second, decide if you need some special skills for dealing with common reactions to your disability.

These approaches help you think about yourself as a person first and then as a person who happens to have a disability. Many social challenges, such as finding a sexual partner, meeting new people, and wanting to be more assertive, are common to all people! Some challenges, such as having a waitress ask your companion, "What does he want to eat?", are directly related to having a disability. More often than not, the challenges you encounter can be resolved by learning general social skills (assertiveness, how to handle anger). The special skills related to your disability can include how to deal with the nondisabled population.

Be an Effective Communicator

People with disabilities need to understand the thinking and actions of the nondisabled world. At times their actions and reactions are frustrating and difficult to understand. All communication involves two parties, and miscommunication also involves two parties. When an interaction or communication is not working, you need to ask two important questions:

- Am I using my best and most effective communication skills?
- Are the other people miscommunicating out of a lack of understanding or a lack of effective communication skills?

If you are using your best skills, go to question two. If the answer to question two is that the others lack information, then you need to educate them. If they are poor communicators, then it is their problem. People with disabilities often think the actions and words of nondisabled people are cruel and intended to be degrading when in fact, the nondisabled people may just be ignorant, not cruel. They mean well but need suggestions for more helpful ways to interact with persons who happen to have disabilities.

When you are doing your best and things are still not going well, the situation may call for special skills and understanding that relate directly to your disability. For example, you must judge when and how to discuss your disability with new friends and potential employers. These skills are learned by experiencing the situations first hand, consulting other people with disabilities, and by learning (reading) about the stereotypes of the nondisabled population to find effective, useful, and productive ways of overcoming those stereotypes. It is not always an easy task, but being a member of a social minority group often requires that you become a teacher of the general population. You didn't ask for that role, but it does come with your wheelchair, crutches, and other paraphernalia. Learning these skills can result in increased self-determination and self-pride!

You Can Work If You Want to Work

Work is a significant part of our lives. It affects us so profoundly, both socially and psychologically, that many people identify "who they are" by their job titles! The other aspects of their self-description (a father, a husband, an organizer) are often secondary. A job can affect how we perceive our status in society. "Oh, I'm just a _____." It influences the kinds of people with whom we associate. For many of us, our work is our life.

As Tom Jackson puts it in *Guerrilla Tactics in the Job Market*, "The degree of satisfaction which you get from your work directly affects the degree of health and vitality in the rest of your life.... The quality of your work experience directly influences or controls the quality of your life experience. Your work and your life are inseparably related."

Having had a spinal cord injury, you may be asking, "Can I work? What kind of job could I do?" The answer is: *YOU CAN WORK IF YOU WANT TO WORK*. W. Mitchell (who became paraplegic in 1975) says in *Options: Spinal Cord Injury and the Future*, "The way I look at it, before I was paralyzed, there were ten thousand things I could do;

ten thousand things I was capable of doing. Now, there are nine thousand. I can dwell on the one thousand, or concentrate on the nine thousand I have left. And, of course, the joke is that none of us in our lifetime is going to do more than two or three thousand of these things in any event."

If job exploration and continuing your education interests you, you should ask to meet with a vocational rehabilitation specialist.

Family and Friends

When an acute spinal cord injury occurs, those people close to you are most likely to be as emotionally shaken up by your injury as you are. They may feel shock (numbness), disbelief, sadness, and anger as they see you move from surviving your injury through your rehabilitation process.

Their reactions may be quite familiar to you, or they may be very unexpected. You may or may not be able to understand the hows and whys of their reactions and actions. In any case, try to remember that this sudden change for you was just as unexpected and unwanted for them. Give yourself and them some time to adjust and think about all of these changes. Some tips on how to help both you and your family and friends during this time of transition are:

1. Try and talk about how all of you feel. By bringing it out into the open, no one has to guess how everyone else is taking it, especially YOU! They love you, and you love them, and that's not a bad place to start.

2. Since your close friends and family may be afraid to bring up the subject for fear of causing you or them more pain, you may have to start the ball rolling. It will be hard, but it may be best in the long run. Timing is very important, however. Adjustment is a healing process, so trust your gut instinct in dealing with certain issues. If either you or your close ones aren't ready to discuss something, let it go for a little while. There will come a time in the natural course of adjustment when you will both feel right about it.

3. Try not to hide all of your feelings. You don't have to be strong for your family and friends. This only makes it harder for them to talk with you.

4. Also, remember that your family and friends are part of society and may have the same misconceptions and attitudes about people with disabilities. When you're able to, try to talk to them about this. You need to teach them the truth. Soon enough, you'll find them educating their friends and families too!

5. If your family lives close to an SCI center, they may want to attend a family support group. Check the bulletin board for day and time.

6. Sometimes, family and friends go overboard trying to do just about everything for you. For some people with disabilities, this becomes a smothering experience. For others, this is merely what they always expect from their close ones. This type of behavior may be O.K., or it may get tiring for both you and your family and friends.

7. Figure out how and with what you'd like to have help. If your family and friends are doing too much, talk to them about it. Let them know how it makes you feel and why you'd prefer that they not do so much for you.

After living with spinal cord injury for a period of time, the feelings you now have about your injury may be very different from those you experienced when you were first injured. You may be more comfortable with this change in your body and what you need to do to keep it healthy.

As you became more experienced in getting around town (either by car, van, or wheelchair), you may have gained a new sense of freedom as well. These challenges have helped you learn and adapt to this new way of life.

Adapting to life with a spinal cord injury is a unique experience. Each individual does it in his or her own way. Whatever way you have chosen is O.K., as long as it keeps you healthy, both in mind and body.

Your family and friends have also adapted to your spinal cord injury. Many have come to realize that you are still the same person they've always loved except for some physical changes. Unfortunately, a few may not have been able to adjust to the new physical you, no matter how much they love you. Some people just can't. Relationships change in everybody's life, no matter if you're disabled or not! Being a spinal cord injured person is a challenging experience that offers a potential for growth.

Being a Parent

You can be a parent if you decide you can or want to be a parent. Many feelings and a great amount of thinking will contribute to that decision. Common feelings may be uncertainty about your ability to provide the physical care and financial support. Fear may arise about how a child will respond to you now that you are in a wheelchair. You may experience feelings of depression or discouragement that cause you to wonder about caring for another person. Or you may experience great joy and satisfaction as you realize your children need and respond to your caring and attention. You may be surprised how accepting and adaptable children are.

As you review your feelings and thinking, it is good to remember that bringing up children is a tough job and that every parent can feel uncertain at one time or another. Although your injury may change how you physically care for a child, it does not create insurmountable barriers. There are many adaptive tools, techniques, and even books that you can explore. Consult your rehabilitation team members for ideas.

When you are making changes because of a spinal cord injury, your child should be included in the process. If you are absent from the home due to a hospital stay, your children, of whatever age, need to have the absence explained at their level of understanding. You and your children need to know that a physical limitation need not change your relationship. Research has shown no difference in emotional and social development between children whose parents have a spinal cord injury and those who don't.

It is also important to remember that your rights as a parent don't change after a spinal cord injury. Custody of your children or your right to seek adoption cannot be denied solely on the basis of your disability.

Specific Thoughts to Keep in Mind

1. Include your children in your rehabilitation program. Find out about visiting hours and passes out of the hospital with your family.

2. Introduce your children and spouse to other parents with SCI. Have your children talk with their children.

3. Include your children in family meetings in and out of the hospital.

4. Continue the discussions with your children about your injury or related feelings after you leave the hospital. Seek out community counseling services that are recommended by your SCIS social worker or psychologist.

5. You can also work closely with your rehab team members about parenting concerns.

Deciding to Become a Parent

As a first step, you may wish to explore your physical capability to have children. Check with your SCIS urologist and doctors. You may wish to consult with your social worker or psychologist if you are thinking about becoming a parent. If you discover you are physically unable to have children, consider adoption or artificial insemination. Take a look at the chapter on "Sexuality." It may also provide some helpful information about this.

Social and Legal Rights

Exercising Your Legal Rights and Responsibilities

People with SCI are entitled to the same constitutional rights as all other U.S. citizens. In addition, many federal laws support the legal rights of citizens with disabilities in the areas of vocational rehabilitation, education, transportation, accessibility, social and medical services, tax exemptions, and social security benefits. Each individual state has various legal rights that are guaranteed. This section identifies some of the major federal laws and shows how you, the voter and the consumer with disabilities, can exercise your rights in a knowledgeable and responsible way. We will start with some general guidelines on how you can assert your rights and get the best results. Next is a journey through the "Land of Laws" with Sam Citizen in order to learn about the legal process and some specific federal laws.

Be an Assertive Citizen

1. Know your basic rights!

2. Vote.

3. Keep a record of your transactions with agencies and programs. Include the following information:

   • Date.
   • Person(s) to whom you talked.
   • Copies of letters, applications, and other paperwork.
   • A file folder for each agency or program is a good idea.

4. If you think your rights have been violated, ask to talk with a supervisor, the administrator, or the person at that agency in charge of grievances relating to civil rights.

5. Learn the appropriate channels for complaints within the particular agency, local and state governments etc.

6. It is your responsibility to:

   • be assertive, not aggressive.
   • learn the established steps for civil rights complaints.
   • listen.

Major Laws and How They Relate to You

There are a number of laws that exist and work for you. Some of the major ones are listed in Table 35.1.

How these relate to you may make more sense if we take a short trip through the Land of Laws. Let's go!

Land of Laws

Federal and state legislatures are elected and then pass laws that affect the lives of citizens.

After a bill is passed and becomes a law, regulations are written. These regulations state how the laws will be carried out by agencies, businesses, and citizens.

Year	Public Law #	Title of Law	Key Provisions
1968	90-480	Architectural Barriers Act	Requires that buildings built with federal funds or leased by the federal government be made accessible.
1970	91-453	Urban Mass Transportation Act	Requires eligible local jurisdictions to plan and design accessible mass-transportation facilities and services.
1973	93-87	Federal and Highway Act	Requires that transportation facilities receiving federal assistance under the act be made accessible; allows highway funds to be used to make pedestrian crosswalks accessible.
1973	93-112	Rehabilitation Act	Prohibits discrimination against qualified handicapped people in programs, services, and benefits that are federally funded; creates Architectural and Transportation Barriers Compliance Board.
1975	94-173	National Housing Act Amendments	Provides for the removal of barriers in federally supported housing; establishes Office of Independent Living in U.S. Department of Housing and Urban Development to serve disabled people.
1978	95-602	Rehabilitation Comprehensive Services and Developmental Disability Amendments	Establishes independent living as a priority for state vocational rehabilitation programs; provides federal funding for independent-living centers.
1980	96-265	Social Security Disability Amendments	Removes certain disincentives to work by allowing disabled people to deduct independent-living expenses in computing income benefits.
1984	98-435	Voting Accessibility for Elderly and Handicapped Act	Provides for access to polling places and ballots and all activities related to voting.
1986	99-435	Air Carrier Access Act	Prohibits discrimination on the basis of disability in the provision of air transportation.
1988	100-430	Fair Housing Amendments Act	Prohibits policies that discriminate on the basis of disability in housing; requires newly constructed multi-family housing to provide accessible units.
1990	101-336	Americans with Disabilities Act	Extends to people with disabilities civil rights similar to those available through the Civil Rights Act of 1964.

Table 35.1. *The law.*

365

Regulations are the rules of our governmental system and directly affect our daily lives. For example, the regulations issued for the Americans with Disabilities Act (ADA) are detailed requirements that will greatly affect both the public and the private sector. Hardly a person in America will be unaffected by the need to comply with this federal mandate.

When regulations are not properly followed or you think the regulations do not insure the rights that you are guaranteed by law, then you can resort to legal action. The court system is set up to uphold laws and prevent unconstitutional regulations.

Civil Rights for Citizens with Disabilities: Americans with Disabilities Act (ADA)

In 1990, the Americans with Disabilities Act became the most significant piece of civil rights legislation since the mid-60s. The ADA is a comprehensive ban on discrimination against people with disabilities and affects almost all areas of daily life. The five titles of the ADA cover employment, state and local governments, public accommodations, telecommunications, and miscellaneous provisions.

The law itself and regulations issued by five federal agencies are very specific as to certain requirements. The Department of Justice, the Department of Transportation, the Equal Employment Opportunity Commission, the Federal Communications Commission, and the Architectural and Transportation Barriers Compliance Board have all published regulations to implement the ADA and provide technical assistance to help people apply the law. The Internal Revenue Service provides two special tax incentives, one a tax deduction for any business to remove barriers, the other a tax credit for small businesses to comply with the ADA.

Activities Affected by the ADA

Title I (Employment). As of July 26, 1992, no employer with more than 25 employees can discriminate against a qualified person with a disability in any area of employment. The same prohibition applies to entities with more than 15 employees after July 26, 1994. This includes hiring, promotion, fringe benefits, sick leave, etc. An employer must make reasonable accommodations to enable an individual with disabilities to perform the essential functions of a job, unless the accommodation causes an undue hardship.

366

The determination of whether a reasonable accommodation poses an undue hardship will depend on the specific circumstances of the employer and the nature of the accommodation needed and will vary in each situation.

Title II (State and Local Governments). The responsibilities of public entities are much the same as they were under § 504 of the Rehabilitation Act. State and local governments and all departments, agencies, and instrumentalities must ensure that their programs are accessible. These requirements apply to all parts of all state and local governments, regardless of whether they receive federal funds. Buses used in public transportation must be equipped with lifts; paratransit must be provided to individuals with disabilities who are unable to use the fixed-route system.

Title III (Public Accommodations). The coverage in Title III will affect almost all private businesses, services, and agencies. A place of public accommodation is a facility operated by a private entity that falls within one of the following categories: place of lodging, such as a hotel; establishment serving food or drink; place of exhibition or entertainment, such as a theater or stadium; place of public gathering, such as a convention center or auditorium; sales or rental establishment; service establishment, such as a bank, dry-cleaner, offices of lawyers, doctors or accountants; station used for transportation; place of public display or collection such as a museum or library; place of recreation, such as a park or zoo; place of education such as private schools; social service establishment such as a senior center, day care center or homeless shelter; place of exercise or recreation such as a gym or golf course.

Places of public accommodation must remove architectural and communication barriers where it is readily achievable to do so. This means that if it is relatively easy and inexpensive to take out a barrier, it must be done. The types of barriers contemplated are steps that can be replaced or supplemented by a ramp; doors that can be widened; hand controls for vehicles; display racks that can be rearranged; accessible parking facilities; accessible bathroom facilities; improved signage. Both landlords and tenants of places of public accommodations are responsible for removal of barriers.

Public accommodations must also offer auxiliary aids to ensure that communication is equivalent to that offered to the general public. For instance, hotels have to provide TDD service and closed caption televisions in a number of rooms; restaurants may have to provide menus in braille or permit a waiter to read the menu to a person with a visual impairment.

Again, as in employment, the public accommodation need not remove a barrier or provide an auxiliary service if it is an undue hardship. As in employment, the obligations of the place of public accommodation will depend on the individual facility.

Private entities that provide transportation services must, depending on the circumstances, acquire accessible vehicles or provide equivalent service to individuals with disabilities. Over-the-road buses such as Greyhound do not have to be accessible until the completion of a study in progress by the Office of Technology Assistance.

Title IV (Telecommunications). This title of the ADA will reform the national telephone system to include people with hearing and speech impairments. Providers of telephone service must provide "relay" service. Relay operators will be middlemen in conversations between individuals using TDDs (telephone device for the deaf) and people using regular phones.

Title V (Miscellaneous). Title V provides that the Architectural and Transportation Barriers Compliance Board (the Access Board) will issue guidelines to ensure that facilities and vehicles are accessible to individuals with disabilities. The ADA Accessibility Guidelines (ADAAG) have been incorporated into regulations issued by the Departments of Transportation and Justice. A study is being performed by the National Council on Disability on accessibility of wilderness areas.

Civil Rights for Citizens with Disabilities: Section 504

Section 504 and its regulations prohibit discrimination against any qualified person on the basis of his or her disability. The regulations apply to every program receiving money from any agency of the federal government. Three very important areas covered by Section 504 are education, employment, and community services. However, because of the comprehensive nature of ADA, most of section 504's regulations are now covered by the ADA.

Getting an Education

Post high-school educational programs and institutions must provide the following accommodations:

Examinations for admission—to higher educational facilities (such as SATs or GREs) must be administered in accessible buildings, and accommodations must be provided for disabled students. Schools and universities cannot make only one building or area accessible, with the intention of segregating students with disabilities from the mainstream.

Housing—generally accepted as the standard of housing for all students, housing must be accessible to students with disabilities and at the same cost as for other students. Programs must be made accessible, and adaptive devices must be made available for students with disabilities. All major renovations and new construction must include functional accessibility. This includes both public and most private colleges and universities.

The Paralyzed Veterans of America has been actively advocating fair housing practices for people with disabilities for more than 40 years. *Fair Housing: How to Make the Law Work For You* is a free guide to recent fair housing legislation, available from the Paralyzed Veterans of America.

Getting Community Resources

Subpart C of the Regulations sets the central requirement of the regulation—*program accessibility*. All new facilities built in whole or in part by federal funds must be constructed so as to be readily accessible to and usable by people with disabilities. Every existing facility need not be made physically accessible, but all agencies must ensure that programs conducted in those facilities are made accessible. While flexibility is allowed in choosing methods, structural changes in such facilities must be made if no other means of assuring program accessibility is available.

Additional Reading

Davis, Martha, Eshelman, Elizabeth R., & McCay, M. *The Relaxation & Stress Reduction Workbook.* Oakland, CA: New Harbinger Publications, 1982.

Dunn, Michael. *Social Relationship and Interpersonal Skills: A Guide for People With Sensory and Physical Limitations.* Fairfax, VA: Institute for Information Studies, 1981.

Fensterheim, Herbert, & Baer, Jean. *Don't Say Yes When You Want To Say No*. New York: Dell, 1975.

Greenwald, Harold. *Direct Decision Therapy*. San Diego, CA: EDITS, 1973.

Lakein, Alan. *How To Get Control of Your Time and Your Life*. New York: Signet, 1973.

Paralyzed Veterans of America. *Fair Housing: How to Make the Law Work for You*. Washington, DC: 1989.

Smith, Manual J. *When I Say No I Feel Guilty*. New York: Bantam, 1985.

Zunin, Leonard, & Zunin, Natalie. *Contact: The First Four Minutes*. New York: Balantine, 1975.

Chapter 36

Sexuality and Spinal Cord Injuries

Sexuality is much more than what happens between two people in bed. When we talk of sexuality, we are talking about how people express themselves, of their maleness or femaleness. People's sexuality is shown in the way they present themselves, in the way they carry themselves, in their body image, and in their grooming habits.

Sex, on the other hand, is the physical interaction of two people. It may or may not be a very intimate experience. It may or may not be with someone of the opposite sex. It does, however, express sexuality.

For many spinal cord injured people, whether male or female, the change in or loss of feeling is one of the biggest impacts. Instead of orgasms being just physical and focused on the genitals, they can be more a state of mind. Many spinal cord injured people say that sex is much more intimate and spiritual than it was prior to their injury. These people have found much pleasure in discovering their own and their partner's bodies in new ways. They do so from touching, caressing, and exploring each other.

This intimacy and pleasure requires open and willing communication. This means talking about what feels good, about how and where to touch, or about being nervous or excited. Talking about things like bladder and bowel function and about how it relates to sex helps a partner to know what to expect.

Excerpted from *Yes, You Can: A Guide to Self-Care for Persons with Spinal Cord Injury*, copyright 1989, Paralyzed Veterans of America (PVA); reprinted with permission. For information on how to obtain a complete copy of this manual or receive a list of other available resources contact the PVA at 1-800-424-8200.

This chapter discusses sexual function, both before and after injury. It will also deal with some myths and attitudes about sex and sexuality, practical things to think about when having sex, and a list of where to look for further information.

Sex After Spinal Cord Injury

Not so long ago, ignorance was a widespread problem in the world. Today, although it is still a major disability for many people, one thing has been learned. Spinal cord injury does not automatically banish a person to "The World That Forgot about Sex." In fact, with a little badgering, society as a whole now can accept that sex, marriage, and being a parent can be part of anyone's life. This means with or without a disability! It is your own choice.

People with SCI like yourself, along with research, have shown two things: You can lead a sexually active life, and you can maintain intimate relationships if you choose to do so. To do this, though, it will be helpful for you to read up on the topics listed below.

- Societal "myths and misconceptions" about sexuality and disability.
- How your injury affects your sexual functioning.
- Personal adjustments you can make to deal with these changes.
- People and places in your community and in your rehab facility that you can turn to if you have more questions.

Myths and Misconceptions

This section presents some *false* notions about sexuality and disability. We will attempt to clear up these untruths and replace them with facts and some basic guidelines.

- *Myth*—It is not fitting for hospital staff to discuss sex with patients.

- *FACT*—Sex is a natural part of life. It deserves equal attention in your rehabilitation program.

- *Myth*—People with disabilities are no longer sexual beings.

- *FACT*—We are all sexual beings. This does not change after spinal cord injury.

After you are discharged from the hospital, you may find that people on the "outside" don't approach you in the same way they did before you were injured. You may also find that new people you meet seem a little uncomfortable or anxious around you. They may not know what to say or how to relate to you. You may not be seen as a sexual person or a potential sex partner. For a time just after your injury, *you* may react to yourself in that same way. This is because many people simply do not see that people with disabilities are still sexual beings.

If you already have a sex partner, you may notice that he or she does not approach you sexually in the same way as before. Likewise, you may be somewhat timid about initiating sex with your partner. If you are, it may come from fear and anxiety about being able to perform sexually with a "new" body. You may not know how to begin or what to expect. That can be very scary. Spinal cord injury sex education is a place to start working out those fears. This, along with good social and communication skills, can help fix this situation.

The onset of paralysis will likely affect your genital function. This does not erase your ability and desire to sexually please and be pleased. You will get to know your body much better than you did before you were injured. You will also learn how to do some sexual acts in new ways. All of this is discussed in more detail in the next section.

- *Myth*—Marriage and parenting are no longer options for the people with SCI.

- **FACT**—People with spinal cord injuries do meet people and fall in love. Marriage often follows.

Women with spinal cord injuries by and large have no trouble getting pregnant.

On the other hand, for men, reproductive functions are more complex. They may be impaired by spinal cord injury. The next section of this chapter will go into detail about this. Keep in mind, though, that there are other means of reproduction. If you wish, you can discuss them with your doctor. (See the "Resources & Counseling Services" section of this chapter.)

Men and women who are spinal cord injured do have success in rearing children and keeping happy households.

In the long run, the effect of spinal cord injury on your sexuality has a lot to do with how you feel about yourself (self-esteem). Your skill and confidence in close relationships make up part of your ability to function sexually. You must accept yourself as a sexual being and use your learned skills. In doing so, you can obtain sexual satisfaction for yourself and your partner. Here are some simple guidelines that might be helpful.

1. The presence of spinal cord injury does not mean the absence of desire.
2. Inability to move does not mean inability to please or be pleased.
3. Absence of sensation does not mean absence of feelings.
4. Loss of genital function and/or sensation does not mean loss of sexuality.

Let's Get Physical!

The physical part of your sexuality may now be different for you because of the nerve damage to your spinal cord. In this section, you will learn about the physical changes that may have occurred since your spinal cord injury.

The Male Sex Organs (See Figure 36.1)

- *Scrotum (SCRO-tum)*—A sack-like piece of skin to house and protect the testes.

- *Testes (TESS-teez)*—These egg-shaped organs produce and secrete the male sex hormone *testosterone (tess-TOSS-ter-own)*. They also produce sperm.

- *Epididymis (epp-i-DID-i-miss)*—A storage place for sperm.

- *Vas Deferens (VASS deaf-air-ENNS)*—One of the narrow tubes through which sperm travels to exit the body.

- *Seminal Vesicles (SEM-i-null VESS-ick-ulls)*—These two small glands add fluid to the sperm.

- *Prostate Gland (PROSS-tate gland)*—A small gland shaped like a walnut that adds more fluid to the sperm. This gland is found just below the bladder. The urethra passes through it.

- *Ejaculatory Duct (ee-JACK-you-lah-tor-ee duckt)*—Close to the time of ejaculation, *semen (SEA-men)* (both the fluid and the sperm) moves through this small passageway. From there it goes into the urethra.

- *Cowper's Gland (COW-purrs gland)*—After a man becomes sexually excited, these two pea-sized glands secrete a small drop of fluid. This fluid allows the sperm safe and easy passage through the urethra.

- *Urethra (your-EETH-rah)*—During ejaculation, this tube acts as a passageway for the sperm to exit the body. It also carries urine out of the body.

- *Penis*—This houses the urethra through which sperm passes. Erection assists in depositing of sperm effectively.

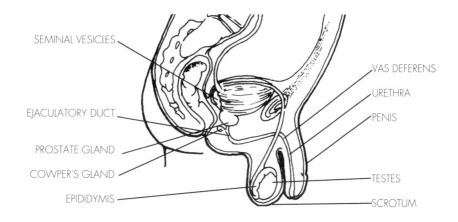

Figure 36.1. The male sex organs

The Female Sex Organs (See Figure 36.2)

- *Labia Majora (LAY-bee-ah mah-JORR-ah)*—("Large lips") These are the larger of the skin folds that surround and protect the vaginal area.

- *Labia Minora (LAY-bee-ah min-ORR-ah)*—("Small lips") These are the smaller skin folds found inside of the larger ones. These lie directly beside the vaginal opening. They can vary in color and size from woman to woman.

- *Clitoris (CLITT-or-iss)*—This projection of skin can vary in size. It is located just above the urinary opening and just below where the tops of the labia minora meet. It is made of the same type of tissues as the penis. Unlike the penis, though, the only purpose of this organ is for pleasure.

- *Vagina (vah-JINE-ah)*—This is a hollow opening into the body. It is about three to five inches long but lengthens and widens with sexual activity. The vagina accepts the penis during sex. It also acts as a passageway in childbirth.

- *Uterus (YOU-turr-uss)*—This is a thick hollow muscle located in the lower abdomen. Its sole purpose is to carry and nurture a child. The *cervix (SURR-vix)* is the opening into the uterus from

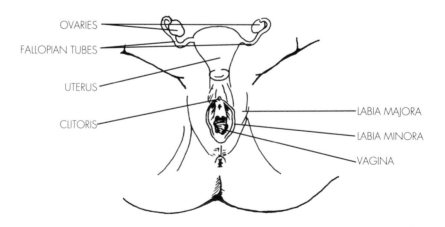

Figure 36.2. The female sex organs.

the vagina. Through it, sperm enters to fertilize the egg and the baby exits to be born.

- *Ovary (OH-vair-ee)*—The ovaries are two small organs that take turns every other month to produce eggs. They also produce and secrete the female sex hormones. These hormones are *estrogen (ESS-tro-jin)* and *progesterone (pro-JESS-turr-own)*.

- *Fallopian Tubes (fall-OPE-ee-an toobs)*—These are two tubes that are attached to the top of the uterus. On the outer ends of the tubes are finger-like pieces of tissue. These "fingers" catch the eggs from the ovaries and pass them down the tube to the uterus. For the most part, it is within these tubes that eggs are fertilized by sperm.

Changes After SCI

The changes after SCI are by and large in *erection, ejaculation, and lubrication*. The lack of, or decrease in, feeling and movement may also change the sexual experience for you.

Erections

There are two types of erections that for the most part occur at just about the same time. Since each is produced through different parts of the spinal cord, we need to speak about them separately.

1. *Psychogenic (SIGH-ko-JENN-ick) Erections*—These erections occur by thinking (fantasy, seeing a good looking person, or reading sexually explicit material) and then becoming sexually excited. If your SCI is in the lower lumbar or sacral area and is incomplete, you may be able to have a psychogenic erection. If you have an incomplete injury above the T12 level, psychogenic erections may still sometimes occur.

2. *Reflexogenic (re-FLEX-o-JENN-ick) Erections*—These erections occur through a reflex mechanism in the sacral part of your spinal cord. Your brain plays no part in getting this type of erection. All you need is an intact functioning reflex system at Sacral two, three, or four segments of the spinal cord. This is present in Upper Motor Neuron (UMN) spinal cord injuries.

Any type of stimulation to the scrotum, penis, or anus may cause this type of an erection. Perhaps you've noticed this when you wash or apply your condom catheter.

If you have difficulty getting erections or the erections you get are less complete or long-lasting than you wish, check out the "Resources & Counseling Services" section of this chapter for some suggestions.

Ejaculation

In order for ejaculation to occur, there must be a fine-tuned coordination of all the different parts of the nervous system.

Think about a defensive play in football When one team member doesn't do what he's supposed to do, the play may not come out as planned. The same thing happens in spinal cord injury. Some nerves cannot do what they used to do. *Therefore, ejaculation may not happen.* (See Figure 36.3.)

Part of the process that allows normal ejaculation is closure of the *bladder neck* so that semen can flow past the bladder and out of the

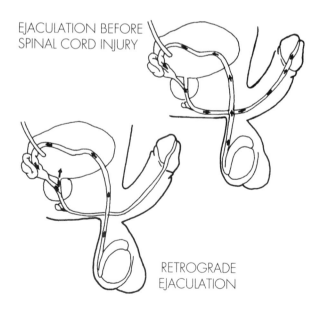

EJACULATION BEFORE
SPINAL CORD INJURY

RETROGRADE
EJACULATION

Figure 36.3. *Ejaculation*

urethra. In many spinal cord injured men, *retrograde ejaculation* occurs. This happens when the bladder neck stays open and semen travels the easy, shorter pathway into the bladder rather than the long distance out of the urethra.

If you have an *incomplete injury*, you're more likely to ejaculate than those men with complete injuries. *But*, some spinal cord injured men defy all knowledge of science and ejaculate a good deal of the time. The best way to check out your ejaculatory status is to try it out. Don't be too impatient. Give yourself a few chances to see if this system still works.

Other Important Information

Pregnancy—The Male Perspective

If you can ejaculate or have any mucus-like fluid from your penis during sexual activity, you *will* need to use birth control if you do not want your partner to get pregnant.

If you want specific details on ejaculation and *fertility* (the ability to father children), ask a member of the rehabilitation team. They'll get you the answers or refer you to someone who will.

Pregnancy—The Female Perspective

It may take spinal cord injured women up to a few months for them to have a period (*menstruate*) again. Once it returns, *you can get pregnant*. If you don't want to get pregnant, you'll need to practice birth control. See the next section or consult a member of the rehab team.

Lubrication

In women, lubrication of the vagina works the same way as erections do in men. An injury to the *sacral* part of the spinal cord may result in lack of lubrication. An injury *above this level* may leave reflex lubrication intact. With an upper motor neuron (UMN) injury, stimulation to the genitals and vagina will most likely cause this reflex. You may also have *psychogenic lubrication* if you were injured *around or below the T12 or L2* level of your spinal cord.

For women who are not able to lubricate, see the section on lubrication in the next section of this chapter for ways to work around this issue.

Diseases

Sexually transmitted diseases (STDs) can affect individuals with SCI as easily as anyone else. In particular, any activities that involve the exchange of blood or semen may place you at risk of contracting the AIDS virus. Use of a condom may decrease the risk. You can contact your nurse-practitioner or doctor or your local AIDS hotline or center or Department of Health, for more information.

There are a number of other STDs that can be contracted by sexually active individuals. If you notice any abnormal discharge or any abnormalities of the skin on your genitalia, consult your nurse-practitioner or doctor immediately.

Sensation

If you have some or no feeling below the level of your injury, you may wonder what sex will be like now. It's true that feeling is ONE (but only ONE) part of the sexual experience. The thing to remember, though, is that this doesn't only come from your sex organs. You still can feel full sexual sensations above the level of your injury. This includes your ears, neck, face, and mouth. Use them and also your other senses to heighten these feelings with the help of the largest sex organ of all—*your brain*.

- *Watch* what your partner is doing.
- *Listen* for sweet nothings.
- *Smell* that favorite scent.

If you have some feeling below your level of injury, explore your body or have someone do it for you. Find out where it feels good. Talk with your partner about what you are feeling.

Changes in the Ability to Move

Partial or complete paralysis below your level of injury may change your ability for certain sexual movement. For some, it may mean changing a few positions in your usual activity. The important aspect to note here is that the loss of movement does not mean you can't enjoy sex. See the next section on practical ways to work around this issue.

Managing Physical Problems Without Stifling Romance

Your needs and desires for sex and intimacy will not change after your spinal cord injury. However, sexual activity now requires some planning. The issue of spontaneous sex may change somewhat as well.

Many people like spontaneity and the freedom to explore themselves and their partner. This can happen if the time is taken to explore your new self, both in body and mind. Your social worker, psychologist, or other rehab team members may have many suggestions about this. All of them are all here to support you in coping with feelings that can come with sexuality and new sexual experience. All you have to do is just let them know if you feel like talking about this.

Things to Think about Before Sexual Activity

1. If bladder control is a problem or concern and you have planned in advance a certain time for sex, decrease your fluid intake three to four hours before sex. Emptying your bladder just before sex may also help.

2. To avoid accidents with your bowels, plan ahead for your bowel program. You may want to do it in the morning or just before intercourse so that it will not be a problem.

3. Making a bath or shower part of foreplay can certainly be fun. It can help take care of unpleasant body odors as well.

4. Because of wheelchairs and concerns with accessibility, you may want to plan where you will have sex. Is your partner's home accessible? Is a hotel more accessible? And so on.

5. If you need to transfer, position, undress, or handle hygiene, will you need help? Some people have attendants do this. Others have partners do it. These activities can always be made part of foreplay.

6. If both you and your partner are disabled, will you need someone to assist you? Some couples may ask an attendant to position them for certain kinds of sexual activities.

7. Sexual loving is always better in a setting that is comfortable for both of you. Don't let the preparation destroy the moment.

Lubrication

Doctors by and large do not advise using Vaseline or any other oil-based substance. This is because it does not dissolve in water and can build up. It is therefore a potential source for infection. Water soluble lubricant jelly is often used.

Erections

It is important to know what kind of erection you can obtain (see above section on this). You can find ways to achieve these erections, and you can teach your partner as well. Prior to sex some people like to discuss with their partner the type of erection they can obtain.

If you have a *reflexogenic* type of erection, it is important to remove the sexual stimulation after you and your partner are finished. If not, the penis can remain erect indefinitely and can cause some medical problems. Be sure to communicate with your partner so you know what each of you is feeling and thinking.

If having a partial or full erection is not easy and you feel it is a major part of your sexual activity, you do have some options. Depending on your case, "penile implants" or an injectable medication that can cause a temporary erection may be an option. An external "penile prosthesis" can also be used. Feel free to discuss these with your physician or other rehab team member.

Women who have a disabled male partner, may want to use *Kegel exercises*. These train women to use pelvic or vaginal muscles to maintain a man's erection or keep a flaccid penis in the vagina. These are listed below.

Kegel Exercises

1. Locate the muscles around the vagina. You can do this by stopping the flow of urine. The muscles that control this flow are the same muscles you flex during Kegel exercises.

2. Insert a finger into the opening of the vagina and contract these muscles. Feel them squeeze your finger.

3. Flex the same muscles for three seconds. Relax. Repeat.

4. Flex and release as quickly as possible; 10 to 25 times. Repeat.

5. Imagine trying to suck something into your vagina. Hold for three seconds.

6. Push out as during a bowel movement, only with the vagina. Hold for three seconds.

7. Repeat exercises 3, 5, and 6 ten times each and exercise four once. This series should be done three times a day. (Adapted from *For Yourself*, pp. 54-55.)

Urinary Appliances

Catheters and other urinary appliances can or may be removed prior to sex. It is your choice. If you do not wish to remove them, there are a few things you may want to consider. For one thing, you can use longer connective tubing with a larger volume "night" bag. This will allow for a bigger area of movement. Check once in a while to make sure the tubing is not pinched or kinked.

Some people prefer to remove their catheters before sex and replace them after sex. With an indwelling (foley) catheter, taking it out may depend on your (or your partner's, or your attendant's) ability to remove and replace it without causing bladder infections.

For men, if taking out a foley is not desired, you can fold the tubing over the end of the penis onto the shaft *after* the penis is erect. The penis and catheter tubing can be inserted into your partner. Some people like to use a prophylactic-type condom. The condom is placed over both the erect penis and the folded-over tubing. If this is done, extra lubrication may be needed around the tubing coming into contact with the penis. This will prevent chafing of the skin.

If you wear an *external (condom) collecting device*, you may wish to remove it. People will often use the bladder voiding methods and wash their penis after taking off the condom.

Women not wishing to remove their foley catheter will often tape the tubing to their stomachs or upper thigh area. If you plan to do this, be sure to use a stretchy type of tape.

If you have an *ostomy*, extra tape may be needed to help prevent the chance of leakage. Avoid direct pressure against the ostomy bag, if you can. This also helps prevent leakage. Colored or decorated ostomy bags are on the market now for those of you who wish to use them.

If you have a *suprapubic catheter*, people often tape the tubing out of the way. If you do, be sure to use a tape that will not pull on your skin.

Leakage and accidents are not the end of the world. They can happen even with all precautions. Even persons without spinal cord injuries sometimes have problems with incontinence. You may want to place a waterproof pad over your mattress. It may also be helpful to keep towels around the bedside in case of accidents.

Spasticity

Some people will use spasticity to help heighten sexual pleasure. In some cases, spasticity can be used to obtain an erection. Some people may use spasticity during sex. Extension of their legs during a heightened moment of pleasure adds to the experience.

Spasticity can also be a hassle during sex. For one thing, spasticity can lead to contractures. This can then prevent certain sexual positions. Your best bet is to maintain your range of motion as outlined by your therapist. During your therapy process, you may also learn to position and move your body in ways that will allow you to control your spasticity.

Positioning

Positioning yourself for sex will be your choice. It will also vary with the type of sexual activity in which you wish to engage. Consult with your doctor for any possible limits. Your therapist may be a good resource of options for positioning during sex. There are also a few books listed at the end of this chapter. They provide pictures and descriptions of sexual positions.

Resources and Counseling Services

These services are a response to the growing number of persons, disabled or not, who want to know more about their sexuality. Sexual counseling is now used by people alone or with their partners.

In recent years, many new resources dealing with sexuality and sexually related concerns have cropped up. Here are a few options on where to go and how to use these resources.

Deciding that you need some professional advice or counseling is not always easy to do. The guidelines below will make it easier for you to find the help you need.

Getting Started

1. On the whole, the hardest part of the process is bringing up the subject and saying what the problem is. Don't get discouraged!

2. Is the problem related to genital function? This includes changes in your ability to have or keep an erection or in vaginal lubrication. If so, consult your doctor or nurse.

3. Is the concern more related to a sexual relationship, lack of one, or a desire to feel better about your sexuality? Consult your social worker, psychologist, or other rehab team member. You can also contact your local mental health center. They may be able to counsel you or refer you to a counselor in your community.

Finding a Good Counselor

While you were in an SCI service, you could get counseling on your sexuality from any member of the staff. Counseling is also there for you through the SCI outpatient clinic when you get out of the hospital. If you do not have access to an SCI clinic and need to find a mental health professional in your own community who can counsel you, be sure that they are the right counselor for you and/or your partner. You may be purchasing their services. A smart consumer needs to know what he or she is buying. Here are a few good questions to ask the counselor:

1. How much experience do you have in sexual counseling?
2. What type of training or professional degree have you received?
3. Have you worked much with clients who have disabilities?

If the counselor has little experience, ask:

4. Do you have an interest in working with clients who have disabilities?
5. Would you be willing to consult the SCI service for more information about spinal cord injuries?
6. How long will I need to see you and how much will it cost?

Some sexual counselors may not have experience with clients who have disabilities. This doesn't mean that they are not good at what they do. More to the point is their willingness to uncover facts about spinal cord injuries when they are needed.

Not all sexual concerns are due to your disability. Sexual and relationship problems can occur in anyone's life!

Additional Resources

Adoption

Adoption is a very real means of having and raising children for those spinal cord injured people who are unable to impregnate their spouse or bear biological children. Adoption agencies and programs can help you decide if it is the right choice for you. These programs can also inform you about legal procedures.

Both married and single persons can apply for adoption. *You cannot be discriminated against because you are a person with a disability.* If you feel you have been denied these services because of your disability, treat this situation the same as any other case of discrimination.

Fertility and Artificial Insemination

For spinal cord injured women, their disability has no affect on their fertility. In the case of men, the ability to impregnate a woman varies with each person. Their fertility can be tested by many methods. It doesn't matter if you can ejaculate or not. There is a chance of having fertile sperm. When in doubt, talk to your doctor or other member of the rehab team.

Artificial insemination, with the sperm of a spouse or an unknown donor, is an option for persons who desire to raise children. This process can involve testing both male and female fertility. You can discuss this option with your physiatrist, urologist, or gynecologist. Some university medical centers have programs of this kind all set up.

External Penile Prostheses

For men who want help with having a fuller erection, an external penile prosthesis is an option. This is a device that fits over the penis. It can create the effect of a full or partial erection. Talk with your doctor, social worker, or psychologist about it. You need to think about whether or not this kind of device will meet your needs and/or the needs of your sexual partner.

Internal Implants

Males unable to achieve an erection may wish to think about the surgical placement of a *prosthesis (pross-THEE-siss)* into the penis. It must be stressed, though, that this process does not restore normal sexual function. Communication and caring are still vital parts of any sexual relationship.

Injectable Medication

For men who are unable to have an erection, a small amount of medication may be injected into the side of the penis to produce an erection lasting about an hour.

Further information may be obtained by consulting your urologist.

Getting More Information

One way to get practical information about the issues discussed in this section is to talk with other people with disabilities. Some communities provide peer support groups or independent living centers. These can help you find a peer who has found a way of sexually adapting to a disability.

If you have questions about resources in your community, your social worker can provide help in finding them.

Books and pamphlets are always a great way to get facts. A few good books and booklets are listed below.

Additional Reading

Barbach, Lonnie. *For Yourself: The Fulfillment of Female Sexuality*. New York: New American Library, 1976.

Cole, T., Chilgren, R., & Mooney, T. *Sexual Options for Paraplegics and Quadriplegics*. Boston: Little, Brown, 1975.

Ferguson, Gregory, M. *Sexual Adjustment: A Guide for the Spinal Cord Injured*. Accent on Living Inc., 1974.

Rabin, Barry J. *The Sensuous Wheeler*. 1980.

Chapter 37

Chronic Pain Management for People with Spinal Cord Injuries

There are two major types of pain—acute or short-lasting, and chronic. Chronic pain is the more challenging to live with and treat. Chronic pain is long-lasting—traditionally defined as occurring for at least six months—is often difficult to cure, and may appear without any tissue damage or physical cause. Researchers have concluded that chronic pain is caused by problems inside the central nervous system—unlike acute pain which is caused by an outside source.

Spinal cord injuries frequently result in chronic pain. A 1987 study estimates that between 11% to 94% of persons with SCI experience such pain.[1] Another study found that pain interfered with daily activities among nearly half of spinal cord injured people.

Unfortunately, despite many recent medical advances, chronic pain due to spinal cord injury is one of the most challenging problems for doctors and chronic pain patients to cope with. In some difficult cases, the treating doctor is left with only one option: Helping the patient understand and cope with the pain.

One physician from Craig Hospital in Englewood CO, well-known for its SCI treatment and rehabilitation program, called chronic pain "extremely difficult to treat particularly, with non-surgical procedures."[2] Two neurosurgeons said that multiple parts of the body's sensory system may be involved in chronic pain and described the search for relief as "a detective story to sort out each culprit associated."[3]

389

Even if managing chronic pain is difficult, there are effective treatments. But before we examine them, we should know the most common causes and types of chronic pain associated with SCI.

Causes

Many researchers believe that chronic pain following SCI originates in the central nervous system. That's why the pain persists even after peripheral sources of acute pain have healed. The pain occurs in the area of the spinal injury where there may be scarred nerve tissue, inflamed membranes and tethered cord.

It's thought that these changes cause the spinal cord to malfunction with abnormal burst firing, altered concentrations of neural chemicals, disturbance of the pain pathways, and other unusual activities.

Types

There are several common types of chronic pain associated with spinal cord injury:

1. Intense, burning pain in a part of the body where sensation may be reduced or gone.

2. A spread-out, aching, crushing sensation in a limb.

3. Recurring, explosive pain with shooting episodes.

4. Phantom limb pain in the stump or phantom limb following amputation.

5. Pain in paralyzed limbs usually made worse by touching or rubbing the skin just above the injury level—or by overfilling the bladder or bowel. Usually develops fairly early after injury.

6. Delayed pain in paralyzed limbs or injury-level skin several years following injury. Often a radiating pain to one or both legs or in the skin just above the injury level.

7. Pain around the abdomen like a tight, squeezing band that produces a bloated sensation that won't go away.

In one group of paraplegics with this delayed-development pain, 60% were found to have a cyst on the spinal cord which required surgery.[3]

Any change in the spinal cord above the injury site is called cystic myelopathy. Factors considered to contribute to this change are arachnoiditis (inflammation of the spinal cord membrane) and tethering of the cord (attachment of the spinal cord to the spinal column itself, restricting movement).

Suspect cystic myelopathy if you have these symptoms along with chronic pain:

- Progressive loss of movement and sensation.
- Increasing spasticity.
- Autonomic hyperreflexia.
- Excessive sweating.
- Horner's Syndrome (lack of sweat, contraction of pupils, rolling of eyes back into sockets, or drooping of eyelids).

If you suspect you have any of these disorders related to cystic myelopathy, see your doctor. Treatment involves neurosurgery and shunting, which is diversion of the cerebrospinal fluid from the spinal cord through a small plastic catheter-like tube. Shunts require regular examinations to check for blockage.

Location

The areas of the body most vulnerable to chronic pain among persons with spinal cord injury are the back, shoulder, elbow and wrist. One study found that during the first six months following injury, 78% of tetraplegics and 35% of paraplegics had shoulder pain. However, examinations six to 18 months after injury found only 33% of the tetraplegics and all of the paraplegics continued to have pain. While the pain did not cause a decrease in movement for most of the paraplegics, it did cause functional disability in 8 of 10 tetraplegics.

Treatment

Many doctors believe a combination of treatments is most effective in combatting chronic pain. This also requires a team approach by specialists skilled in each area such as physicians, surgeons, rehabilitation nurses, physical/occupational/recreational therapists, and psychologists. Usually, physicians prefer to start with the most conservative types of treatment before moving on to surgery or more risky treatments.

General Health

Rehab doctors and nurses treat problems such as urinary infections, breathing difficulties, pressure sores, etc., and also educate the person on ways to improve overall health. If the person with SCI can achieve a feeling of well-being, the body's natural painkillers (opiates or endorphins) may increase and help reduce the pain.

Drugs

Pain medications can be divided into two major types: Non-narcotic and narcotic.

Non-narcotic drugs. Antidepressants, anticonvulsants, and antipsychotic medications fall into this category. There is disagreement over whether these drugs provide effective pain relief. There are no scientific studies proving that this category of drugs works well to relieve chronic pain. Nevertheless, many people appear better able to cope with chronic pain when treated with these drugs.

One case study[1] published in 1992, however, reported that a combination of an anticonvulsant (carbamazepine) and an antidepressant (amitriptyline) was effective. The two drugs together reduced the pain reported by a 33-year-old woman who is a C8-level tetraplegic (quadriplegic). Neither drug given alone was as effective.

The doctors theorized that the two medications may work on different parts of the woman's pain—or that the two drugs in combination had an additive effect.

If you are experiencing a difficult case of chronic pain, you might ask your doctor to read the report in the Archives of Physical Medicine & Rehabilitation, Vol. 73, March 1992. You and your doctor need to consider the side effects of the drugs, however, such as dry mouth, constipation, nausea, drowsiness, dizziness, visual disturbances, and the rare side effect from carbamazepine of bone marrow depression.

Researchers have found that higher doses of antidepressants aren't more beneficial. In fact, just the opposite has been found. Lower than normal doses are more effective in relieving pain, and taking such medications in lower doses means there is less chance of experiencing side effects.

Steroids are another potent substance that relieves pain. Steroids reduce inflammation, improve appetite, and improve general well-being but you should ask about possible side effects[4]. While minor side effects are possible from steroid injections, serious side effects are common with long-term steroid use.

Narcotic drugs. Unless the patient has a terminal illness, use of these potent substances has been considered unacceptable until just recently. Doctors feared side effects, possibility of increased drug tolerance (meaning more and more is needed to have the same effect), dependence or even addiction.

While these dangers need to be considered, Thomas E. Balazy, M.D., of Craig Hospital says narcotic drugs do have a place in treatment of chronic pain.[2] However, because of the traditional taboos against their use, narcotic drug treatment often has been "too little too late."

Methadone is considered the narcotic of choice for chronic pain, Dr. Balazy says. Given by mouth, methadone is rated three times as effective as morphine, codeine and other similar drugs. Another advantage is that methadone doesn't dull the mind as do some other narcotics. In addition, methadone is relatively inexpensive.

However, some medical experts believe that narcotics are rarely effective except in addicting doses.

There are adverse side effects to be weighed by the doctor as well as the person with chronic pain such as respiratory depression, sedation, constipation, antidiuretic tendencies, and reduced sex drive and/or potency.

If you are required to use narcotics to get pain relief, you probably will want to plan on tapering off the dosage as your mental outlook improves and your physical activity increases.

One approach to chronic pain relief involves injecting small doses of narcotics into the skin or spine to attack the pain near the source. This relief lasts longer and reduces some side effects such as respiratory or circulation problems. A surgically-implanted device that will automatically give the person doses of painkillers shows promise after early tests.

TNS

Transcutaneous nerve stimulation (transcutaneous means through the skin) is a medical term that includes many types of therapy: massage, manipulation, exercise, vibration, laser, acupuncture, accupressure, and low frequency electric current (TENS).

One of the most important types of therapy for chronic SCI pain is transcutaneous electrical nerve stimulation (TENS).TENS uses low levels of electricity applied to the pain area to block or reduce transfer of nerve pain signals.

TENS units include small battery-powered, portable devices that can be worn for regular use. Larger clinical units powered by AC electricity are available for long-term, stationary use in medical offices.

TENS is reported effective in about 30-40% of people with chronic pain. But the treatment usually provides relief only for the symptom rather than the cause. (An exception is healing chronic skin ulcers and improving blood circulation in cases of pain caused by lack of good circulation). One study found TENS to be least successful for central origin pain and peripheral neuropathy (diseases of the smaller nerves).[5] But TENS has been found to be effective in treating accidental or surgical trauma, and can reduce the need for narcotic treatments.

While TENS isn't addictive, there are precautions in its use. Skin reactions or burns can occur, particularly with skin having no sensation or with people unable to communicate or understand. People with heart problems are at even greater risk, especially those with pacemakers. Implanted metal can distort or concentrate the electrical current.

Acupuncture

Acupuncture may also block or reduce pain signals. It has been reported to be successful in treating spasms, tension, migraine headaches and phantom limb pain. Muscle and skeletal problems (such as arthritis but not rheumatoid, and bursitis) seem to respond best to acupuncture treatment as does acute pain. But a thorough knowledge of the acupuncture points of the body is required, and placement of the needle—whether electrical or not—must be very accurate. Although chronic pain may not be cured by acupuncture treatment, some medical experts believe it may be worth trying because of the low rate of complications.

Nerve Blocks

Nerve blocks are used for chronic pain therapy, diagnosis and prognosis. Blocking the nerve pathways can be done though injection of substances like alcohol into the nerve or by applying heat or cold.

Similarly, freezing a peripheral nerve stops the flow of pain signals but doesn't change the structure of the nerve. Finally, small thermal lesions (burns) made surgically in the nerve can permanently interrupt the flow of pain signals. Unfortunately, relief of chronic pain by nerve injections usually are only temporary.

Nerve blocks also are used for diagnosis of an injury and prognosis, whereby the neurosurgeon can test the effects of surgery to see whether or not it gives the patient the relief he or she wants. The person can experience the effects of the interruption of the nerve signals (denervation) before deciding to go ahead with surgery.

Diet

In the early 1960s, a Swedish researcher found that peripheral pain results from an acid increase in the surroundings of the nerve endings.[6] The finding led him to believe that if he could reduce this acid content, the pain would be reduced. This researcher (Olov Lindahl) has treated pain sufferers by giving them alkaline-ash food and alkaline medications by mouth. Over 20 years, about 70% of patients were reported pain-free within 2-6 months.

His medication consists of a mixture of potassium salts and calcium magnesium with lactate, citrate, or carbonate. At the same time, he asks the person to eliminate acid-ash foods such as meat, fish and other animal products, bread, sugar, salt, coffee, tea, chocolate, cereals, beans, apples, citrus fruits, alcohol and tobacco. He advises the person to stop taking acidic medications such as aspirin, and encourages the eating of alkaline-ash food such as vegetables.

The treatment has worked on premenstrual syndrome and rheumatoid arthritis but this researcher, Olov Lindahl, didn't report any studies involving spinal cord injuries. Results may take a considerable time, such as several months or even years.

While Lindahl's study showed improvement in pain due to diet changes, the patients were observed for only one month. That raises the possibility, he says, that the improvement could be due to the initial one-week fasting by all patients—which has been shown to improve rheumatoid arthritis.

Surgery

A fairly recent surgical development in the treatment of chronic pain in spinal cord injuries is the DREZ (dorsal root entry zone) operation.

Dorsal roots are nerve branches radiating from the spinal cord in the back or chest area.

Until this surgical technique was introduced in 1975, pain caused by disconnection of the dorsal roots from the spinal cord due to injury was difficult to relieve. However, few hospitals or surgeons perform this surgery.

The DREZ surgery is used in the case of avulsion injury (tearing away of the tissue or nerves). Lesions are burned into the dorsal root area with a thermal electrode or a laser to stop the pain signals and relieve the pain.

Severe long-term pain from avulsion injury occurs in 10% of patients.[3] Symptoms of an upper avulsion injury are a limp, sensationless arm with pain usually in the hand and fingers, especially the thumb and index fingers. Pain is of two types: An aching, crushing sensation in the limb, and a second type, an intermittent, shooting, explosive pain. A similar injury is associated with gunshot wounds in the lower spine or with fractures of the pelvis. If you're experiencing these types of pain, ask your doctor about the DREZ procedure.

Chemical "removal" of nerve portions is used to treat pain and spasticity of paraplegia, multiple sclerosis, and other neurological problems.

Finally, surgical nerve blocks through creation of lesions using electric probes can relieve pain which otherwise won't respond to treatment.

Electrical Stimulation

Stimulation of peripheral nerves has been used successfully to relieve pain that couldn't be relieved by surgery or temporary nerve block. Usually the person who got relief from this method had responded to TENS treatment. For deafferentation (nerve interruption) which may occur in spinal cord injury, stimulation of the spinal cord rather than peripheral nerves is used for pain in the lower extremities.

The technique involves implanting an electrode next to the affected nerve. Excellent or good long-term pain relief has been reported in 25% of patients, and an additional 50% obtained partial relief. One study reported satisfactory results in 50% of a small group of persons with spinal cord injuries. The traditional means of activating the electrode has been with a battery and pulse generator unit that is worn or carried. Recently, lithium-powered generators that can be fully implanted in the body have been developed. However, when the battery dies, another surgery is required with the fully implantable system.

A related pain-relieving technique is deep brain stimulation. This technique involves implanting electrodes in the brain, and in some cases the patient needs to be awake to help determine correct placement. Again, a trial stimulation is used before permanently hooking up the system. The best results (67% to 73% success) for pain associated with interrupted nerveways have been obtained in patients with peripheral nerve disorders including partial spinal cord injuries. In most cases, persons with complete spinal cord injuries had poor results from deep brain stimulation.

Severe complications are not common with deep brain stimulation but complications include sometimes fatal blood vessel breaks inside the brain, infection, and temporary eye movement disorder. Removal of an electrode implanted deep in the brain for repair is considered more dangerous than the original insertion.

Physical Treatment

Physical treatment tackles problems that aggravate the chronic pain. Therapists and physicians treat through range of motion and stretching exercises to reduce spasticity, joint contractures, joint inflammations, spinal alignments problems, or muscle atrophy (weakening and shrinking).

Changes in your wheelchair, sitting posture, and seat cushion may be recommended to prevent pain, pressure sores, scoliosis (curvature of the spine), joint contractures, and other problems. In addition, the therapist aims to improve your overall physical condition through aerobic exercises and to improve the efficiency of movement in your wheelchair. Finally, therapists recognize the therapeutic value of recreational exercise in managing pain through diversion of attention from the pain itself.

Psychosocial

Some studies have found that pain may increase depending on the person's mental state. One study showed that persons with spinal cord injuries who were angry reported more severe pain, and that those who were more accepting of their pain reported lower levels of pain severity. In this study[7], anger was associated with severe pain more often than was depression or anxiety.

Other studies in this field have concluded that older people with higher verbal intelligence, high levels of anxiety, and a negative psychosocial environment experience greater pain.[8] So it seems that controlling your anger, anxiety, and negative feelings may help reduce chronic pain.

Some types of behavioral control have been found to be effective in pain control. Researchers have found that imagining a pleasant or distracting event (emotive imagery) can be effective in pain management. A number of studies have shown that preparing patients for pain and giving them a sense that they can exert some degree of control over the sensation will raise their pain threshold or tolerance. Patients who were given descriptions of the pain, its type and how long it might last asked for less pain medication in a post-surgery recovery room. Other behavioral techniques such as relaxation, deep and slow breathing, diversion of attention, and changing the painful sensation through fantasy have been shown to be effective.[11]

Chronic pain is challenging to treat and live with. But there are methods of relief available. You should realize that a number of treatments may be called for, however, and that none may be 100% effective. Your chances of finding relief are better if you are an active partner with your doctor or therapist in searching for the most effective treatments.

Chronic Pain Terminology

Arachnoiditis (a-rack'-noyd-i-tus). Inflammation of one of the three membranes covering the spinal cord and brain. The membrane resembles a spider's web. Arachnoiditis has been associated with use of oil-based contrast substances in neural examinations.

Avulsion (ah-vul'-shun). Tearing away of a portion of tissue or nerve.

Cord Cyst (kord sist). A sac-like growth on the spinal cord sometimes associated with spinal cord injury. To relieve the pain, neurosurgeons may try to create permanent drainage, or block the pain through burning lesions at key points in the nerves.

Cordotomy (kor-dot'-uh-me). Surgically dividing a portion of the spinal cord.

Cystic Myelopathy (sis'-tick mi-il-op'-ah-the). Cystic changes in the spinal cord from the area of injury upward. Examples are arachnoiditis and tethering of the cord (connection of the cord to the spinal column bones which restricts movement).

Deafferentation (dee-af-fur-en-tah'-shun). Refers to sensory nerve fibers that have been interrupted or eliminated.

Denervation Pain (dee-nerve'vay-shun). Caused by an abnormality in the normal nerve signals to the brain and a resulting lack of equilibrium in the dorsal horn. Frequently found in paraplegics, or others with sensation loss.

Dorsal Horn (door'-sol horn). The horn-shaped portion of the spinal cord made up of the front column and the back column of the cord. Often involved in chronic pain.

Dysesthesia (dis-thez'-i-uh). Impairment of any sense, especially sense of touch. Also refers to unpleasant sensation caused by normal stimuli.

Peripheral Pain (purr-riff'-fur-ul). Pain in the branches of the nerve system in extremities or other body regions away from the spinal cord. Not central pain.

Psychosocial (sigh'-ko-so-shal). Relating to the mind and social influences.

TENS (transcutaneous electrical nerve stimulation). Sending electric current through the skin to relieve pain.

Tetraplegic (tett'-ruh-plegic). Medical term for quadriplegic.

TNS (transcutaneous nerve stimulation). Many different forms of therapy using through-the-skin stimulation to provide pain relief. Includes mechanical, heat, electrical, and chemical methods. Examples: Massage, manipulation, exercise, vibration, laser, acupuncture, and low-frequency electric current.

For Further Reading

This text is intended to present an overview on chronic pain management. If you'd like to research the subject in greater detail here are some suggested readings:

1. **Function-limiting Dysesthetic Pain Syndrome Among Traumatic Spinal Cord Injury Patients: A Cross-sectional Study.** Pain, 1987, 29:39-48. G. Davidoff, E. Roth, M. Guarracina, J. Sliwa, G. Yarkony.

2. **Clinical Management of Chronic Pain in Spinal Cord Injury.** Thomas E. Balazy, M.D. The Clinical Journal of Pain, 1992; 8:102-110.

3. **The Neurosurgeon and Chronic Pain.** B.S. Nashold, Jr., and Brian P. Brophy. Handbook of Chronic Pain Management, 1987, Elsevier Science Publishers B.V.

4. **Management of Chronic Pain: the Anesthetist's Role.** Mark Mehta and Menno E. Sluijter. Handbook of Chronic Pain Management, 1987, Elsevier Science Publishers B.V.

5. **Transcutaneous Electrical Stimulation for Pain: Efficacy and Mechanisms of Action.** 1982. J.N. Campbell and D.M. Long. In: N.H. Hendler, D.M. Long and T.N. Wise (Eds.), Diagnosis and Treatment of Chronic Pain, Wright, Boston, pp.90-91.

6. **Dietary Factors in Chronic Pain Management.** Olov Lindahl. Handbook of Chronic Pain Management, 1987, Elsevier Science Publishers B.V.

7. **Psychosocial Factors in Chronic Spinal Cord Injury Pain.** Jay Summers, Michael Rapoff, George Varghese, Kent Porter and Richard Palmer. Handbook of Chronic Pain Management, 1987, Elsevier Science Publishers B.V.

8. **Psycho-social Aspects of Chronic Pain in Spinal Cord Injury.** Pain, 1980 8:355-366. J.S. Richards, R.L. Meredith, C. Nepomuceno, P.R. Fine, G. Bennett.

9. **Chronic Pain.** Anthony Love & Connie Peck. Health Care: A Behavioural Approach. 1986. Grune & Stratton Australia.

10. **Self-Medicating Practices for Managing Chronic Pain After Spinal Cord Injury.** Maria Radwanski. Rehabilitation Nursing. Nov-Dec. 1992; 17:312-317.

11. **Behavioral Assessment of Chronic Pain.** Mary C. White, Laurence A. Bradley, and Charles K. Prokop. Behavioral Assessment in Behavioral Medicine. 1985. Springer Publishing Co.

The Research and Training Center on Independent Living

Information in this chapter is from *Chronic Pain Management*, part of the Secondary Conditions Prevention & Treatment series of booklets written and produced quarterly by the Research and Training Center on Independent Living, and supported by a grant from the Education Training Foundation under the aegis of the Paralyzed Veterans of America. Other available titles include:

- Spasticity
- Joint Problems
- SCI and Aging
- Pressure Sores
- Urinary Tract Infections
- Chronic Fatigue

Contact the Research and Training Center on Independent Living for a complete list of publications and ordering information.

Training Director
Research and Training Center on Independent Living
University of Kansas
4089 Dole Center
Lawrence KS 66045-2930
(913) 864-4095

Chapter 38

Spinal Cord Injuries: Science Meets Challenge

After days of cramming for college mid-term exams while holding down a full-time job as a security guard, Marc Miller needed a break. So Miller and two friends made the rounds of three Richmond, Va., nightspots before going their separate ways at evening's end.

"I was more tipsy than normal, but I felt fine. I drove out of the parking lot where we had left our cars, and reached over to roll down the passenger window. That's the last thing I remember," Miller recalls. "It was so quick. Suddenly my whole life was changed."

In that instant, his '84 Toyota pickup truck had crossed to the other side of the road, slamming into a telephone pole. On that April 1989 evening, Miller went from carefree college student to paraplegic, joining the 10,000 Americans paralyzed by spinal cord injury each year. After a two-month hospital stay, he returned to college, earning an associate degree in architectural engineering. Now 26, he works full-time as an engineering technician, and lives in Richmond with his wife, Kimberly, 24, whom he met on the job.

"I'm lucky. I have a good job, I play wheelchair basketball, I can still have sex, and I found someone I really love. I couldn't have made it without my friends and family. I wasn't very close to my mother before the accident; now we're really close. I also got very close to my faith in God. Being in a wheelchair gives you a different perspective," he says. "But life is harder. You battle bladder infections. If you get sick, it's harder. I get irritated more easily, and occasionally I

FDA Consumer, July/August 1993.

get depressed. Life is more of a struggle. It's a struggle to get in and out of cars—just driving to Hardees for an iced tea is exhausting."

Comebacks like Miller's would have been unheard of as recently as the World War II era, when 90 percent of spinal cord-injured patients died. It wasn't until the late 1960s and early 1970s that survival rates began approaching 90 percent, primarily due to advances in handling bladder problems. Today, estimates of the number of people living with spinal cord injuries vary from 200,000 to 500,000.

Spinal Cord Complex

Spinal cord injury is devastating because of the complexity, delicacy and importance of the spinal cord itself. Containing more than 20 million nerve fibers, it is the major conduit for transmitting motor and sensory information between brain and body. It runs vertically within the spinal column, composed of 33 vertebrae separated by rubbery disks.

The nerve signals that travel the spinal cord help regulate sensation, movement, and bodily functions, such as bladder control. When the spinal cord's axons (long fibers that nerve cells send out) are damaged, paralysis can result. Axons transmit nerve signals from cell to cell, so when they're destroyed the cells can't communicate, causing loss of functions controlled by the affected cells.

Spinal cord injury affects a number of body functions. Bladder control is usually impaired, and sometimes completely destroyed. Some people retain involuntary reflexes that help empty the bladder, but others have completely flaccid bladder muscles. Urine left in the bladder breeds infection, which can become chronic and cause kidney damage. Bowel management is another challenge, since messages from brain to bowel to empty don't get through, and anal sphincter muscle control is lost. Then there are skin problems like bedsores, common to wheelchair patients.

The location of a spinal cord injury helps determine the level of disability: The higher the injury on the spinal cord, the more extensive the paralysis. Injury above the C7 vertebra results in quadriplegia—impaired function in arms, trunk, legs, and pelvic organs. Paraplegia results from damage done to the thoracic, lumbar or sacral regions of the spinal cord. Although arm function is spared, the trunk, legs, and pelvic organs may be involved, depending on the level of injury.

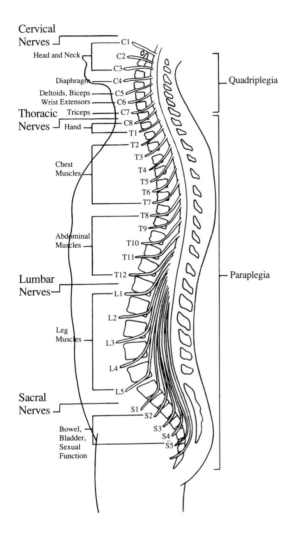

Figure 38.1. Paralysis Locations. The higher the injury on the spinal cord, the more extensive the paralysis. Injury above the C7 vertebra results in quadriplegia, impairing function in arms, trunk, pelvic organs, and legs. Damage to the thoracic, lumbar or sacral spinal cord regions results in paraplegia, in which arm function is retained while—depending on the level of injury—trunk, legs, or pelvic organs may be affected.

Advances Bring Hope

For many years; medical experts considered extensive recovery of body function after spinal cord injury hopeless. This is because in most mammals, nerve cells of the central nervous system (brain and spinal cord) show little evidence of being able to regenerate when damaged. But today, researchers and clinicians alike share optimism about improvements for people with spinal cord injuries. Electrical stimulation of muscles, use of restorative devices, drug therapy advances, and advances in nerve regeneration research are bringing hope to an area long deemed hopeless.

"Since the Vietnam war, there have been significant clinical advances as research centers across the country learned how to care for severely debilitated quadriplegic patients," says Paul R. Beninger, M.D., M.S., acting director for the Food and Drug Administration's division for general and restorative devices. "For example, use of automated wheelchairs became commonplace after the Vietnam war, and the pulmonary care of patients improved."

FDA regulates devices like motorized wheelchairs, but does not regulate accessories like mechanized van lifts for wheelchairs. A stair-climbing motorized wheelchair FDA approved three years ago is a recent advance in devices for patients with spinal cord injuries. The sophisticated chair has sensors that monitor the steepness of stairs, altering both position and speed depending on incline. But the chair is expensive (about $20,000) and heavy; home stairways need inspection to verify their capability for handling the weight.

Muscle Stimulators

Muscle stimulators using electrical currents that stimulate muscles to contract, especially FES systems (functional electrical stimulation), have been the focus of much media attention. Some FES systems under development are enabling paralyzed people to walk again. Such systems operate as a kind of complex prosthetic device, meaning that although the stimulation can cause muscles to contract and legs to move, it is a kind of "artificial" walking, since no actual movement has been regained by the patient and there is no sensation of movement.

Other FES systems stimulate nerves to give hand movement so quadriplegic individuals without hand function can feed themselves.

But FES systems are not without drawbacks: They aren't for everyone, they're costly and still largely experimental, and surgery to implant electrodes is required, which can pose possible complications.

Stimulators aren't just for walking or movement. For example, FDA-approved phrenic nerve stimulators allow people with high-level spinal cord injuries to breathe without respirators. (The phrenic nerve goes from the spinal cord to the diaphragm, and activating it causes the diaphragm to contract). But again, there are use limitations; the phrenic nerve has to be healthy. Robert F. Munzner, Ph.D., chief of FDA's neurological devices branch, estimates that only a few hundred people nationwide can use the device.

According to Marie A. Schroeder, a physical therapist and chief of FDA's restorative devices branch, many muscle stimulators have been cleared for marketing, but not specifically for functional purposes.

"For example, if some muscles are not totally paralyzed and doctors want to see how much improvement in movement or feeling someone will get, they may use a stimulator to maintain range of motion to help provide muscle reeducation, until they see how much voluntary control the patient gains," she explains. "But using stimulators for functional purposes gets into the investigational area. The only functional use of a muscle stimulator that has been cleared are those stimulators that might be used for a patient with a localized nerve injury—for example, a patient who can't lift his foot up. However, we consider the stimulation of muscles needed for the purpose of walking to be investigational."

Physicians surveyed say electrical stimulation is not being widely used on a routine basis because the technology is not yet "user-friendly." William O. McKinley, M.D., director of spinal cord injury and rehabilitative medical services at The Medical College of Virginia, notes that devices that assist paralyzed patients in coming to a standing position, for example, are "very expensive, very time-consuming to learn, and usefulness has to be determined on a patient-by-patient basis."

Many other uses of stimulators are not common or remain investigational. For example, although stimulators that offer pain prevention and electro-ejaculation to collect sperm to enable paralyzed men to become fathers are used clinically, their use is not widespread.

F. Terry Hambrecht, M.D., head of the neural prosthesis program at the National Institutes of Health's National Institute of Neurological Disorders and Stroke, says such systems are still technologically limited, but he is optimistic about the future.

"The problem now is that we're in the Model-T stage. We don't yet have the sophistication and reliability we need," he admits. "But there's no doubt in my mind that eventually functional stimulation devices will be developed for spinal cord-injured patients. We're funding quite a few projects for people who are paralyzed."

Hambrecht says one current project involves electrode implantation to restore bladder and sexual function to paralyzed men and women. He anticipates the first implants will be done within five years.

Drug Treatment

Muscle stimulators have provided drama, but the steroid methyl-prednisolone, experts say, has actually changed the face of clinical treatment for people with spinal cord injuries. A recent report of a 1985 to 1989 study of 487 patients, funded by the National Institute of Neurological Disorders and Stroke, showed that patients given high doses of this cortisone-like drug within eight hours of injury regained an average of 20 percent of lost motor and sensory function. Experts cite the study as the first evidence that a medication can improve the outcome of spinal cord injury, and today the drug is widely used for acute spinal cord injury.

Surgeons use the potent drug, which was approved some years ago by FDA as an anti-inflammatory agent and is also approved to treat swelling around the brain, to manage acute attacks of multiple sclerosis and for a variety of allergic conditions.

Wise Young, M.D., Ph.D., part of the methylprednisolone study team, is a professor of neurosurgery, physiology and biophysics and director of the neurosurgery research lab at New York University Medical Center. Young points out that the drug does not enable patients to immediately "leap out of bed." Beneficial effects are usually not apparent until at least six weeks after the drug is administered. Yet he believes the use of the drug is a landmark development.

"It has changed the attitude of doctors toward spinal cord injury. They no longer see it as a hopeless condition, and patients are rushed to hospitals earlier," he explains. "It also has tremendous implications for chronic spinal cord injury, since the finding that you only need a few axons to get function back means you don't have to regenerate as many axons."

"Currently there are over two dozen drugs reported to be neural-protective in animals," Young says. "The leap that was made in 1990 was between absolutely no hope to some hope. There is a real sense of optimism now; it's not a matter of if, but when, a drug will be available to aid regeneration of the spinal cord."

Treatments Under Study

Another drug under study is GM-1 ganglioside. Fred H. Geisler, M.D., Ph.D., a neurosurgeon at the Chicago Neurosurgical Center, headed a team at the University of Maryland Shock Trauma Center in Baltimore that studied 34 people with paralyzing spinal cord injuries in a placebo-controlled, double-blind, randomized study.

The study results were reported in the June 27, 1991, *New England Journal of Medicine*. Within three days of injury, 16 of Geisler's patients began daily injections of GM-1 for 18 to 32 days, while the rest received placebo injections. Patients given GM-1 had improved recovery of motor functions in the arms, and later in the legs. About half of the improvement occurred at the two-month mark. Most of the improvements happened within four months of patients' receiving GM-1 injections, but some improvements continued for up to one year after GM-1 treatment.

Researchers theorize that GM-1 ganglioside, naturally present in cell membranes of the spinal cord and brain, helps protect against additional nerve cell death after spinal cord injury and also stimulates nerve-fiber growth and repair.

"We saw some major improvements....In many cases, people were walking where they could not ambulate at all before," Geisler says. He is now heading a new study of this investigational drug, following 166 patients given GM-1 at 22 medical centers in North America. Geisler says the goal is to enroll 720 patients.

Neural grafting, or transplantation of tissue into the brain and spinal cord, is still highly experimental. Possible sources of grafting material include genetically engineered cells, human fetal tissue, and other tissues from a patient's own body. Neural grafts are being tested in animal models of brain and spinal cord injury to find out if they can induce growth or replace damaged areas.

Other Improvements

Other factors besides drug advances and technology are improving the outlook for people with spinal cord injuries. Car accidents by far remain the number one cause of spinal cord injuries (47.7 percent), followed by falls, gunshot wounds, and recreational sports, particularly diving accidents. Spinal cord injury happens mostly to young people, and mostly to males (82 percent).

MCV's McKinley says improvements in on-site emergency medical management, with better-trained technicians skilled in stabilizing the spine to prevent further injury, means doctors are seeing more patients with "non-complete" injuries, or injuries where some function and motor sensation is preserved.

"We are also doing a better job of educating people in how-to protect against spinal cord injury, such as wearing seat belts, buying cars with air bags, and not diving into shallow water," he says.

In rehabilitation, the emphasis remains on regaining as much functional ability as possible.

"Chronic patients and rehabilitation are the real challenge. Research is exciting and potentially part of the future, but it still has a long way to go," McKinley says, pointing out that helping patients through the adjustment period after injury remains challenging. "They need to know how to self-catheterize, how to detect bladder infections," he says. "Are the doors at home wide enough for a wheelchair? Do they need a ramp?"

McKinley says the first thing newly injured patients ask about is their ability to walk, but questions about sexuality are not far behind.

"Paralysis can affect the ability to have an erection.... But with adaptations, sexual relations are very possible. So I tell patients yes, it's possible, but different. Loving and caring and other means of sexual gratification take on new priority for injured patients," he explains.

Hope and patience may be the most important factors regarding the future treatment of spinal cord-injured people. Hope comes from optimism about recent advances in treatment, but research complexity and funding issues make patience necessary as well.

"For at least the last decade, research papers have shown that spinal cord injuries can be improved, or that the amount of injury can be decreased," Geisler says. "My hope is that lab findings will be able to move to the clinical area."

Marc Miller, like many people with spinal cord injuries, is both optimistic and philosophical about the treatment advances.

"I think in the next 10 years they will find treatments that reduce the impact of spinal cord injuries. But I think it's important for people to remember that we're just normal folks who can't walk," he says. "I have a better grasp of who I am now; being in a wheelchair gives you a different perspective. I'm not disabled, I just can't walk. I play wheel-chair basketball, I want to learn to water ski and to snow ski....I just want to do all I can do now."

For More Information

The American Paralysis Association, an organization dedicated to eliminating paralysis, provides a 24-hour toll-free information and referral hot line, at (1-800) 526-3456. The hot line helps callers search for support and resources on everything from sexual concerns to selecting a rehabilitation facility.

The National Spinal Cord Injury Association also provides information and resource help at (1-800) 962-9629.

— by Audrey T. Hingley

Audrey T. Hingley is a writer in Mechanicsville, Va.

Chapter 39

Milestones in Spinal Cord Injury Research

Searching for a Cure

The American Paralysis Association (APA), based in Springfield, New Jersey, is a national nonprofit organization that encourages and supports research to find a cure for paralysis caused by spinal cord injury (SCI) and other central nervous system disorders. Since its inception in 1982, APA has strategically invested more than $11 million worldwide in research activities designed to speed progress toward a cure.

APA has funded the research of more than 250 investigators around the world and has become a driving force in the spinal cord research field. It provided long-term support for the small cadre of scientists who, beginning in the 1980's, chose to carve out their careers in the spinal cord, contrary to the prevailing wisdom of the time. It badgered, coaxed and cajoled, and demanded that scientists whose interests were in the brain and peripheral nervous system turn their attention to the spinal cord. APA has provided seed money for much of the seminal research that has culminated in the recent breakthroughs in the field.

A Major Step Forward

"The only way to eliminate [diseases and neurological afflictions like spinal cord injury paralysis] is through a long-term commitment

Information in this chapter is compiled from several documents produced by the American Paralysis Association: "APA Backgrounder," "Milestones," and *Progress in Research*, Spring 1996; reprinted with permission.

413

to research," states Arthur D. Ullian, chairman of the National Campaign to End Neurological Disorders, in his remarks to the House of Representatives in February 1995.

Today, APA makes one-year grants of $30,000 to encourage bright young scientists to tackle issues relevant to repairing the damaged spinal cord, to entice well-established investigators to apply their expertise to the spinal cord, and to enable researchers to develop pilot data for novel, sometimes risky, ideas.

APA believes, however, that spinal cord research can be encouraged to move more quickly than it presently is, that there are many scientific leads but insufficient leadership and focus, and that there are too few, widely-scattered financial resources. To expedite the search for effective treatments for spinal cord injury, APA is working toward expanding its traditional research program. The APA Consortium on Spinal Cord Injury was established to help stimulate research on repair of the chronically damaged spinal cord. The APA Consortium will strive to achieve three objectives: a) characterizing the injured and uninjured cords at the cellular and molecular levels; b) identifying ways to promote recovery of nerve cell function and axon regrowth; and c) investigating strategies to replace nerve cells destroyed by the injury. The APA Consortium pools the expertise and scientific tools of eight world-class neuroscientists and focuses them strategically and cohesively on the problem.

To increase public awareness of spinal cord injury, APA has created a Home Page on the Internet (http://www.apa.uci.edu/paralysis), a three-tiered resource targeted to lay, clinical and scientific audiences. Users will find a wealth of general information on APA and spinal cord injury, extensive research data on projects funded by APA, and a clinical reference guide.

As the number of spinal cord injured individuals increases yearly, by an average of 11,000, so do their care and coping costs and so, too, does the need to focus ever more sharply on neuroscience research. When APA was founded, there was virtually no hope for a paralysis cure. Today, thanks in large part to the Association, that "dogma" is no longer true. Progress in the neurosciences has simply exploded in this "Decade of the Brain," and the promise of treatments and cures for a whole host of diseases and afflictions is real. Sadly, however, the dollars available for neuroscience research have not kept pace with the astounding progress of recent years.

The Need for Hope

APA was started by a handful of people, all of whom had a personal interest in spinal cord injury paralysis. They were either injured themselves or had loved ones who were. They were visionaries in the sense that they refused to accept the "dogma" that damage to the spinal cord is irreparable. With an equally pioneering handful of scientists, they set about to change the status quo. Their goal was to prove the medical community wrong and bring hope to all spinal cord injured individuals. Today, hope has indeed replaced indifference, so that Martin E. Schwab, Ph.D., a prominent neuroscientist at the University of Zurich, Switzerland, and a member of APA's Science Advisory Council, can state that, "A treatment for spinal cord injury is on the horizon."

APA is currently challenged on two fronts. It must continue as a driving force in the spinal cord research field and ensure that the federal government, the nonprofit sector and the corporate world bring sufficient dollars to bear on the neurosciences. APA believes success will bring effective treatments for spinal cord injury paralysis—and a cure.

Milestones

Key Events in the Diagnosis of Spinal Cord Injury Paralysis and the Search for a Cure

2500 B.C. Spinal cord injury is described as "an ailment not to be treated"—found on an Egyptian surgical papyrus.

1830's. Anatomist Theodor Schwann finds evidence of rabbit sciatic regeneration below a cut nerve. The peripheral nervous system cells that make the myelin wrapping around axons are named Schwann cells in his honor. These cells, transplanted to the damaged spinal cord, are eventually thought to help repair nerves whose wrapping has been lost due to injury.

1890. Santiago Ramón y Cajal, the father of modern neuroscience, describes the nervous system and its individual nerve cells. He reports that although mammalian CNS nerves try to regenerate, they do not get far. He blames their failure to regrow on the hostile environment of the CNS.

415

World War II. Individuals begin to survive the initial stages of spinal cord injury with the advent of neurosurgery and bacteria-killing drugs that control formerly fatal lung, bladder and skin infections.

Sir Ludwig Guttmann pioneers a centralized rehabilitation approach to SCI individuals. His Stoke Mandeville Hospital in England becomes a model for the worldwide development of SCI centers.

1951. Nobel Prize winner Rita Levi-Montalcini and Viktor Hamburger, discover a nerve growth factor (NGF). NGF is needed for the survival of nerves, enhanced regeneration in lower animals and the "rescue" of certain nerve cells in mammalian brains after injury.

1969. Regeneration research gets a huge boost when Geoffrey Raisman shows electron microscopic proof that new synapses (connections) form in the adult rat brain after injury. It had always been thought that the CNS was "hard wired" and lacked plasticity (the ability to adapt following trauma). Raisman's work shows that the CNS actually could "reorganize" itself after injury and form new connections.

1981. Albert Aguayo proves that axons in the rat could regrow in the central nervous system (CNS) through a peripheral nerve graft. However, once on the other side of the graft, back in the hostile CNS environment, the regenerating axons stop almost immediately.

1988. Martin Schwab discovers two myelin-associated proteins that inhibit growth in the damaged mammalian spinal cord, a revolutionary finding. Until now, it was believed that the cord's inability to regenerate was due only to the absence of nerve growth factors.

1990. "Decade of the Brain" declared by the United States Congress.

Martin Schwab induces nerve regeneration in the rat spinal cord by blocking damaging proteins with an antibody called IN-1. With this treatment, regenerating axons grow about 11 millimeters; without treatment, they do not grow even one millimeter.

The first effective treatment for acute SCI is identified. Clinical trials show that neurologic recovery in Human spinal cord injuries improves by an average 20% if large doses of the steroid methylprednisolone (MP) are administered within eight hours of injury.

1992. First human clinical trials of the nerve-boosting drug 4-aminopyridine (4-AP) are held. 4-AP allows nerve signals to pass along axons which have lost their "insulation wrapping" due to injury. These early trials show that in some chronically paralyzed patients, 4-AP can increase the ability of axons to conduct signals and thus restore some lost function after injury.

1994. Fred Gage reports that skin cells, genetically engineered to secrete growth factors and neurotransmitters, cause massive regeneration of sensory nerve cells in the spinal cord. Genetically engineered cells with growth factors believed to cause regeneration of movement controlling cells are now being tested.

Wise Young organizes the first multi center, animal spinal cord injury (SCI) study using a standardized rodent model, treatment protocols and behavioral recovery scale to test drug therapies, to identify viable SCI treatments and reduce the average 11-year wait for FDA approval.

Martin Schwab reports dramatic regrowth of nerves in partially severed rat spinal cords after treatment with a combination of the antibody IN-1 and the growth-promoting factor NT-3.

1995. The American Paralysis Association Consortium on Spinal Cord Injury is organized to help stimulate research on repair of the chronically damaged spinal cord. The APA Consortium focuses on three objectives: a) characterizing the injured and uninjured cords at the cellular and molecular levels; b) identifying ways to promote recovery of nerve cell function and axon regrowth; and c) investigating strategies to replace nerve cells destroyed by the injury. The collaboration pools the expertise and scientific tools of a number of neuroscientists and focuses them strategically and cohesively on the problem of chronic spinal cord injury.

Progress in Research

Axonal Growth and Recovery of Function after Spinal Cord Injury in Rats

After treatment with a molecule to neutralize growth-blocking proteins in the spinal cord, a group of rats with acute mid-thoracic spinal cord lesions recently recovered specific reflex and locomotor functions. The study demonstrates that brain stem spinal and corticospinal axons will regenerate and undergo anatomical plasticity in an environment in which inhibitory influences are decreased and that the anatomical growth is associated with improved motor function.

This groundbreaking research was reported in the November 30, 1995 issue of *Nature* by an international team of researchers led by APA Science Advisory Council members Barbara S. Bregman, Ph.D. of Georgetown University Medical Center in Washington, D.C. and Martin E. Schwab, Ph.D. of the Brain Research Institute in Zurich.

At the time of injury, half the rats received a sham treatment and half were treated with IN-1, an antibody to myelin-associated inhibitory proteins found in the spinal cord. Under normal conditions, these inhibitors stop regeneration. IN-1, characterized by Schwab several years ago, allows the axon to grow.

The rats were allowed to recover for four to six weeks and then underwent extensive behavioral testing for analysis of reflex and locomotor function.

Testing showed that 80 percent of the IN-1-treated animals recovered a reflex known as contact placing, a foot placement in response to light skin contact. This is significant because such a reflex depends on an intact corticospinal pathway and suggests that this pathway was regenerated after treatment. Other tests of locomotor function also showed improvements in the IN-1-treated animals.

To test whether newly grown cortical fibers actually contributed to recovery of function, the scientists removed cells of origin of the corticospinal pathway bilaterally. The result was a loss of contact placing ability, indicating that the corticospinal pathway had contributed to the recovered movement.

Schwab and Bregman are currently studying a combination treatment of the IN-1 antibody with NT-3, a growth factor that appears to boost axon regeneration. Bregman's lab is also exploring the effects of transplants of fetal spinal cord tissue in combination with the neurotrophin and IN-1 treatment, and Schwab is investigating the effects of delayed IN-1/NT-3 treatment in rats with chronic injuries.

APA Director of Research Susan Howley said, "We are extremely optimistic about the implications of this research, particularly in the context of moving the field closer to everyone's goal of developing treatments to promote and enhance function after spinal cord injury. It is especially gratifying and significant that APA provided support for the investigators' early work which culminated in these remarkable studies."

For More Information

For more information about the APA, contact:

American Paralysis Association
500 Morris Avenue
Springfield, NY 07081
(201) 379-2690
(800) 225-0292

Internet address: http://www.apa.uci.edu/paralysis

Chapter 40

What's New in Spinal Cord Injury Cure and Treatment Research

When someone sustains a spinal cord injury (SCI), one of the most difficult issues to deal with is that there is no "cure" at the present time. One would think that, with the "explosion in scientific knowledge" we hear about almost every day, **someone** would be doing **something** to find a cure for people with SCI. If we can achieve the impossible in other areas, like transplanting entire organs and organ systems from one person to another and isolating human genes, why can't we figure out why the spinal cord does not repair itself and then do something to correct this biological problem? Compared to a lot of the scientific puzzles that **have** been solved, it shouldn't be all that difficult...

There are really two separate issues involved in this assumption:

1. Is the scientific question, "Why won't the spinal cord regenerate?" easy to answer?

2. What's being done to find a cure?

Let's look at these issues and put them into the context of what scientists have been doing about SCI over the past half century.

Before World War II, an injury to the spinal cord was considered to be a fatal condition. If you did not die as a direct result of the injury, you probably would die within a few weeks or months from

National Spinal Cord Injury Association, 545, Concord Avenue, Suite 29, Cambridge. MA 02138; (617) 441-8500, August 1995.

complications, such as a kidney infection, respiratory problems, or badly infected skin sores.

Fortunately, an improved understanding of SCI led to better patient management, enabling many people to survive their injuries and the initial period afterwards. In addition, the discovery of penicillin and sulfa drugs made common, but life-threatening complications like kidney and skin infections manageable conditions rather than potential killers.

Because the spinal cord carries vital information to the brain, the muscles and many organs, the fact that SCI is now a survivable injury is a miracle itself. However, this miracle leads to another pressing need—to find a way to reverse, or at least diminish, the devastating physical effects of the injury.

The Search for a Cure

The 1980's and 1990's have been an exciting time for people interested in spinal cord injury repair and regeneration. Both in terms of treatment techniques and general knowledge about nervous system function, the progress that has occurred in recent years is encouraging.

The search for a cure involves one of the most complex parts of the human body. The spinal cord is an integral part of the body's most specialized system, the central nervous system (CNS). The CNS consists primarily of the brain and spinal cord.

A major role of the spinal cord is to carry messages to and from all parts of the body and the brain. Some of these messages control sensation, such as knowing your finger is touching a hot stove, while others regulate movement. The spinal cord also carries messages that regulate autonomic functions such as heart rate and breathing—over which we generally do not exert voluntary control.

The spinal cord carries these messages through a network of nerves which link the cells of the spinal cord to target cells in all other systems of the body. An individual nerve cell is called a *neuron*, each with receptive branching fibers called *dendrites*. The *axon*, carrying an output signal, extends from the cell body, and is covered by a protective fatty substance called a *myelin sheath* which helps the impulse travel efficiently.

A nerve impulse from one neuron is picked up by the dendrite of the next nerve cell in the pathway at a specialized connection called a *synapse*. An electrochemical reaction causes the impulse to "jump" across the synapse and the signal stimulates the second nerve cell and the impulse then travels down its axon. The message is picked up and transmitted by a series of neurons until the connection is complete.

There are millions of nerve cells within the spinal cord itself. Some of these lower motor neurons receive motor commands from the brain and send their signals directly to the muscles. Other spinal cord neurons form relay pathways for information travelling up or down the length of the spinal cord. Still other spinal cord neurons remain intact and form intricate circuits below the level of injury. Because cells below the injury are no longer under voluntary control, they cannot be utilized as effectively and may cause unintentional movements such as spasms.

Regeneration

Most of the cells in the human body have the ability to repair themselves after an injury. If you cut your finger, often you have a visible laceration for a few days or weeks, followed by the formation of a scar. In time, you may not be able to tell that the cut had occurred. This indicates that skin cells regenerate, just like cells in the blood vessels, organs and many other tissues. *Peripheral nerves* (nerve fibers outside the brain and spinal cord), such as those located in your fingertips, also regenerate, although this process is different from that in the skin and other organs.

For years, scientists have focused on the big mystery: "Why doesn't the central nervous system regenerate?" This question is even more perplexing because we know that central nerves in lower animal species **can** regenerate. There are no definite answers to this mystery yet, but scientists are exploring the questions in many ways.

Basic Cell Research

An important avenue of research is to look at normal cell function in the CNS of mammals. Scientists investigating this area of research are attempting to identify and describe cellular interactions in properly working systems. In addition, they are working with SCI models in an attempt to identify and explain what occurs after an injury.

Through cell research, scientists are trying to identify the following:

1. What substances are present in the CNS which "switch off" CNS nerve growth in mammals?

It has been shown that regeneration occurs in lower animals, as well as in mammalian fetuses in the very early stages of development. At some point in development, the cells appear to lose the ability to regenerate. This loss may be related to the maturation of the nerve cells or to changes in other nervous system cells past which axons must regenerate.

2. What growth inhibiting factors, present in the CNS of mammals, prevent nerve cells from regenerating and reestablishing connections (synapses)?

    Scientists have identified some proteins in the myelin sheath surrounding spinal cord axons which inhibit nerve cell growth. Additionally, other regeneration-inhibiting proteins have been identified on the surfaces of cells that form the nervous system equivalent of a "scar." Some scientists believe that nerve cells can be encouraged to regrow and re-establish functional synapses by removing or altering this cellular "scar." Antibodies generated against some of these proteins can neutralize the inhibitors and allow growth to occur. The ability of central nerves to regenerate in lower animals is thought to be due to the lack of inhibitors in their CNS.

3. Can growth stimulating substances be introduced into the mammalian CNS to encourage nerve growth and synapse development?

    Investigators are attempting to alter the environment around the injury site to encourage nerve cell growth and repair. As described above, our peripheral nerves can regenerate. This is due to the presence of cell proteins that stimulate rather than inhibit nerve growth. When these cells or the factors they produce such as "growth factors" that nourish nerve cells are introduced into the CNS, central nerve regrowth can occur. Finding ways to effectively introduce these cells or substances to achieve functional recovery is a major goal of "cure" research today.

Development of New Therapeutic Approaches

Ongoing research using animal models to test possible new therapies is progressing more rapidly than ever before. This type of research takes several forms that can best be explained as they apply to solving certain types of damage that result from SCI. There are three major classes of damage to neural tissues that have been identified, each requiring a different therapeutic approach:

1. **Death of nerve cells within the spinal cord.** Because nerve cells lose the ability to undergo cell division as they mature into the highly specialized forms that make up our nervous systems, the death of nerve cells due to injury presents a difficult problem. No functional connections can be established if the nerves no longer exist. Therefore, *replacement of nerve cells* may be required.

2. **Disruption of nerve pathways.** When the long axons carrying signals up and down the spinal cord are cut or damaged to the point where they break down after an injury, the parents nerve cells and axons often survive up to the point where the injury occurred. In this case, *regeneration of damaged axons* is a real possibility to re-establish connections of nerve circuits.

3. **Demyelination or the loss of the insulation around axons.** Animal studies and recent studies of human specimens have established that in some types of SCI, the nerve cells and axons may not be lost or interrupted, but that the loss of function may be due to a loss of myelin sheaths. As described above, myelin sheaths provide insulation so that electrochemical signals are carried efficiently down the long, thin axons. This type of damage may be the most amenable to treatment because rewiring of complex circuits may not be needed and *remyelination of axons* is known to be possible.

Although specific human injuries may involve any or all types of damage just described, therapies developed to combat any one of them might restore important functions. The "cure" for spinal cord injury may take the form of multiple strategies, each in turn restoring functions that make important improvements in the quality of life for a spinal cord injured individual.

The approach to "cure" research then, is to concentrate on techniques that hold the promise of repairing specific types of spinal cord damage. With the explosion of efforts and progress in the fields of Neuroscience and Molecular Biology (sometimes called genetic engineering), the scope of possible new therapies is wider than ever before.

Replacement of Nerve Cells. Mature nerve cells cannot divide to heal a wound as skin cells can. Replacement of nerve cells requires transplantation of new nerve cells into the site of the injury with the hope that they will mature and integrate themselves into the host nervous system. One approach is to transplant healthy CNS cells from the same animal species. Researchers have been unanimous in their agreement that transplantation of adult nerve tissues does not work, while embryonic or fetal transplantation can be quite successful. The embryonic tissues do grow and develop, and scientists hope that they will form circuits that will return important functions to areas below the injury. Research to date has not supported the hope that host axons would use these grafts as "bridges" across the injury site. An important consideration is that if fetal tissue transplants prove successful in animal models, transferring this approach to human beings will involve important ethical considerations regarding donor tissues and other important questions about immune rejection of cells transplanted from one individual to another.

Another approach that may avoid some of those problems is the use of genetic engineering to manufacture "cell lines" that would work as nerve cells after grafting. This approach involves inserting segments of DNA (genes) into fetal nerve cells that allow the cells to divide indefinitely, creating an ongoing supply of donor tissue. The use of purely neuronal cell lines diminishes the chances of immunological rejection of the grafts. Recently, rodent cell lines have been developed that stop dividing after transplantation (so there is no risk of tumor formation), and that mature into very specialized nerve cells. Research has not yet shown that these cells can restore function after spinal cord injury.

Very recently, scientists have learned that some cells of the adult CNS can be stimulated to divide and develop into new nerve cells. This exciting finding has opened up new possibilities for cell line development without a need for fetal tissue donors.

Regeneration of Damaged Axons. Nerve cells in both the central and peripheral nervous systems are associated with helper cells called *neuroglial cells*. After injury, the CNS helper cells largely inhibit regeneration, while those of the peripheral nerves, the *Schwann cells*, stimulate regeneration, even in humans. Scientists are attempting to isolate these cells from peripheral nerves and transplant them into the spinal cord to induce regeneration by providing an altered, supportive environment. In this strategy, a SCI individual could act as their own donor, since Schwann cells can be obtained from biopsies of peripheral nerves in adults.

Schwann cells, nerve cells and some other cells make proteins known to nourish nerve cells called "growth factors." By introducing these factors into injury sites alone or in combination with grafts, researchers hope to stimulate additional nerve regeneration and promote the health of nerve cells. This approach has been shown to stimulate CNS regeneration, including growth of axons from nerve cells within the spinal cord and those from the brain that send their long axons down the spinal cord. Significant restoration of function has not yet been achieved.

Another technique is to genetically alter cells so that they produce large amounts of growth factors and to introduce these into the injury site. While nerve fibers have been stimulated to grow by such grafts, this type of research is in its very early stages. Cells making many types of factors will have to be tested and functional recovery carefully demonstrated.

Remyelination of Axons. Schwann cells are also the cells in peripheral nerves that form myelin sheaths. They are not usually found in the brain or spinal cord where another neuroglial cell, the *ogliodendrocyte*, is responsible for making myelin. Researchers have shown that Schwann cells grafted into the brain can myelinate central axons. When the loss of myelin is an important part of injury, implanting Schwann cells could stimulate remyelination and thereby restore function.

Another approach involves a drug called 4-aminopyridine (4-AP), which may help demyelinated nerves conduct signals. Animal studies show that a very small percent of healthy, myelinated axons can be enough to carry on important functions in the spinal cord, even in the face of damage to surrounding nerve cells. Helping nerve fibers that have lost myelin to conduct impulses should improve function after injuries that extensively damage myelin sheaths but do not disrupt nerve connections. This research is also in its very early phases.

Summary of Basic Science Research

As you can see by the facts detailed above, the problem of CNS response to injury is incredibly complex. No one theory or approach will overcome all of the effects of SCI, and many scientists now believe that the "cure" will not be found in a single approach, but rather in a combination of techniques. Consequently, it is important for all possible research areas to be addressed so our overall knowledge about how the system works may eventually lead to a cure for SCI.

What about the "imminent breakthroughs" you hear about regularly in the press? It must be remembered that there is a vast difference between a "scientific breakthrough" and a "clinical breakthrough." While scientific discoveries occur quite frequently, clinical (treatment) ones do not. Public announcements of scientific progress help to keep the attention and funding focused on finding solutions to the problems caused by SCI but new scientific breakthroughs generally do not lead to immediate treatment applications.

Research in SCI Treatment

Drug Treatments for New Injuries

*Note: It is important to realize these drugs are **not** a cure for chronic (long-term) spinal cord injuries. It is heartening to note, however, that treatments finally are available to lessen the severity of some acute injuries.*

Research has shown that all damage in SCI does not occur instantaneously. Mechanical disruption of nerves and nerve fibers occurs at the time of injury. Within 30 minutes, hemorrhaging is observed in the damaged area of the spinal cord and this may expand over the next few hours. By several hours, inflammatory cells enter the area of spinal cord injury and their secretions cause chemical changes that can further damage nervous tissue. Cellular content of nerve cells killed by the injury contribute to this harmful chemical environment. This process may go on for days or even weeks.

Hope lies, therefore, in treatments that could prevent these stages of progressive damage. Drugs that protect nerve cells following injury are now available to lessen the severity of some injuries. Other drugs and combinations of drugs are currently being tested in both animal and clinical trials.

Methylprednisolone

Few treatment approaches have raised as much hope as the announcement by the National Institute of Health that the steroid, methylprednisolone, reduces the degree of paralysis if administered shortly after spinal cord injury.

In clinical trials, an extremely high dosage of methylprednisolone was used in a **double-blind study** (neither patients nor doctors knew who was getting the experimental drug). The improvement in some patients was so remarkable that the National Institutes of Health felt it was important to "break the code" (i.e., determine who was getting the drug and who was not) so more patients could potentially be helped.

Overall, the trial showed that while the methylprednisolone treated group retained significantly more function than the placebo group, subjects in both groups experienced chronic loss of function due to their injuries.

Methylprednisolone is effective **only** if used in high doses within eight hours of acute injury. It is hypothesized that this drug reduces damage caused by the inflammation of the injured spinal cord and the bursting open of the damaged cells. The contents of the damaged cells are believed to adversely affect adjacent cells. High doses of methylprednisolone can lead to side effects, such as suppression of the immune system, but no serious problems have been reported when it is used over a short term as in this study.

Because the success of the methylprednisolone trial had changed the "standard of care" in the United States, subsequent drug trials are now testing the effectiveness of other drugs in combination with methylprednisolone administration. Thus, to demonstrate significant effectiveness, new treatments will have to surpass the functional sparing effects seen with methylprednisolone alone.

Simultaneously, researchers are cooperating to conduct a large multi-center animal study to test the effect of other drugs with or without methylprednisolone.

Tirilizade

Similar positive results to those of methylprednisolone have been achieved in animal studies using another steroid, *tirilizade mesylate* (Freedox®). This drug, which acts like methylprednisolone, also appears to be effective only if administered within a few hours after injury. From initial animal studies, it appears that this drug may cause less side effects than methylprednisolone. Clinical trials are ongoing.

A large clinical trial with humans is currently underway comparing 48 hour treatment of methylprednisolone with or without added tirilizade. Study results are anticipated to be available in late 1995.

GM-1 Ganglioside

Once again, the announcement of a new treatment approach has raised interest and hope in the SCI community. In a small study, the experimental drug Sygen®), or GM-1 Ganglioside, was given within 72 hours of injury and then continued for up to 32 days. Neurological assessments were conducted up to one year after the treatment. Individuals who received Sygen® showed significantly more functional recovery than those who received a placebo.

Currently, a large scale multi-center clinical trial of GM-1 is ongoing with a targeted completion date of 1996-1997. In the current study, all patients receive the "standard" dose of methylprednisolone. In earlier studies, a standard dose of methylprednisolone was not given.

There are two theories about how GM-1 Ganglioside may act on spinal cord tissue. The first is that it performs some type of damage control by reducing the toxicity of amino acids released after spinal cord tissue is injured. The "excitatory" amino acids cause cells to die and increase the damage caused by the initial injury. The second theory suggests there may be a neurotrophic effect, somehow encouraging the growth of injured neurons. Neither of these theories have been scientifically proven yet.

Sygen® has not yet been approved for clinical use in this country by the Food and Drug Administration (FDA). It has only been used in a limited number of experiments. Sygen® was provided recently to injured football player Dennis Byrd and approximately 65 other patients through an open-label protocol. Although this protocol is no longer in effect, the large double-blind, multi-center trial in acute SCI mentioned above is well underway.

Surgery

Clinical studies are being conducted by surgeons to determine the optimum time for surgery to relieve pressure on the spinal cord after spinal cord injury. Additionally, the use of delayed decompressive surgery is being investigated in cases of chronic SCI.

Preventing new injuries during spinal surgery

Intraoperative monitoring techniques have been developed to protect healthy nerve roots during spinal stabilization procedures. Scientists tested, first on animals then on humans, a technique that assists surgeons in the placement of metallic hardware for stabilization of the spine. The technique which utilizes nerve stimulation and muscle responses has been shown to effectively predict and allow the prevention of nerve damage during surgery in the lumbosacral spinal column.

Treatments for Chronic Spinal Cord Injury and Its Complications

Functional Electrical Stimulation. FES uses implanted or external electrodes to stimulate paralyzed nerves so that arms and legs can be used for improved function. Over the past decade, three primary applications for FES have been developed: FES for exercise; FES for **upper extremity** (hand/arm) function; and FES for **lower extremity** (leg function.) FES is discussed in detail in Fact Sheet No. 9, Functional Electrical Stimulation: Clinical Applications.

Omentum Transposition. One controversial treatment for SCI is Omentum Transposition. The omentum is a band of tissue in the abdomen of mammals which provides circulation to the intestines.

A surgical procedure is used to partially detach the omentum, tunnel it under the skin and suture it in place at the injury site. The omentum tissue, which is rich in blood vessels, may supply the damaged nerve cells with vital oxygen. It is believed that the omentum tissue may also secrete chemicals that stimulate nerve growth, as well as have the ability to soak up fluids to reduce pressure which can damage nerve cells.

Initial animal trials seem to show some functional improvement if the operation is completed within 3 hours of injury. Little or no improvement is shown when the procedure is done 6-8 hours post injury. This research, however, has never been scientifically documented.

The on-going clinical trial for people who have had a SCI for months or years has recently been cancelled. Many scientists believe it is premature for human trials, since the results of the earlier research have not been sufficiently documented.

Biomedical engineering. Scientists in the field of biomedical engineering developed mechanical devices that use today's computer technology to assist individuals in activities of daily life. Examples of the types of devices under research and development are environmental control devices, electronic hand grip devices, and walking devices.

Spasticity/Pain. The complications of spasticity and pain are common in spinal cord injury. Spasticity that is severe enough to cause problems with mobility and self care, that contributes to skin breakdown, and that causes pain is reported in a number of cases of SCI.

Studies in the treatment of spasticity are investigating pharmacological agents, intrathecal baclofen, and spinal cord stimulation. In addition to drugs that have been available for some time (baclofen, valium, dantrium) the use of tizanidine has recently been explored. FDA approval of tizanidine is expected in late 1995.

The problem of pain occurs in approximately 50% of all cases of SCI. Five to thirty percent characterize the pain as disabling. Pharmacologic agents as well as surgical interventions such as the DREZ (dorsal root entry zone) procedure, cordotomy and cordectomy are under investigation for the treatment of severe causes of pain from SCI.

Male Fertility. In most SCI men, the ability to have an ejaculation and to father a child naturally is diminished. In fact, ten years ago, doctors were telling newly injured SCI men that they would not be able to father their own children. With advances made in procedures to assist men in obtaining an ejaculation as well as advances in assistive reproduction technology, SCI men now have the potential to become biological fathers. Vibratory stimulation and electroejaculation are procedures that have been investigated and are currently available to assist men in obtaining ejaculations.

Obtaining the ejaculation is only part of the fertility problem in SCI men, however, the semen from SCI men most often contains a lower than normal percent of motile sperm. Questions that researchers hope to be able to answer with investigations on the quality of sperm of SCI men are: what happens to semen quality following SCI? and how successful is artificial insemination and other reproductive technology using semen from SCI men?

Technology and research are making it possible for spinal cord injured men to consider options regarding their fertility and is providing a more encouraging answer to the question, "Will I be able to have children?"

Alternative Therapies. Various controversial treatments for SCI have come and gone over the years, but none have proved to be effective in reversing the damage to the spinal cord that occurs in spinal cord injury. Often alternative therapies are very difficult to evaluate because of the unscientific nature in which the treatments are introduced to the human population. Many alternative therapies have no documented scientific evidence to substantiate their effectiveness. Currently, examples of treatments that fall into this category are the use of Sygen® (GM-1) in chronic injuries and omentum transposition.

Summary of Treatment Research

Over the last several years there has been progress in the treatment of acute SCI to limit damage and preserve function. Treatment of chronic SCI presents a greater challenge, as damage that has already occurred must be corrected and then reversed.

It is entirely possible that, given appropriate financial support, many of the complex problems of SCI one day will be solved. Until that day arrives, it is important to urge the federal government to provide broad-based support for basic science research so the fundamental questions about how and why the CNS acts the way it does can be answered. A cure or new treatments are possible only if scientists receive the support necessary to continue their work in this important area.

For further Information on Freedox® clinical trials, contact: Upjohn Company, 929 Lawrence Court, N. Bellmore, NY 11710, 516-486-5276.

For further Information on Sygen® clinical trials, contact: Fidia Pharmaceutical Corp., 1401 I Street, NW, #900, Washington, DC 20005, 202-371-9898.

For further Information about FES applications, contact: the F.E.S. Information Center, 25100 Euclid Avenue, Suite 105, Cleveland, OH 44117, 800-666-2353.

For further Information about The Miami Project, contact: The Miami Project, 1600 Northwest 10th Avenue, R-48, Miami, FL 33136, 1-800-STAND-UP.

Suggested Readings:

Books

Maddox, Sam, (1992): *The Quest for Cure: Restoration of Function After Spinal Cord Injury.* Paralyzed Veterans of America, 801 18th Street, N.W., Washington, DC 20006.

U.S. Department of Health and Human Services, National Institutes of Health, The NINDS Research Program, (1989): *Spinal Cord Injury.* NIH-NINDS, Building 31A, Room 8A16, 9000 Rockville Pike, Bethesda, MD 20892.

Newsletters/Magazines

International Spinal Research Trust Newsletter, International Spinal Research Trust, Nicholas House—River Front, Effield, Middlesex, England.

Paraplegia: International Journal of the Spinal Cord, Churchill-Livingston of Edinbourough London, Subscription Manager, Journal Department, Longman Group, 4th Avenue, Harlow Essex CN19 SA, UK.

Paraplegia News, monthly research column, Paralyzed Veterans of America, 801 18th Street, NW, Washington, DC 20006.

Progress in Research and Walking Tomorrow, the American Paralysis Association, P.O. Box 187, Short Hills, NJ 07078.

SCI Life, National Spinal Cord Injury Association quarterly publication.

The Project: News from the Miami Project to Cure Paralysis, Miami Project, 1600 NW 10th Avenue, R-48, Miami, FL 33136.

Manuscripts/Articles

Neural Grafting, Repairing the Brain and Spinal Cord, New Developments in Neuroscience, Congress of the United States, Office of Technology Assessment, Superintendent of Documents, U.S. Government Printing Office, Washington, DC 20402-9325.

Bracken, M., (May, 1990). A Randomized Controlled Trial of Methylprednisolone or Naloxone in the Treatment of Acute SCI, *The New England Journal of Medicine*, 322(20) pp. 1405.

Bunge, R.P., et al. (1991). Regeneration of Axons from Human Retina In Vitro, *Experimental Neurology*, 112:243-251.

Bunge, R.P., et al. (1991). Isolation and Functional Characterization of Schwann Cells Derived from Adult Peripheral Nerve, *Journal of Neuroscience*, 11:2433-2442.

Bunge, R.P., et al. (1992). Sygeneic Schwann Cells Derived from Adult Nerves Seeded in Semipermeable Guidance Channels Enhance Peripheral Nerve Regeneration, *The Journal of Neuroscience*, 12(9): 3310-3320.

Bunge, R.P. (1994). Clinical implications of recent advances in neurotrauma research. In: *The Neurobiology of Central Nervous System Trauma*,(Salzman, S.K., Faden, A.I., Eds.). Oxford University Press, pp 329-339.

Calancie, Blair, et al. (1992). Intraoperative Evoked EMG Monitoring in an Animal Model, A New Technique for Evaluating Pedicle Screw Placement, *Spine*, Volume 17, No. 10; 1229-1235.

Calancie, Blair, et al. (1994). Involuntary stepping after spinal cord injury, *Brain*, 117; 1143-1159.

Geisler, F.H. et al. (June, 1991). Recovery of Motor Function After Spinal Cord Injury—A Randomized, Placebo-Controlled Trial with GM-I Ganglioside, *The New England Journal of Medicine*, 324(26) 1829-1838.

Guenard, V., Xu, X.M., Bunge, M.B. (1993). The use of Schwann cells transplantation to foster central nervous system repair, *Seminars in the Neurosciences*, 5;410-411.

Onifer, S.M., Whittemore, S.R., and Holets, V.R. (1993). Variable morphological differentiation of a raphe-derives neuronal cell line following transplantation in adult rat CNS, *Experimental Neurology*, 122;130-142.

Travis, John, (October 1992). Spinal Cord Injuries: New Optimism Blooms for Developing Treatments, *Science*, Volume 258, pp 218-220.

This factsheet was prepared with the assistance of Dr. Cheryl Chanaud of the National Institutes of Health and Dr. Naomi Kleitman and Marie Amador, RN, CRRN of the Miami Project to Cure Paralysis. This factsheet is offered as an information service and is not intended to cover all treatments nor research in the field, nor is it an endorsement of the methods mentioned herein. Any information you may have to offer to further update this factsheet would be greatly appreciated. The National Spinal Cord Injury Resource Center (NSCIRC) provides information and referral on any subject related to spinal cord injury. Contact the resource center at 1-800-962-9629.

Chapter 41

Disability and Social Security

Who Should Read This Chapter?

You should, if you want to know more about the various kinds of disability benefits available from Social Security. This chapter will tell you who is eligible, how to apply, and what you need to know once benefits start.

We pay disability benefits under two programs: the Social Security disability insurance program and the Supplemental Security Income (SSI) program. The medical requirements for disability payments are the same under both programs and a person's disability is determined by the same process. While eligibility for Social Security disability is based on prior work under Social Security, SSI disability payments are made on the basis of financial need. And there are other differences in the eligibility rules for the two programs. This chapter deals primarily with the Social Security disability program. For information on SSI disability payments, refer to the section, "A Word about Supplemental Security Income," at the back of this chapter, or ask for the booklets, *SSI* (Publication No. 05-11000) and *Working While Disabled ... How Social Security Can Help* (Publication No. 05-10095).

Please Note: This chapter provides a general overview of the disability program. The information it contains is not intended to cover all provisions of the law. For specific information about your case, contact Social Security.

SSA Pub. No. 05-10029, January 1992.

Introduction to Disability and Social Security

Disability is something most people don't like to think about. But the chances of your becoming disabled are probably greater than you realize. In fact, studies show that one out of four young workers will become disabled some time during their lifetime.

It's a fact that, while most people spend time working to succeed in their jobs and careers, few think about ensuring that they have a safety net to fall back on should the unthinkable happen. This is where Social Security comes in. We pay cash benefits to people who are unable to work for a year or more because of a disability. Benefits continue until a person is able to work again on a regular basis and a number of work incentives are available to ease the transition back to work.

What We Mean by "Disability"

It's important that you understand how Social Security defines "disability." That's because different programs have different bases for determining disability. Some programs may pay for partial disability or for short-term disability. Social Security does **not**.

Disability under Social Security is based on your inability to work. You will be considered disabled if you are unable to do any kind of work for which you are suited, and only if your inability to work is also expected to last for at least a year or to result in death.

Some consider this a strict definition of disability, and it is. The program assumes that working families have access to other resources to provide support during periods of short-term disabilities, including workers compensation, insurance, savings, and investments. It is designed to provide a continuing income to you and your family when you are unable to do so. Benefits continue as long as you remain disabled.

Who Can Get Social Security Disability Benefits

You can receive Social Security disability benefits at any age. If you are receiving disability benefits at age 65, they become retirement benefits, although the amount remains the same. Certain members of your family may also qualify for benefits on your record. They include:

- Your unmarried son or daughter, including a stepchild, adopted child, or, in some cases, a grandchild. The child must be under 18 or under 19 if in high school full time.

- Your unmarried son or daughter, 18 or older, if he or she has a disability that started before 22. (If a disabled child under 18 is receiving benefits as a dependent of a retired, deceased, or disabled worker, someone should contact Social Security to have his or her checks continued at 18 on the basis of disability.)

- Your spouse who is 62 or older.

- Your spouse at any age if he or she is caring for a child of yours who is under 16 or disabled and also receiving checks.

Certain family members may qualify for disability benefits if you should die. They include:

- Your disabled widow or widower 50 or older. The disability must have started before your death or within 7 years after your death. (If your widow or widower caring for your children receives Social Security checks, she or he is eligible if she or he becomes disabled before those payments end or within 7 years after they end.)

- Your disabled ex-wife or husband who is 50 or older if the marriage lasted 10 years or longer.

Disability Benefits for Children

In recent years, there has been a growing concern about whether parents are aware of the disability benefits that are available for their disabled children. More than 475,000 children under 18 who have disabilities currently receive such benefits; many suffer some form of mental retardation, others from various childhood conditions. We recently changed the way we decide if a child is disabled, generally making it easier for children to qualify.

SSI disability benefits are payable to people of any age with a disability, including children. For more information, ask Social Security for the booklets, *SSI* (Publication No. 05-11000) and *Social Security*

439

and SSI Benefits For Children With Disabilities (Publication No. 05-10026).

Social Security dependents benefits are payable to children under 18 if a parent is receiving retirement or disability benefits or is deceased. These benefits may also be paid to children 18 or older who were disabled before age 22. Benefits will continue into their adult years as long as they remain disabled.

How Much Work You Need for Social Security Benefits

To qualify for Social Security disability benefits, you must have worked long enough and recently enough under Social Security. You earn up to a maximum of 4 credits per year. The amount of earnings required for a credit increases each year as general wage levels rise. Family members who qualify for benefits on your work record do not need work credits.

The number of work credits needed for disability benefits depends on your age when you become disabled.

- **Before age 24**—You need 6 credits in the 3-year period ending when your disability starts.

- **Age 24 to 31**—You need credit for having worked half the time between 21 and the time you become disabled. For example, if you became disabled at age 27, you would need credit for 3 years of work (out of 6 years).

- **Age 31 or older**—You need to have the same number of work credits as you would need for retirement, as shown in the following chart. Also, you generally must have earned at least 20 of the credits in the 10 years immediately before you became disabled.

Signing Up for Disability

How to Apply

You should apply at any Social Security office as soon as you become disabled. (You may file by phone, mail, or by visiting the nearest office.) However, Social Security disability benefits will not begin

Born After 1929, Become Disabled At Age	Born Before 1930, Become Disabled Before 62	Credits You Need
31 through 42		20
44		22
46		24
48		26
50		28
52		30
53		31
54		32
55		33
56		34
57	1986	35
58	1987	36
59	1988	37
60	1989	38
62 or older	1991 or later	40

Table 41.1. Credits needed for Social Security disability benefits.

until the 6th full month of disability. This "waiting period" begins with the first full month after the onset of your disability.

The claims process for disability benefits is generally longer than for other types of Social Security benefits—from 60 to 90 days. It takes longer to obtain medical information and to assess the nature of the disability in terms of your ability to work. However, you can help shorten the process by bringing certain documents with you when you apply. These include:

- The Social Security number and proof of age for each person applying for payments. This includes your spouse and children, if they are applying for benefits.

- Names, addresses, and phone numbers of doctors, hospitals, clinics, and institutions that treated you and dates of treatment.

- A summary of where you worked in the past 15 years and the kind of work you did.

- A copy of your W-2 Form (Wage and Tax Statement), or if you are self-employed, your Federal tax return for the past year.

- Dates of any prior marriages if your spouse is applying.

Do not delay filing for benefits just because you do not have all of the information you need. The Social Security office will be glad to help you.

Who Decides If You Are Disabled

After helping you complete your application, the Social Security office will review it to see if you meet the nondisability requirements of the law. These include such factors as whether you have worked long enough and recently enough to qualify for disability benefits, your age, and, if you are applying for benefits as a family member, your relationship to the worker. The office will then send your application to the Disability Determination Services (DDS) office in your State. There, a decision will be made as to whether you are disabled under the Social Security law.

In the DDS office, a team consisting of a physician (or psychologist) and a disability evaluation specialist will consider all the facts in your case and decide if you are disabled. They will first make every reasonable effort to get medical evidence from your doctors and from hospitals, clinics, or institutions where you have been treated. The Government pays a reasonable charge for any medical reports that it needs and requests. If the DDS team has difficulty getting a medical report, you may be asked to help obtain it. You do not need to ask your doctor for a report before you apply for disability benefits. But, if you have copies of your medical reports available, it may take us less time to process your claim.

On the medical report forms, your doctors or other sources are asked for a medical history of your condition: What is wrong with you and when it began; how the condition limits activities; what the medical tests have shown; and what treatment has been provided. They are also asked for information about your ability to do work-related activities, such as walking, sitting, lifting, and carrying. They are **not** asked to decide whether you are disabled.

Additional medical information may be needed before the DDS team can decide your case. If it is not available from your current medical sources, you may be asked to take a special examination called a "consultative examination." Your doctor or the medical facility where you have been treated is the preferred source to perform this examination. Social Security will pay for the examination or any other additional medical tests you may need, and for certain travel expenses related to it.

The rules in the Social Security law for determining disability differ from those in other Government and private programs. However, a decision made by another agency and the medical reports it obtains may be considered in determining whether you are disabled under Social Security rules.

Once a decision on your claim is reached, you will receive a written notice from the Social Security Administration. If your claim is approved, the notice will show the amount of your benefit and when payments start. If it is not approved, the notice will explain why.

How We Determine Disability

You should be familiar with the process we use to determine if you are disabled. It's a step-by-step process involving five questions. They are:

1. **Are you working?** If you are and your earnings average more than $500 a month, you generally cannot be considered disabled.

2. **Is your condition "severe"?** Your impairments must interfere with basic work-related activities for your claim to be considered further.

3. **Is your condition found in the list of disabling impairments?** We maintain a list of impairments for each of the major body systems that are so severe they automatically mean you are disabled. If your condition is not on the list, we have to determine if it is of equal severity to an impairment on the list. If it is, your claim is approved. If it is not, we go to the next step.

4. **Can you do the work you did previously?** If your condition is severe, but not at the same or equal severity as an

impairment on the list, then we must determine if it interferes with your ability to do the work you did in the last 15 years. If it does not, your claim will be denied. If it does, your claim will be considered further.

5. **Can you do any other type of work?** If you cannot do the work you did in the last 15 years, we then look to see if you can do any other type of work. We consider your age, education, past work experience, and transferable skills, and we review the job demands of occupations as determined by the Department of Labor. If you cannot do any other kind of work, your claim will be approved. If you can, your claim will be denied.

If Your Claim Is Denied

If your claim is denied, or if you disagree with any other decision we make, you may appeal the decision. The Social Security office will help you complete the paperwork.

There are four levels of appeal. If you disagree with the decision at one level, you may appeal to the next level. You have 60 days from the time you receive the decision to file an appeal to the next level. We assume that you receive the decision 5 days after the date on it, unless you can show us that you received it later.

Reconsideration. Your file is reviewed by persons other than those who made the original decision.

Hearing. If the reconsideration decision is still unfavorable, you may apply for a hearing before a judge. If you are appealing a decision that you are no longer medically disabled, you may also request that we continue your benefits while you wait for a decision.

Appeals Council. The Appeals Council will review your case if it feels that there is an issue that the judge did not address. If it denies your review, or you otherwise disagree with its decision, you may appeal to a Federal Civil Court.

United States District Court. Again, you have 60 days from the day you received the notice of the decision to appeal to a Federal Court.

When Your Claim Is Approved

Your First Check

Once a decision is made that you are disabled, you will receive your first Social Security disability check dating back to the 6th full month from the onset of your disability. You also will receive a booklet describing your responsibilities as a Social Security beneficiary: *When You Get Social Security Disability Benefits — What You Need To Know* (Publication No. 05-10153). You should read this booklet carefully and keep it in a safe place with your other valuable papers in order to refer to it whenever questions arise.

How Much You Will Get from Social Security

The amount of your monthly disability benefits is based on your lifetime average earnings covered by Social Security. If you would like an estimate of your disability benefit, all you have to do is call or visit Social Security and ask for it. We'll send you a form you can use to get a *Personal Earnings and Benefit Estimate Statement.*

How Other Payments Affect Benefits

Eligibility for other government benefits can affect the amount of your Social Security disability benefits.

Other Disability Benefits. Social Security benefits may be affected if you are also eligible for workers' compensation (including black lung) or for disability benefits from certain Federal, State, local government, Civil Service, or military disability programs. Total combined payments to you and your family from Social Security and any of these other programs generally cannot exceed 80 percent of your average current earnings before becoming disabled.

Government Pension Offset. If you are a disabled widow or widower or the spouse of a disabled worker, a "government pension offset" may reduce your Social Security payment. The offset applies if you become eligible for a Federal, State, or local government pension based on your own work not covered by Social Security. The amount of your Social Security spouse's benefit may be reduced by two-thirds of the amount of your government pension.

There are some exceptions when the offset would not apply. For more information, call or visit Social Security to ask for a free copy of the factsheet, *Government Pension Offset* (Publication No. 05-10007).

Pension From Work Not Covered By Social Security. If you become disabled and entitled to a Social Security disability benefit and you also receive a monthly pension based on work not covered by Social Security, your disability payment will be smaller than normal. That's because we use a different formula to figure the Social Security benefit of people who get other public pensions.

For more information, call or visit Social Security to ask for a free copy of the factsheet, *A Pension From Work Not Covered By Social Security* (Publication No. 05-10045).

Benefits May Be Taxed

A relatively small number of people may have to pay Federal income taxes on their Social Security benefits. This usually happens only if your total income is high. At the end of the year, you will receive a Social Security Benefit Statement (Form SSA-1099) showing the amount of benefits you received. The statement is to be used for completing your Federal income tax return if any of your benefits are subject to tax. You may use the Internal Revenue Service Publication 915 for additional information on the tax.

You Can Get Medicare If You're Disabled

You will be automatically enrolled in Medicare after you have been getting disability benefits for 2 years.

There are two parts to Medicare—hospital insurance and medical insurance. Hospital insurance helps pay hospital bills and some follow-up care. The taxes you paid while you were working financed this coverage, so it's premium free if you're eligible. The other part of Medicare, medical insurance, helps pay doctors' bills and other services. You pay a monthly premium for this coverage if you want it. Almost everybody has both parts of Medicare.

If you get Medicare, and have little income or resources, you should know about a program that can save you money on out-of-pocket medical costs. The program is called the "Qualified Medicare Beneficiary" program, or QMB. For more information, call a Social Security office to ask for the factsheet, *You Should Know About QMB* (Publication No. 05-10079).

Reviewing Your Disability

Your benefits will continue as long as you are disabled. However, your case will be reviewed periodically to see if you are still disabled. The frequency of the reviews depends on the expectation of recovery.

- If medical improvement is "expected," your case will normally be reviewed within 6 to 18 months.
- If medical improvement is "possible," your case will normally be reviewed no sooner than 3 years.
- If medical improvement is "not expected," your case may be reviewed no sooner than 7 years.

What Can Cause Benefits to Stop

There are two things that can cause us to decide that you are no longer disabled and to stop your benefits.

Your benefits will stop if you work at a level we consider "substantial." Usually, average earnings of $500 or more a month are considered substantial.

Your disability benefits would also stop if we decide that your medical condition has improved to the point that you are no longer disabled.

You must promptly report any improvement in your condition, your return to work, and certain other events as long as you are receiving benefits. These responsibilities are explained in the booklet you will receive when benefits start.

Going Back to Work

Benefits While You Work

If you're like most people, you would rather work than try to live on disability benefits. There are a number of special rules that provide cash benefits and Medicare while you attempt to work. We call these rules "work incentives." You should be familiar with these disability work incentives so that you can use them to your advantage.

If you are receiving Social Security disability benefits, the following rules are among the work incentives that apply:

- **Trial Work Period**—For 9 months (not necessarily consecutive), you may earn as much as you can without affecting your benefits. (The 9 months of work must fall within a 5-year period before your trial work period can end.) A trial work month is any month in which you earn more than $200. After your trial work period ends, your work is evaluated to see if it is "substantial." If your earnings do not average more than $500 a month, benefits will generally continue. If earnings do average more than $500 a month, benefits will continue for a 3-month grace period before they stop.

- **Extended Period of Eligibility**—For 36 months after a successful trial work period, if you are still disabled, you will be eligible to receive a monthly benefit without a new application for any month your earnings drop below $500.

- **Deductions for Impairment-Related Expenses**—Work expenses related to your disability will be discounted in figuring whether your earnings constitute substantial work.

- **Medicare Continuation**—Your Medicare coverage will continue for 39 months beyond the trial work period. If your Medicare coverage stops because of your work, you may purchase it for a monthly premium.

For more information about Social Security's work incentives, ask for a copy of the booklet, *Working While Disabled ... How Social Security Can Help* (Publication No. 05-10095).

A Word about Supplemental Security Income

As we stated earlier, the medical requirements for disability payments are the same for Social Security and SSI, and a person's disability is determined by the same process for both programs. But there are some differences between Social Security and SSI that you should know about. These include:

- No disability waiting period is required under SSI. Because SSI payments are based on financial need, the presumption that a person has resources to handle short-term health problems does not exist.

- Under SSI, you may qualify for an immediate disability payment if your condition is obviously disabling and you meet the SSI income and resource limits.

- Different work incentive rules apply to SSI recipients. The major difference is that cash benefits and Medicaid continue as long as the SSI income limits are not exceeded (the "substantial" income level discussed in "Going Back to Work" does not apply). Another important rule permits money to be set aside for up to 48 months for a work goal. Other special rules apply to blind persons, disabled students, and people with disabilities who work in sheltered workshops.

Some work incentive rules are the same for Social Security disability and SSI. These include the work expenses exclusion and the continuation of benefits while in a vocational rehabilitation program.

For more information about SSI disability payments, ask for the publications, *SSI* (Publication No. 05-11000) and *Working While Disabled ... How Social Security Can Help* (Publication No. 05-10095).

For More Information

For more information or to apply for benefits, call or visit Social Security. It's easiest to call Social Security's toll-free telephone number. The number is 1-800-772-1213. You can speak to a representative 7 a.m. to 7 p.m. on business days.

The Social Security Administration treats all calls confidentially—whether they're made to our toll-free number or to one of our local offices. We also want to ensure that you receive accurate and courteous service. That is why we have a second Social Security representative listen to some incoming and outgoing telephone calls.

Other Booklets Available

Social Security has a number of publications that contain information about other Social Security programs. Contact Social Security to get a free copy of any of these publications. They include:

- *Understanding Social Security* (Publication No. 05-10024)—A comprehensive explanation of all the Social Security programs.

- *Retirement* (Publication No. 05-10035)—Explains Social Security retirement benefits.

- *Survivors* (Publication No. 05-10084)—Explains Social Security survivors benefits.

- *Medicare* (Publication No. 05-10043)—Explains Medicare hospital insurance and medical insurance.

- *SSI* (Publication No. 05-11000)—Explains this program, which provides a basic income to people who are 65 or older, disabled, or blind and have limited income and resources.

- *Social Security And SSI Benefits For Children With Disabilities* (Publication No. 05-10026)—Explains benefits available to children with disabilities.

All these publications are available in Spanish.

Chapter 42

Information for the Air Traveler with a Spinal Cord Injury

Introduction

For years, access to the nation's air travel system for persons with disabilities was an area of substantial dissatisfaction, with both passengers and the airline industry recognizing the need for major improvement. In 1986 Congress passed the Air Carrier Access Act, requiring the Department of Transportation (DOT) to develop new regulations which ensure that persons with disabilities will be treated without discrimination in a way consistent with the safe carriage of all passengers. These regulations were published in March 1990.

The DOT regulations, referred to here as the Air Carrier Access rules, represent a major stride forward in improving air travel for persons with disabilities. The rules clearly explain the responsibilities of the traveler, the carriers, the airport operators, and contractors, who collectively make up the system which moves over one million passengers per day. (These rules do not apply to foreign airlines.)

The Air Carrier Access rules are designed to minimize the special problems that travelers with disabilities face as they negotiate their way through the nation's complex air travel system from origin to destination. This is achieved:

New Horizons: Information for the Air Traveler with a Disability, 2nd ed. U.S. Department of Transportation, July 1995.

- By recognizing that the physical barriers encountered by passengers with disabilities can frequently be overcome by employing simple changes in layout and technology.

- By adopting the principle that many difficulties confronting passengers with hearing or vision impairments will be relieved if they are provided access to the same information that is available to all other passengers.

- Through training of all air travel personnel who come in day-to-day contact with persons with disabilities, to understand their needs and how they can be accommodated quickly, safely, and with dignity.

This guide is designed to offer travelers with disabilities a brief but authoritative source of information about the Air Carrier Access rules: the accommodations, facilities, and services that are now required to be available. It also describes features required by other regulations designed to make air travel more accessible.

The guide is structured in much the same sequence as a passenger would plan for a trip: the circumstances he or she must consider prior to traveling, what will be encountered at the airport, and what to expect in the transitions from airport to airplane, on the plane, and then airplane to airport.

Planning Your Trip

The New Traveling Environment

The Air Carrier Access rules sweep aside many restrictions that formerly discriminated against passengers with disabilities:

- A carrier may not refuse transportation to a passenger solely on the basis of a disability.

- Air carriers may not limit the number of individuals with disabilities on a particular flight.

- All trip information that is made available to other passengers also must be made available to passengers with disabilities.

- Carriers must provide passage to an individual who has a disability that may affect his or her appearance or involuntary behavior, even if this disability may offend, annoy, or be an inconvenience to crew-members or other passengers.

There are a few exceptions:

- The carrier may refuse transportation if the individual with a disability would endanger the health or safety of other passengers, or transporting the person would be a violation of FAA safety rules.

- If the plane has fewer than 30 seats, the carrier may refuse transportation if there are no lifts, boarding chairs or other devices available which can be adapted to the limitations of such small aircraft by which to enplane the passenger. Airline personnel are not required to carry a mobility-impaired person onto the aircraft by hand.

- There are special rules about persons with certain disabilities or communicable diseases. These rules are covered in the section entitled "At the Airport."

- The carrier may refuse transportation if it is unable to seat the passenger without violating the FAA Exit Row Seating rules. See the section "On the Plane."

There are new procedures for resolving disputes:

- All carriers are now required to have a Complaints Resolution Official (CRO) immediately available (even if by phone) to resolve disagreements which may arise between the carrier and passengers with disabilities.

- Travelers who disagree with a carrier's actions toward them can pursue the issue with the carrier's CRO on the spot.

- A carrier that refuses transportation to any person based on a disability must provide a written statement to that person within 10 calendar days, stating the basis for the refusal. The statement must include, where applicable, the basis for the carrier's opinion that transporting the person could be harmful to the safety of the flight.

- If the passenger is still not satisfied, he or she may pursue DOT enforcement action.

Getting Advance Information about the Aircraft

Travelers with disabilities must be provided information upon request concerning facilities and services available to them. When feasible this information will pertain to the specific aircraft scheduled for a specific flight. Such information includes:

- Any limitations which may be known to the carrier concerning the ability of the aircraft to accommodate an individual with a disability;

- The location of seats (if any) with movable aisle armrests and any seats which the carrier does not make available to an individual with a disability (e.g., exit rows);

- Any limitations on the availability of storage facilities in the cabin or in the cargo bay for mobility aids or other equipment commonly used by an individual with a disability;

- Whether the aircraft has an accessible lavatory.

Normally, advance information about the aircraft will be requested by phone. Any carrier that provides telephone service for the purpose of making reservations or offering general information must provide comparable services for hearing-impaired individuals, utilizing telecommunications devices for the deaf (TDDs), or text telephones (TTs). The TTs shall be available during the same hours that the general public has access to regular phone service. The response time to answer calls on the TT line shall also be equivalent to the response time available to the general public. Charges for the call, if any, shall be the same as charges made to the general public.

When Advance Notice Can Be Required

Airlines may not require passengers with disabilities to provide advance notice of their intent to travel or of their disability except as provided below. Nonetheless, letting the airline know in advance how they can help you will generally result in a smoother trip.

Carriers may require up to 48 hours advance notice and one hour advance check-in from a person with a disability who wishes to receive any of the following services:

- Transportation for an electric wheelchair on an aircraft with fewer than 60 seats;

- Provision by the carrier of hazardous materials packaging for the battery of a wheelchair or other assistive device;

- Accommodations for 10 or more passengers with disabilities who travel as a group;

- Provision of an on-board wheelchair on an aircraft that does not have an accessible lavatory for persons who can use an inaccessible lavatory but need an on-board chair to do so.

Carriers are not required to provide the following services or equipment, but should they choose to provide them, they may require 48 hours advance notice and a one hour advance check-in:

- Medical oxygen for use on board the aircraft;
- Carriage of an incubator;
- Hook-up for a respirator to the aircraft's electrical supply;
- Accommodations for a passenger who must travel on a stretcher.

Carriers may impose reasonable, nondiscriminatory charges for these optional services.

Where a service is required by the rule, the airline must ensure that it is provided if appropriate notice has been given and the service requested is available on that particular flight. If a passenger does not meet advance notice or check-in requirements, carriers must make a reasonable effort to accommodate the requested service, providing this does not delay the flight.

If a passenger with a disability provides the required notice but is required to fly on another carrier (for example, if the flight is cancelled), the original carrier must, to the maximum extent feasible, provide assistance to the second carrier in furnishing the accommodation requested by the individual.

It must be recognized that even when a passenger has requested information in advance on the accessibility features of the scheduled aircraft, carriers sometimes have to substitute a different aircraft at the last minute for safety, mechanical or other reasons. It must also be recognized that the substitute aircraft may not be as fully accessible—a condition that may prevail for a number of years. On-board wheelchairs must be available on many aircraft, but it will take a number of years before movable aisle armrests are available on all aircraft with over 30 seats. Similarly, while accessible lavatories must be built into all new wide-body aircraft, they will be put into existing aircraft only when such aircraft are undergoing a major interior refurbishment.

When Attendants Can Be Required

Carriers may require the following individuals to be accompanied by an attendant:

- A person traveling on a stretcher or in an incubator (for flights where such service is offered);

- A person who, because of a mental disability, is unable to comprehend or respond appropriately to safety instructions from carrier personnel;

- A person with a mobility impairment so severe that the individual is unable to assist in his or her own evacuation from the aircraft;

- A person who has both severe hearing and severe vision impairments which prevent him or her from receiving and acting on necessary instructions from carrier personnel when evacuating the aircraft during an emergency.

The carrier and the passenger may disagree about the applicability of one of these criteria. In such cases, the airline can require the passenger to travel with an attendant, contrary to the passenger's assurances that he or she can travel alone. However, the carrier cannot charge for the transportation of the attendant.

The airline can choose an attendant in a number of ways. It could designate an off duty employee who happened to be traveling on the same flight to act as the attendant. The carrier or the passenger with a disability could seek a volunteer from among other passengers on the flight to act as the attendant. The carrier could provide a free ticket to an attendant of the passenger's choice for that flight segment. In the end, however, a carrier is not required to find or furnish an attendant.

The attendant would not be required to provide personal service to the passenger with a disability other than to provide assistance in the event of an emergency evacuation. This is in contrast to the case of the passenger that usually travels accompanied by a personal attendant, who would provide the passenger whatever service he or she requests.

If there is not a seat available on the flight for an attendant, and as a result a person with a disability holding a confirmed reservation is denied travel on the flight, the passenger with a disability is eligible for denied boarding compensation.

For purposes of determining whether a seat is available for an attendant, the attendant shall be deemed to have checked in at the same time as the person with the disability.

At the Airport

Airport Accessibility

Until recently, only those airport facilities designed, constructed, or renovated by or for a recipient of federal funds had to comply with federal accessibility standards. Even at federally-assisted airports, not all facilities and activities were required to be accessible. Examples are privately-owned ground transportation and concessions selling goods or services to the public. (The accessibility features for over 500 airports are covered in a publication of the Airports Council International entitled Access Travel: Airports—A Guide to the Accessibility Of Terminals. It may be obtained by writing the Consumer Information Center, Pueblo, CO 81009.) As a result of the Air Carrier Access rules, and the Americans with Disabilities Act of 1990 (ADA) and implementing regulations, these privately-owned facilities must also be made accessible.

In general, airports under construction or being refurbished must comply with the ADA Accessibility Guidelines (ADAAG) and other regulations governing accessibility in accordance with a timetable established in the ADA. Thus, while there are still many changes to be made, the accessibility of most airports is improving. With few exceptions, the following services should be available in all air carrier terminals within the next few years:

- Accessible parking near the terminal;

- Signs indicating accessible parking and the easiest access from those spaces to the terminal;

- Accessible medical aid facilities and travelers aid stations;

- Accessible restrooms;

- Accessible drinking fountains;

- Accessible ticketing systems at primary fare collection areas;

- Amplified telephones and text telephones (TTs) for use by persons with hearing and speech impairments (there must be at least one TT in each terminal in a clearly marked accessible location);

- Accessible baggage check-in and retrieval areas;

- Jetways and mobile lounges that are accessible (at airports that have such facilities);

- Level entry boarding ramps, lifts or other means of assisting an individual with a disability on and off an aircraft;

- Information systems using visual words, letters or symbols with lighting and color coding, and systems for providing information orally;

- Signs indicating the location of specific facilities and services.

Moving Through the Airport

To make travel easier for an individual with a disability, major airports will be required to make the following services accessible under new rules being put into effect in the next several years:

- Shuttle vehicles, owned or operated by airports, transporting people between parking lots and terminal buildings;

- People movers and moving walkways within and between terminals and gates.

All carrier facilities must currently include one accessible route from an airport entrance to ticket counters, boarding locations and baggage handling areas. These routes must minimize any extra distance that wheelchair users must travel compared to other passengers to reach these facilities. Outbound and inbound baggage facilities must provide efficient baggage handling for individuals with a disability, and these facilities must be designed and operated so as to be accessible. There must be appropriate signs to indicate the location of accessible services.

Carriers cannot restrict the movements of persons with disabilities in terminals or require them to remain in a holding area or other location while awaiting transportation and other assistance.

Curbside baggage check-in (available only for domestic flights) may be helpful to passengers with a disability.

Passenger Information

Carriers must ensure that individuals with disabilities, including those with vision and hearing impairments, have timely access to the same information provided to other passengers, including (but not limited to) information on:

- ticketing;
- scheduled departure times and gates;
- change of gate assignments;
- status of flight delays;
- schedule changes;
- flight check-in;
- checking and claiming of luggage.

This information must be made available upon request. A crew member is not required to interrupt his or her immediate safety duties to supply such information.

A copy of the Air Carrier Access rules must be made available by carriers for inspection upon request at each airport.

As previously noted, any carrier that provides telephone service for the purpose of making reservations or offering general information shall also provide TT service. This service for people with speech and hearing impairments must be available during the same hours that the general public has access to regular phone service, with equivalent response times and charges.

Security Screening

An individual with a disability must undergo the same security screening as any other member of the traveling public.

If an individual with a disability is able to pass through the security system without activating it, the person shall not be subject to special screening procedures. Security personnel are free to examine an assistive device that they believe is capable of concealing a weapon or other prohibited item. If an individual with a disability is not able to pass through the system without activating it, the person will be subject to further screening in the same manner as any other passenger activating the system.

Security screening personnel at some airports may employ a handheld device that will allow them to complete the screening without having to physically search the individual. If this method is still unable to clear the individual and a physical search becomes necessary, then at the passenger's request, the search must be done in private.

If the passenger requests a private screening in a timely manner, the carrier must provide it in time for the passenger to board the aircraft. Such private screenings will not be required, however, to a greater extent or for any different reason than for other passengers. However, they may take more time.

Medical Certificates

A medical certificate is a written statement from the passenger's physician saying that the passenger is capable of completing the flight safely without requiring extraordinary medical care.

A disability is not sufficient grounds for a carrier to request a medical certificate. Carriers shall not require passengers to present a medical certificate unless the person:

- Is on a stretcher or in an incubator (where such service is offered);

- Needs medical oxygen during flight (where such service is offered);

- Has a medical condition which causes the carrier to have reasonable doubt that the individual can complete the flight safely, without requiring extraordinary medical assistance during the flight; or

- Has a communicable disease or infection that has been determined by federal public health authorities to be generally transmittable during flight.

If the medical certificate is necessitated by a communicable disease (see next section), it must say that the disease or infection will not be communicable to other persons during the normal course of flight, or it shall state any conditions or precautions that would have to be observed to prevent transmission of the disease or infection to others.

Carriers cannot mandate separate treatment for an individual with a disability except for reasons of safety or to prevent the spread of a communicable disease or infection.

Communicable Diseases

As part of their responsibility to their passengers, air carriers try to prevent the spread of infection or a communicable disease on board an aircraft. If a person who seeks passage has an infection or disease that would be transmittable during the normal course of a flight, and that has been deemed so by a federal public health authority knowledgeable about the disease or infection, then the carrier may:

- Refuse to provide transportation to the person;

- Require the person to provide a medical certificate stating that the disease at its current stage would not be transmittable during the normal course of flight, or describing measures which would prevent transmission during flight;

- Impose on the person a condition or requirement not imposed on other passengers (e.g., wearing a mask).

If the individual has a contagious disease but presents a medical certificate describing conditions or precautions that would prevent the transmission of the disease during the flight, the carrier shall provide transportation unless it is not feasible to act upon the conditions set forth in the certificate to prevent transmission of the disease.

Getting On and Off the Plane

The Safety Briefing

FAA regulations require that carrier personnel provide a safety briefing to all passengers before takeoff. This briefing is for the passengers' own safety and is intended for that purpose only.

Carrier personnel may offer an individual briefing to a person whose disability precludes him or her from receiving the information presented in the general briefing. The individual briefing must be provided as inconspicuously and discretely as possible. Most carriers choose to offer this briefing before other passengers board the flight if the passenger with a disability chooses to pre-board the flight. A carrier can present the special briefing at any time before takeoff that does not interfere with other safety duties.

Carriers may not 'quiz' the individual about the material presented in the briefing, except to the same degree they quiz all passengers about the general briefing. A carrier cannot take any adverse action against the passenger on the basis that, in the carrier's opinion, the passenger did not understand the safety briefing.

Safety briefings presented to passengers on video screens must have an open caption or an insert for a sign language interpreter, unless this would interfere with the video or would not be large enough to be seen. This requirement takes effect as old videos are replaced in the normal course of business.

Handling of Mobility Aids and Assistive Devices

To the extent consistent with various FAA safety regulations, passengers may bring on board and use ventilators and respirators, powered by non-spillable batteries. Assistive devices brought into the cabin by an individual with a disability shall not count toward a limit on carry-on items.

Persons using canes and other assistive devices may stow these items on board the aircraft, consistent with safety regulations. Carriers shall permit passengers to stow wheelchairs or component parts of a mobility device under seats, or in overhead compartments.

Carriers must permit one folding wheelchair to be stowed in a cabin closet, or other approved priority storage area, if the aircraft has such areas and stowage can be accomplished in accordance with FAA safety regulations. If the passenger using it pre-boards, stowage of the wheelchair takes priority over the carry-on items brought on by other passengers enplaning at the same airport (including passengers in another cabin, such as First Class), but not over items of passengers who boarded at previous stops.

When stowed in the cargo compartment, wheelchairs and other assistive devices must be given priority over cargo and baggage, and must be among the first items unloaded. Mobility aids shall be returned to the owner as close as possible to the door of the aircraft (consistent with DOT hazardous materials regulations) or at the baggage claim area, in accordance with whatever request was made by the passenger before boarding.

If the priority storage accorded to mobility aids prevents another passenger's baggage from being carried, the carrier shall make its best efforts to ensure the other baggage arrives within four hours.

On certain aircraft, some assistive devices will have to be disassembled in order to be transported (e.g., electric wheelchairs, other devices too large to fit in the cabin or in the cargo hold in one piece). When assistive devices are disassembled, carriers are obligated to return them to passengers in the condition that the carrier received them (e.g., assembled).

Carriers must transport battery-powered wheelchairs, except where cargo compartment size or aircraft airworthiness considerations do not permit doing so. Electric wheelchairs must be treated in accordance with both DOT regulations for handling hazardous materials, and DOT Air Carrier Access regulations, which differentiate between spillable and nonspillable batteries:

Spillable Batteries. If the chair is powered by a spillable battery, the battery must be removed unless the wheelchair can be loaded, stored, secured, and unloaded always in an upright position. When it is possible to load, store, secure, and unload with the wheelchair always in an upright position and the battery is securely attached to the wheelchair, the carrier may not remove the battery from the chair.

Nonspillable batteries. It is never necessary under the DOT hazardous materials regulations to remove a nonspillable battery from a wheelchair before stowing it. There may be individual cases, however, in which a carrier is unable to determine whether a battery is spillable or nonspillable. DOT has issued new rules that require new nonspillable batteries to be marked as such effective September 1995.

The carrier may remove a particular unmarked battery from the mobility aid if there is reasonable doubt that it is nonspillable, and it cannot be loaded, stored, secured and unloaded always in an upright position. An across-the-board assumption that all batteries are spillable is not consistent with the Air Carrier Access Rules.

A nonspillable battery may be removed where it appears to be damaged and leakage of battery fluid is possible.

Determining the Battery Type. Compliance with DOT rules on the marking of nonspillable batteries is sufficient to identify a battery as nonspillable for this purpose. In the absence of such markings, carrier personnel are responsible for determining, on a case-by-case basis, whether a battery is nonspillable, taking into account information provided by the user of the wheelchair.

- The battery of a wheelchair may not be drained.

- When DOT hazardous materials regulations require detaching the battery from the wheelchair, the carrier shall upon request provide packaging for the battery that will meet safety requirements.

- Carriers may not charge for packaging wheelchair batteries.

- Carriers may require passengers with electric wheelchairs to check in one hour before flight time.

- If a passenger checks in less than one hour before flight time, the carrier shall make a reasonable effort to carry his or her wheelchair unless this would delay the flight.

- Carriers must allow passengers to provide written instructions concerning the disassembly and assembly of their wheelchairs.

Carriers may not require a passenger with a disability to sign a waiver of liability for damage or loss of wheelchairs or other assistive devices. The carrier may make note of any pre-existing defect to the device.

On domestic trips, carriers' maximum liability for loss, damage or delay in returning assistive devices is twice the liability limit established for passengers' luggage under DOT regulations. As of the publication of this booklet, the current limit for liability on assistive devices is $2,500 per passenger (i.e., two times the $1,250 limit for luggage). (As with any passenger baggage, this limit may be increased through Excess Valuation coverage purchased through the individual airline. The passenger should also check his or her homeowners or renters insurance to determine whether it provides additional coverage.)

This expanded liability does not extend to international trips, where the Warsaw Convention applies. For most international trips (including the domestic portions of an international trip) the current liability is approximately $9.07 per pound for checked baggage and $400 per passenger for unchecked baggage.

Boarding and Deplaning

Properly trained service personnel who are knowledgeable on how to assist individuals with a disability in boarding and exiting must be available if needed. Equipment used for assisting passengers must be kept in good working condition.

Boarding and exiting most medium and large-size jet aircraft is almost always by way of level boarding ramps or mobile lounges, which must be accessible. If ramps or mobile lounges are not used, a lifting device (other than a device used for freight) must be provided to assist persons with limited mobility safely on and off the aircraft.

Lifting devices have recently become available for certain small commuter aircraft. The Department of Transportation is evaluating what approaches are viable to ensure that these devices become widely available.

Carriers do not have to hand-carry passengers on and off aircraft with fewer than 30 seats, if this is the only means of getting the person on and off the aircraft. Carrier employees may do so on a strictly voluntary basis.

In order to provide some personal assistance and extra time, the air carrier may offer a passenger with a disability, or any passenger that may be in need of assistance, the opportunity to pre-board the aircraft. The passenger has the option to accept or decline the offer.

On connecting flights, the delivering carrier is responsible for providing assistance to the individual with a disability in reaching his or her connecting flight.

Carriers cannot leave a passenger unattended for more than 30 minutes in a ground wheelchair, boarding chair, or other device in which the passenger is not independently mobile.

On the Plane

Aircraft Accessibility

Prior to the enactment of the Air Carrier Access Act of 1986, accessibility requirements for aircraft were very limited. The rules implementing that law require that new aircraft delivered after April 1992 have the following accessibility features:

- For aircraft with 30 or more passenger seats:

  —At least one half of the armrests on aisle seats shall be movable to facilitate transferring passengers from on-board wheelchairs to the aisle seat;

  —Carriers shall establish procedures to ensure that individuals with disabilities can readily obtain seating in rows with movable aisle armrests;

  —An aisle seat is not required to have a movable armrest if not feasible or if a person with a disability would be precluded from sitting there by FAA safety rules (e.g., an exit row).

- For aircraft with 100 or more seats:

  —Priority space in the cabin shall be provided for stowage of at least one passenger's folding wheelchair. (This rule also applies to aircraft of smaller size, if there is a closet large enough to accommodate a folding wheelchair.)

- For aircraft with more than one aisle:

  —At least one accessible lavatory (with door locks, call buttons, grab bars, and lever faucets) shall be available which will have sufficient room to allow a passenger using an on-board wheelchair to enter, maneuver, and use the facilities with the same degree of privacy as other passengers.

Aircraft with more than 60 seats must have an operable on-board wheelchair if

- There is an accessible lavatory, or

- A passenger provides advance notice that he or she can use an inaccessible lavatory but needs an on-board chair to reach it even if the aircraft predated the rule and has not been refurbished (see below).

An aircraft delivered before April 1992 does not have to be made accessible until its interior is refurbished. At that time the relevant accessibility features shall be added.

Airplanes in the commercial fleet have their seats replaced under different schedules depending on the carrier. At the time when all seats are being replaced on an aircraft with 30 or more passenger seats, half of the aisle seats must be equipped with movable aisle armrests. This shall be done on smaller aircraft to the extent it is not inconsistent with structural, weight, balance, operational or interior configuration limitations.

Similarly, all aircraft undergoing replacement of cabin interior elements or lavatories must meet the accessibility requirements for the affected features, including cabin storage space for a folding wheelchair, and an on-board wheelchair if there is an accessible lavatory (unless prohibited by structural, weight, balance, or configuration limitations)

Seat Assignments

An individual with a disability cannot be required to sit in a particular seat or be excluded from any seat, except as provided by FAA safety rules, such as the FAA Exit Row Seating rule. For safety reasons, that rule limits seating in exit rows to those persons with the most potential to be able to operate the emergency exit and help in an aircraft evacuation. The carrier cannot deny transport, but may deny specific seats to travelers who are less than age 15 or lack the capacity to act without an adult, or who lack sufficient mobility, strength, dexterity, vision, hearing, speech, reading or comprehension abilities to perform emergency evacuation functions. The carrier may also deny specific seats to persons with a condition or responsibilities, such as caring for small children, that might prevent the person from performing emergency evacuation functions, or cause harm to themselves in doing so.

A traveler with a disability may also be denied certain seats if:

- The passenger's involuntary behavior is such that it could compromise safety of the flight and the safety problem can be mitigated to an acceptable degree by assigning the passenger a specific seat rather than refusing service;

- The seat desired cannot accommodate guide dogs or service animals.

In each instance, carriers are obligated to offer alternative seat locations.

Service Animals

Carriers must permit dog guides or other service animals with appropriate identification to accompany an individual with a disability on a flight. Identification may include cards or other documentation, presence of a harness or markings on a harness, tags, or the credible verbal assurance of the passenger using the animal.

If carriers provide special information to passengers concerning the transportation of animals outside the continental United States, they must provide such information to all passengers with animals on such flights, not simply to passengers with disabilities who are traveling with service animals.

Carriers must permit a service animal to accompany a traveler with a disability to any seat in which the person sits, unless the animal obstructs an aisle or other area that must remain clear in order to facilitate an emergency evacuation, in which case the passenger will be assigned another seat.

In-Cabin Service

Air carrier personnel shall assist a passenger with a disability to:

- Move to and from seats as a part of the boarding and exiting process;

- Open packages and identify food (assistance with actual eating is not required);

- Use an on-board wheelchair when available to enable the passenger to move to and from the lavatory;

- Move to and from the lavatory, in the case of a semi-ambulatory person (as long as this does not require lifting or carrying by the airline employee);

- Load and retrieve carry-on items, including mobility aids and other assistive devices stowed on board the aircraft.

Carrier personnel are not required to provide assistance inside the lavatory or at the passenger's seat with elimination functions. The carrier personnel are also not required to perform medical services for an individual with a disability.

Charges for Accommodations Prohibited

Carriers cannot impose charges for providing facilities, equipment, or services to an individual with a disability that are required by DOT's Air Carrier Access regulations. They may charge for optional services, however, such as oxygen and accommodation of stretchers.

Personnel Training

Carriers must provide training on passengers with disabilities for all personnel who deal with the traveling public. This training shall be appropriate to the duties of each employee and will be designed to help the employee understand the special needs of these travelers, and how they can be accommodated quickly, safely, and with dignity. The training must familiarize employees with:

- The Department of Transportation's rules on the provision of air service to an individual with a disability;

- The carrier's procedures for providing transportation to persons with disabilities, including the proper and safe operation of any equipment used to accommodate such persons;

- How to respond appropriately to persons with different disabilities, including persons with mobility, sensory, mental, and emotional disabilities.

Compliance Procedures

Each carrier must have at least one Complaints Resolution Official (CRO) available at each airport during times of scheduled carrier operations. The CRO can be made available by telephone.

Any passenger having a complaint of alleged violations of the Air Carrier Access rules is entitled to communicate with a CRO, who has authority to resolve complaints on behalf of the carrier.

If a CRO receives a complaint before the action of carrier personnel has resulted in violation of the Air Carrier Access rules, the CRO must take or direct other carrier personnel to take action to ensure compliance with the rule. The CRO, however, does not have authority to countermand a safety-based decision made by the pilot-in-command of an aircraft.

If the CRO agrees with the passenger that a violation of the rule occurred, he must provide the passenger a written statement summarizing the facts and what steps if any, the carrier proposes to take in response to the violation.

If the CRO determines that no violation has occurred, he must provide the passenger a written statement summarizing the facts and reasons for the decision or conclusion.

The written statement must inform the interested party of his or her right to pursue DOT enforcement action if the passenger is still not satisfied with the response. If possible, the written statement by the CRO must be given to the passenger at the airport; otherwise, it shall be sent to the passenger within 10 days of the incident.

Carriers shall establish a procedure for resolving written complaints alleging violations of any Air Carrier Access rule provision. If a passenger chooses to file a written complaint, the complaint should note whether the passenger contacted the CRO at the time of the alleged violation, including the CRO's name and the date of contact, if available. It should include any written response received from the CRO. A carrier shall not be required to respond to a complaint postmarked more than 45 days after the date of an alleged violation.

A carrier must respond to a written complaint within 30 days after receiving it. The response must state the airline's position on the alleged violation, and may also state whether and why no violation occurred, or what the airline plans to do about the problem. The carrier must also inform the passenger of his or her right to pursue DOT enforcement action.

Any person believing that a carrier has violated any provision of the rule may contact the following office:

Department of Transportation
Aviation Consumer Protection
Division, C-75
400 Seventh Street, S.W.
Washington, D.C. 20590
(202) 366-2220
TT (202) 755-7687

In Conclusion

Our work is not yet done. At the time of publication of this booklet, there remained a number of accessibility issues unresolved. These include:

- Accessible terminal transportation systems;
- Boarding chair standards;
- Substitute transportation for persons unable to board small aircraft;
- Accessible lavatories on narrow body aircraft;
- Open captioning for in-flight movies and videos;
- TT service on aircraft.

There are many others.

The Department of Transportation, along with groups representing people with disabilities and the air carrier industry, is dedicated to eliminating these barriers with all possible speed.

Chapter 43

Assistive Technology
for People with
Spinal Cord Injuries

Introduction

Technology plays an important role in every aspect of daily life. To get from one place to another, most people use automobiles or public transportation. Mothers with small children use baby carriages or strollers to assist them in carrying their children around the mall. Televisions are equipped with remote controls for ease of operation, and electric can openers and garage door openers are convenience tools that have become commonplace in our society. All of these devices have one thing in common: they are used to assist us in accomplishing everyday activities.

Technology plays an even more significant role in the life of someone with a severe disability such as a spinal cord injury (SCI). SCI can have a major effect on virtually all aspects of one's life. Products and devices designed to increase an individual's level of function and independence can be instrumental in providing a person with SCI the highest possible level of function after injury.

The physical effects of SCI are varied. Depending upon the level and severity of injury, it can affect the ability to walk or to use one's arms and hands, to drive, and to control physical functions such as

This guide was researched and written by Lynn Halverson and Katherine Belknap and produced by ABLEDATA. ABLEDATA is funded by the National Institute on Disability and Rehabilitation Research (NIDRR), under contract number HN-92026001 and is operated by Macro International Inc. Copyright 1996, Macro International Inc. Reprinted with permission.

473

bowel and bladder control or to have sexual relations. A number of excellent publications discussing the effects of SCI are available and are referenced below.

This *Informed Consumer Guide* is designed to provide an introduction to the many types of products and devices people with SCI can use in order to function more independently in their daily activities. People with new injuries may assume that certain activities cannot be performed any longer because of the disability. In many cases, however, devices have been developed to allow people with SCI to do the same things they did before the injury. Adaptive devices have been developed to enable people with SCI to participate in almost every type of sporting or recreational activity. Cars and vans can be modified to enable someone in a wheelchair to drive or be a passenger while remaining in a wheelchair or transferring to a standard car seat.

The first step toward getting the types of products that one needs is to know the right questions to ask, and to know that appropriate products exist. This Guide, therefore, can help people with SCI arrive at that "first step" toward greater independence and self-sufficiency after a spinal cord injury.

How to Use This Guide

This Guide describes the types of products that may be used by people with SCI to maximize their physical capabilities. Detailed information about specific products in each category discussed below can be found in ABLEDATA, a database of information about more than 22,000 products for people with disabilities. ABLEDATA also produces Fact Sheets and Informed Consumer Guides on specific categories of technology. Included are the *Informed Consumer Guide to Wheelchair Selection* and the *Informed Consumer Guide to Accessible Housing,* as well as individual Fact Sheets on *Powered Wheelchairs, Manual Wheelchairs, Wheelchairs for Children, Aquatic Sports, Cycling,* and *Adaptive Winter Sports.* Additional information also is included in this Guide about other available resources to describe individual product areas or to accomplish specific tasks.

Assistive Technology

Personal Mobility

One of the major consequences of SCI is its effect upon a person's ability to walk. Some people with SCI are able to walk with the assistance of braces and crutches. Others may need—or choose to use— a manual wheelchair. Still others may require or prefer some sort of powered mobility device, such as a scooter (a three- or four-wheeled cart) or powered wheelchair. Deciding what type of mobility device to use is based upon a number of factors: medical diagnosis; personal lifestyle; cost of the device; and personal preference.

For someone who has recently sustained a spinal cord injury, a functional evaluation by physical therapists and other rehabilitation professionals is an important part of the process for determining the individual's best options. For someone who has had a spinal cord injury for a number of years, the best sources of information on products available often are other consumers who have practical experience with the product(s) being considered.

Wheelchairs. The majority of people with spinal cord injuries use a wheelchair at some point in their lives as a mode of personal mobility. For some this may mean using a powered wheelchair, while others may find a standard manual chair or a lightweight or sport chair more suitable. Selecting the appropriate wheelchair from the many options available often is an overwhelming task to someone with a new injury. However, there are a number of excellent resources available to assist with this task, and both wheelchair prescribers and current wheelchair users can provide helpful advice on features or products to consider, as well as "problem" products to avoid.

Information Resources

A Guide to Wheelchair Selection: How to Use the ANSI / RESNA Wheelchair Standards to Buy a Wheelchair. Peter Axelson, Jean Minkel, Denise Chesney. Paralyzed Veterans of America. 202/872-1300. 1994.

Choosing a Wheelchair System. Department of Veterans Affairs, 1990. Department of Veterans Affairs, Veterans Health Services and Research Administration, Washington, DC 20420. Clinical Supplement #2, Journal of Rehabilitation Research and Development, March 1990. FREE.

How to Select and Use Manual Wheelchairs. A. Bennett Wilson. Accent on Living, P.O. Box 700, Bloomington, IL 61702. 1993. Tel: 800/787-8444.

Informed Consumer Guide to Wheelchair Selection. ABLEDATA, Macro International. 800/227-0216. 1994. Contact the office for pricing information.

ABLEDATA Fact Sheets on *Manual Wheelchairs*, *Powered Wheelchairs*, *Wheelchairs for Children* (1994) and *Scooters* (1996). ABLEDATA, 8455 Colesville Road, Suite 935, Silver Spring, MD 20910. Contact the office for pricing information.

Seating Systems. In general, wheelchair users also must use a specialized seating system to ensure adequate support and protection of soft tissues. Selection of an appropriate seating system is of utmost importance to someone with SCI in order to avoid pressure sores, a risk for those unable to change position or who have diminished sensation. The seating system must be selected along with the wheelchair to ensure that the two systems are compatible and provide the best support possible to the user.

Seating systems come in many different styles and formats, depending upon the user's needs and personal preference. The simplest and least expensive systems are foam cushions, generally three- to five-inches thick and covered with fabric. These may be flat foam or contoured to more closely match the shape of the user. Cushions are also available in air, flotation, gel, and water models. The variety of cushions provide different levels of support and require varying levels of maintenance. Also available are hybrid cushions, combining the best characteristics of several types of cushions, such as foam and gel.

Depending upon the nature and extent of the disability caused by SCI, some individuals may require complete seating systems. These types of systems assist those who lack sufficient strength or balance to sit upright or have difficulty maintaining proper positioning. Components may include seats, backs, pelvic and hip supports, and or leg and foot supports.

As with other kinds of assistive technology, first-time decisions should be made in consultation with therapists and other rehabilitation professionals to be certain that the system selected best meets the needs of the user.

Crutches. Some people with spinal cord injuries are able to walk with the aid of braces and crutches. Two basic styles of crutches are available, depending upon an individual's level of injury and degree of mobility. Traditional under-arm crutches are preferred by some users, while fore-arm or Canadian-style crutches provide an alternative.

Walkers. Walkers are metal frames designed to provide support and stability while walking. For someone with SCI, walkers often are used in conjunction with braces or crutches to provide stability and support while ambulating. Walkers may be folding or fixed and they may be height-adjustable. They may or may not be equipped with wheels on the front or all four legs. A variety of specialty walkers are available as well, including stair walkers and walkers with seats. Accessories such as platform arm supports and carrying aids help adapt walkers to more fully provide the user with independence.

Driving and Transportation

Transportation often plays a key role in determining whether or not an individual will be able to work, go to school, or participate in recreational activities. For people who are able to drive, specialized products are available to operate an automobile or van with hand controls. Special access options, such as lifts or ramps for vans and wheelchair tie-down systems to stabilize wheelchairs inside a moving vehicle also are available. The following categories of automotive adaptive equipment and other transportation-related devices, selected from the ABLEDATA Thesaurus, are available.

Driving Controls. People with limited or no use of their lower limbs use hand controls to accelerate, brake, and shift gears. These controls may be mounted on the steering column or they may be comprised of a ring system on the steering wheel, allowing the driver to keep both hands on the wheel. Hand controls are available from a number of different companies and meet a variety of user needs. Many hand controls are designed not to interfere with operation of the vehicle by drivers who are not disabled.

Automobile Accessories. An assortment of accessory items, including wheelchair and transfer lifts, handles to assist in transfers from a wheelchair to car, car door openers, and swivel seats are available to drivers and passengers with disabilities.

477

Van Accessories. In addition to the standard accessory items available for automobiles, specialty accessories are also available. Raised van tops, tie-down systems, and transfer bars designed specifically for vans can be purchased to make driving or riding in a van safer and more comfortable for someone with SCI.

Van Lifts and Ramps. Full-sized and mini-vans can be fitted with a variety of ramps and lifts. Lifts may be attached to the side door or to the rear door, and some newer models are designed to require less space and/or to leave part of the door free to accommodate passengers who are not in wheelchairs.

Some wheelchair users find ramps a preferred method of access. A variety of ramp systems are available including two-track and wider one-piece models. These ramps may be permanently installed such that they fold up or slide under the van floor; or they may be portable to allow for use with more than one vehicle.

Raised ceilings or lowered floors often are used in conjunction with a lift or ramp to equip a van to accommodate a person in a wheelchair.

Information Resource

"Van Lifts: The Ups and Downs and Ins and Outs." A. Perr and K. Barnicle. *TeamRehab Report* (Vol. 4 No. 4, June 1993), pp. 49-53. Presents information on how to select an appropriate wheelchair lift for a van, noting that safety and function are the two top priorities when choosing the best type of lift. Other factors include cost, ability to use the lift, size of the user, wheelchair size, locations where the lift will be used, and how else the van will be used.

Wheelchair Carriers and Loaders. Specialized wheelchair carriers can be attached to the outside of a car or van to carry wheelchairs from one location to another. Some carriers are combined with loaders, lifting and storing the chair on the car's bumper. Other loaders enable the wheelchair to be lifted into a car trunk or onto a roof rack.

Making Your Home Accessible

Many people discover that their homes are not fully accessible to them after they have sustained a spinal cord injury. Doorways may be too narrow to accommodate a wheelchair; hallways may not provide sufficient turning room; bedrooms may be located up a flight of stairs. It may seem that the only option is to sell the home and move to one that is wheelchair accessible, and for some this may be a preferred option. In some cases, however, it may be possible to make renovations to an existing home, enabling one to remain there indefinitely. Some homes may simply require the installation of assistive devices such as special door hinges, elevating and lowering cabinets, electronic faucets, and a stair lift to make the home more accessible and "user friendly" to someone in a wheelchair.

Information Resources

Informed Consumer Guide to Accessible Housing. ABLEDATA, 1995. Contact the office for pricing information.

Home Modification Resource Guide. NARIC, 1994. FREE

Special Section: Home Improvements, *Paraplegia News*, November 1994. Vol 48, No. 11, pp. 27-32.

Managing Your Environment

A spinal cord injury that causes quadriplegia can limit a person's ability to use arms or hands for such everyday tasks as picking up a telephone, typing, writing, or operating electrical entertainment equipment such as a television or VCR. There are a number of devices available, however, that can assist one with these tasks. Both products designed for the general public—such as speaker phones or universal remote controls—and assistive devices designed especially for people with limited hand and arm function are available. Included are specialized telephones, assistive writing and typing devices, computers, safety and security systems, and environmental controls. Many of these systems are voice-activated, eliminating the need to use one's hands. Additional alternative input modes are also available.

Staying in Shape

Sports and recreation are important both as leisure activities and as ways to stay in shape mentally and physically. Some activities can be done without any adaptations or special equipment. Others require specialized equipment or modifications to accommodate wheelchair users, and the range of options open to people with SCI is expanding almost daily. Whether you are interested in fitness, skiing, cycling, basketball, rugby, tennis, hunting, or some other activity, there are products, facilities and people able to assist you in participating in the recreational activity of your choice.

Sports. The competitive sports arena is alive and well for athletes with spinal cord injuries or other disabilities. If a sport is available to an able-bodied person, the likelihood is high that it is available also to someone with a spinal cord injury. Athletes with disabilities participate regularly in the Boston Marathon and other running events, with wheelchair division times recorded along with other divisions. Wheelchair basketball, quad rugby, archery, bowling, tennis, snow and water skiing, and just about every other sport can be played by someone who uses a wheelchair. In many cases, the key to competition is access to the appropriate equipment, whether it is a lightweight wheelchair or the newest skiing equipment. Specialized wheelchairs have been developed specifically for use in various sports, including racing, wheelchair sports, and basketball.

Information Resources

Before trying to locate specialized equipment, it may be helpful to contact one of the many organizations or publications that keep track of sports and recreation opportunities for people with disabilities. Two excellent resources are **National Handicapped Sports**, an organization for people with disabilities, and *Sports 'n Spokes*, a bi-monthly magazine that features sports and recreation opportunities for all people with disabilities.

Disabled Sports USA
451 Hungerford Drive
Suite 100
Rockville, MD 20850. 301/217-0960

Sports 'n Spokes
PVA Publications
5201 North 19th Avenue, Suite 111
Phoenix. AZ 85015. 602/246-9426

Fitness. For people interested in developing an exercise program, the following three videos may be helpful:

Nancy's Special Workout features occupational therapist Nancy Sebring. This program is geared to the wheelchair user, both children and adults. The 45 minute routine starts with a warm-up, moves to a vigorous cardiovascular workout and ends with a cool-down. Aviano USA, 1199-K Avenida Acaso, Camarillo, CA 93012. 805/484-8138.

Also available from Aviano USA is *Keep Fit While You Sit*, for advanced workouts. It has been designed to increase circulation, respiratory capacity, flexibility, muscle tone and strength and is endorsed by the American Paralysis Association.

Anybody Can Sit and Be Fit was developed by Martha Rounds, who has had 30 years in the field of health and fitness. This 20-minute routine is for people who need to sit while exercising. The program involves the arms and upper body and some leg lifts to help burn calories, increase circulation and relieve muscle tension. Accent on Living, P.O. Box 700, Bloomington, IL 61702. 800/787-8444.

Adaptive exercise equipment is also available for people with SCI. Included are pulley weights, complete weight systems designed to be used by persons seated in a wheelchair, recumbent exercise bikes, and exercise cycles designed to be "pedaled" with the arms. Some of these products feature power systems for assisted exercise.

With any exercise program, it is advisable to consult with a physician before undertaking new activity, whether using a video or adaptive exercise equipment.

Standing Aids. Health care professionals often recommend that people with SCI stand several times per day to improve cardiovascular fitness, prevent bone deterioration, and exercise muscles. Standing frames and stand-up wheelchairs provide the support needed to accomplish this activity.

Hobbies and Recreation. A wide range of products is available to enable people with SCI to engage in the hobby or recreational activity of their choice. From music to gardening; from photography to fishing; from boating to flying, assistive technology is available.

Personal Care

For many people, the ability to be as independent as possible in personal care activities is of paramount importance. There are many devices that have been developed to enable people with limited physical function to perform personal care activities with little or no assistance from others. Products are available in the following categories:

Bathing and Showering
Clothing
Dressing
Eating
Grooming and Hygiene
Health Care
Holding
Reaching
Sexual Aids
Smoking
Toiletting
Transferring

For those with new injuries, consultation with an occupational therapist will be helpful in determining the kinds of assistance required and the best products to help meet those needs.

Making Your Workplace Accessible and Usable

With the variety of adaptive devices available for almost any worksite, many people who have sustained spinal cord injuries have been able to return to their previous positions after their rehabilitation is completed. Whether in an office setting, a warehouse, or on the farm, to mention just a few examples, there are adaptive products and information resources available to make the return to work easier.
Product categories include:

Computers
Agricultural Equipment
Office Equipment
Tools
Desks
Specialized Work Stations

General Resources on Spinal Cord Injury

For more information on spinal cord injury in general, the following publications are recommended:

Spinal Cord Injury: A Guide for Patient and Family. Phillips, L, et al, New York, NY: Raven Press, 1987. 290 pp.

This practical guide addresses in straightforward laypersons' terms the many medical, social and psychological issues that face people with spinal cord injuries and their families. Co-authored by physicians, lay experts, and a rehabilitation engineer who himself sustained a spinal cord injury, the book clearly explains how spinal cord injuries occur, what happens to the body after injury, and where to go for help. It also describes current research being done to find ways of improving function after a spinal cord injury. A glossary of terms and a list of publications are included. 1987. Raven Press, 1185 Avenue of the Americas, New York, NY 10036. ISBN 0-88167275-0 (Order Code 1732) Tel: 212/930-9500.

Spinal Network: The Total Resource for the Wheelchair Community, Second Edition. Maddox, S. Boulder, CO: Spinal Network, 1993. 568 pp.

One of the most comprehensive resources available for the SCI community, this book offers detailed medical information on spinal cord injuries, covers sports and recreation, travel, substance abuse, sex and romance, fashion, survival on the farm, horticulture, fund raising, history of wheelchairs, cushions, driving, disability rights, legal and financial issues; includes list of resources for the person with SCI, including associations, assistive groups, contacts, state groups, and Canadian provincial groups. Personal perspectives on SCI and many references for further information are included. Available from Miramar Communications, P.O. Box 8987, Malibu, CA 90265-8987. 800/543-4116.

How to Live with a Spinal Cord Injury. Written by a person with paraplegia, this guide includes information about dealing with disability on a day-to-day basis. Available from: Accent on Living, P.O. Box 700, Bloomington, IL 61702. 800/787-8444.

An Introduction to Spinal Cord Injury. This pamphlet provides basic information about spinal cord injury, suggested additional readings, and a glossary of terms. Available from: Paralyzed Veterans of America (PVA), 801 Eighteenth Street, NW Washington, D.C. 20006. 800/424-8200, 202/872-1300.

Fact Sheets on Spinal Cord Injury. The National Spinal Cord Injury Association, a national membership organization for people with spinal cord injuries, publishes a series of fact sheets on spinal cord injury. Topics include: What is Spinal Cord Injury?; Spinal Cord Injury Statistical Information; The Importance of Basic Science in Research; Sexuality After Spinal Cord Injury; and many other topics. A complete publications list describes the NSCIA Fact Sheets series as well as other publications available through the association. Available from: National Spinal Cord Injury Association, 545 Concord Avenue, Suite 29, Cambridge, MA 01801. 800/962-9629 or 617/935-2722.

Yes, You Can! is an easy-to-read guide to self-care for people with spinal cord injuries. Prepared by the staff of a spinal cord injury rehabilitation center, it covers issues such as attendant care; bowel and bladder management; psychosocial adjustment; recreation; skin care; and driving. It is available in English or Spanish. Available from: Paralyzed Veterans of America (PVA),801 Eighteenth Street, NW, Washington, D.C. 20006. 800/424-8200 or 202/872-1300.

Funding Sources

Funding for wheelchairs and other assistive devices, is dependent upon an individual's eligibility for medical, social services, income support or vocational assistance from any of a number of different resources. Depending upon the terms of the policy, some medical insurance providers cover a portion of the cost of some devices with a doctor's prescription and justification of medical need. Additional funding sources include community agencies, community organizations and churches.

Further information on resources and methods of funding assistive devices is available from the Assistive Technology Funding & Systems Change Project, a project of the National Institute on Disability and Rehabilitation Research (NIDRR) run by the United Cerebral Palsy Associations, Inc. Individuals requiring information and technical assistance on funding may call 800/827-0093 (voice) or 800/833-8272

(TT) or fax 404/919-8305. Information about resources is also available in an ABLEDATA *Fact Sheet on Funding Assistive Technology*.

Conclusion

A new spinal cord injury can mean major changes in lifestyle, but with the appropriate medical and informational resources and assistive technology, it may be possible to engage in the same activities as before the injury.

For those seeking information on assistive technology and information about more than 21,000 products for people with disabilities. ABLEDATA can be reached by calling 800/227-0216 or 301/588-9284. Information specialists are on hand to assist callers locate the information they need. For a small fee, ABLEDATA can provide patrons with computer printouts of information on specific wheelchairs listed in the database. Costs are determined by the size of the database search requested.

ABLEDATA also has a series of Fact Sheets on assistive devices. Included is the *Funding Assistive Technology* Fact Sheet discussed above. Other titles include *Manual Wheelchairs*, *Powered Wheelchairs*, *Wheelchairs for Children*, and the *Informed Consumer Guide to Wheelchair Selection*. Contact the ABLEDATA office for a complete list of titles and prices.

ABLE INFORM is a computer bulletin board service (BBS) that allows computer users to search ABLEDATA themselves and to download information obtained from those searches. ABLE INFORM can be accessed via modem at 301/589-3563 (8-1-n), or through the Internet. (Telnet to FedWorld.gov, select option G, select option 1, then select system #115 to connect.) There is no charge to use the BBS, although callers from outside the metropolitan Washington, D.C. area will be charged by their telephone company for a long distance call when calling on commercial telephone lines.

Most ABLEDATA publications are available in a variety of accessible formats, including large print, Braille, on cassette, and computer diskette. For additional copies or for more information, contact ABLEDATA, 8455 Colesville Road, Suite 935, Silver Spring, MD 20910-3319. 800/227-0216 or 301/588-9284 (both lines are voice/text telephone), or call ABLE INFORM, our electronic bulletin board system (BBS) at 301/589-3563 with modem settings 2400-9600 baud, 8-N-1.

Chapter 44

The National Spinal Cord Injury Hotline and Other Resources for People with Spinal Cord Injuries

National Spinal Cord Injury Hotline

(800) 526-3456

Mission

The Hotline is a toll-free information and referral service available to individuals who have sustained a traumatic spinal cord injury (SCI) and their families. The office hours are Monday-Friday, 9:00 am-5:00 pm, EST (24 hours for new injuries). Established in 1984, the Hotline has received more than 40,000 calls, addressed by the staff of medical professionals and health administrators.

Some staff members have a spinal cord injury, which can assist in discerning questions. The hotline facilitates the callers' search for support and resources by referring them to others who have personal experience (peer volunteers) or to professionals with expertise in SCI. Referrals to resources include rehabilitation facilities, SCI literature and spinal cord injury organizations.

The Hotline works with people to find answers to questions ranging from therapeutic programs to house modifications, from medical equipment to sports and recreation. The Hotline is able to provide

"National Spinal Cord Injury Hotline: The Facts," nd, financially supported by the Paralyzed Veterans of America; and "Spinal Cord Injury: A NARIC Resource Guide," ©1995 KRA Corporation; both reprinted with permission.

direction to the myriad of questions facing a family following a paralyzing injury.

Population

The Hotline serves individuals who have sustained a traumatic spinal cord injury resulting in paralysis. Common terms are quadriplegia (involvement of the upper and lower extremities) and paraplegia
(involvement of the lower extremities). The primary causes of these
injuries are motor vehicle accidents, sports accidents, gunshot wounds,
and falls. The SCI Hotline also works with professionals who provide
a service to the disabled population.

Need

The impact of SCI is devastating. It is a tragic experience that prompts
questions, concerns and a seemingly endless state of confusion. Where
can individuals and their families turn to receive information to deal
with the countless challenges that they must face when one becomes
paralyzed?

Professional support given by a knowledgeable staff will help families organize, prioritize and clarify important information. The Hotline
staff, with the peer support network, can make this overwhelming
period easier.

Peer Support

"The Connection" is a group of individuals across the country who
volunteer for the Hotline as peer contacts. They agree to provide support and assistance to others in their geographic area who have concerns related to their injury. The frustration and fear associated with
a new paralyzing injury are often allayed when communicating with
a peer contact, "someone who has been there." These people combine
their own personal experience with knowledge of area resources and
organizations. Callers often will request a Peer contact in their locale.

National Spinal Cord Injury Hotline

The National Spinal Cord Injury Hotline is financially supported by
the Paralyzed Veterans of America. For more information contact:

National Spinal Cord Injury Hotline
2200 N. Forest Park Ave.
Baltimore MD 21207
(401) 448-6623 Voice
(401) 448-6627 Fax
(800) 526-3456 Hotline

A NARIC Resource Guide for People with Spinal Cord Injuries and Their Families

Each year in the United States an estimated 6,000-8,000 people survive a spinal cord injury. People who recently have sustained a spinal cord injury (SCI) often have many questions about what happens when a spinal cord injury occurs and where to get the information needed to live with a spinal cord injury. After an injury occurs, the person with SCI must relearn many everyday activities, depending upon the level and extent of the injury.

The purpose of this resource guide is to identify some of the major publications (books, magazines, and newsletters), organizations, and other resources assisting people with SCI (from the point of injury onward, focusing on specific aspects of SCI). In this guide it is not possible to solve specific dilemmas, but it is possible to provide a solid introduction to the resources that currently do exist.

General Resources

Spinal Network: The Total Resource for the Wheelchair Community. Maddox, S., 1993. c/o Miramar. 23815 Stuart Ranch Road, Malibu, CA 90265, (800) 543-4116. Cost: $37.95 (plus $5 shipping), $39.95 (plus $5 shipping) for the edition that lays flat when opened.

One of the most comprehensive resources available for the SCI community, this book offers detailed medical information on spinal cord injuries, covers sports and recreation, travel, substance abuse, sex and romance, fashion, survival on the farm, horticulture, fundraising, history of wheelchairs, cushions, driving, disability rights, legal, and financial issues. Also included is a list of resources for the person with SCI, including associations, assistive groups, contacts, state groups, and Canadian provincial groups. Personal perspectives on SCI and many references for further information are included.

Spinal Cord Injury: A Guide for Patient and Family. Phillips, L., et al. New York, NY: Raven Press, 1987. 290 pp. Available from: Raven Press, 1185 Avenue of the Americas, New York, NY 10036. ISBN 0-88167-275-0 (Order Code 1732); (212) 930-9500. Cost: $39 (hardback); $17 (paperback).

This practical guide addresses in straightforward laypersons' terms the many medical, social, and psychological issues that face people with spinal cord injuries and their families. Coauthored by physicians, lay experts, and a rehabilitation engineer who sustained a spinal cord injury, the book clearly explains how spinal cord injuries occur, what happens to the body after injury, and where to go for help. It also describes research being conducted to improve function after a spinal cord injury. A glossary of terms and a list of publications are included.

How to Live with a Spinal Cord Injury. 1989. Available from: Accent on Living, P.O. Box 700, Bloomington, IL 61702. (800) 787-8444. Cost: $6.95 (plus $2 shipping & handling).

Written by a person with paraplegia, this guide includes information about dealing with disability on a day-to-day basis.

An Introduction to Spinal Cord Injury. Available from: Paralyzed Veterans of America (PVA), 801 - 18th Street NW, Washington, DC 20006. (800) 424-8200, (202) 872-1300. Cost: free.

This pamphlet provides basic information about spinal cord injury, suggested additional readings, and a glossary of terms.

Factsheets on Spinal Cord Injury. Available from: National Spinal Cord Injury Association, 545 Concord Avenue, Suite 29, Cambridge, MA 02138. (800) 962-9629, (617) 441-8500. Cost: free to members; $3 per Factsheet to nonmembers.

The National Spinal Cord Injury Association (NSCIA), a national membership organization for people with spinal cord injuries and diseases, publishes a series of fact sheets on spinal cord injury. Topics include: *What Is Spinal Cord Injury?, Spinal Cord Injury Statistical Information, What's New in SCI Research?, Sexuality After Spinal Cord Injury*, and many other topics. A complete publications list describes the NSCIA Factsheets series as well as other publications available through the association.

490

Bowel and Bladder Care Resources

Bowel Management: A Manual of Ideas and Techniques, by Raymond C. Cheever and Charles D. Elmer, R.P.T. Available from: Accent on Living. (Contact information above.) Cost: $3.50 (plus .85 shipping & handling).

This booklet includes considerations such as frequency, timing, diet, water intake, exercise, use of laxatives, and successful approaches used at several different rehabilitation centers.

Urinary Tract Infections. Available from: the Research and Training Center (RTC) on Independent Living, University of Kansas. Life Span Institute, 4089 Dole, Lawrence, KS 66045-2930. (913) 864-0592. Cost: $2.

Urinary Tract Infections was developed by the RTC on Independent Living at the University of Kansas with grant funds from the Paralyzed Veterans of America Education and Training Foundation. This 12-page pamphlet explains urinary tract care and treatment in lay language. It describes alternative bladder-emptying methods and discusses problems that can arise in someone with a spinal cord injury.

Overcoming Bladder Disorders, Rebecca Chalker and Kristene Whitmore, MD. Available from Accent on Living. Cost: $11 (plus $1.25 shipping & handling).

This fact-filled guide draws on the latest research, surveys, and first-person accounts to provide up-to-date information on diagnosis, treatment, and prevention of urinary system disorders.

Children's Resources

Rebecca Finds a New Way: How Kids Learn, Play, and Live-with Spinal Cord Injuries and Illnesses. (1994). Written for children to help them understand that others with spinal cord injuries have the same needs. Available from: In Touch with Kids Network at the National Spinal Cord Injury Association (Contact information above). Cost: $3.50; free to children with SCI.

Speedway Sam, A book about spinal cord injury for children. Available from: UAB Spain Rehabilitation Center, RTC Training Office, 1717 6th Avenue South, Birmingham, AL 35233-7330. (205) 934-3283. Cost: $3.50.

A book designed to help children learn about SCI, SCI prevention, and positive attitudes toward people with disabilities. Can be used as a coloring book.

Resources for Personal Care/Daily Living for People with Spinal Cord Injuries

Yes, You Can! Available from: Paralyzed Veterans of America. (Contact information above). Cost: $9.50 (plus $2.50 shipping & handling). Available in English or Spanish.

Yes, You Can! is an easy-to-read guide to self-care for people with spinal cord injuries. Prepared by the staff of a spinal cord injury rehabilitation center, this guide covers issues such as attendant care, bowel and bladder management, psychosocial adjustment, recreation, skin care, and driving.

Exercise Resources

Nancy's Special Workout. Available from: Avenues Unlimited, Inc. 1199 K Avenida Acaso, Camarillo, CA 93012. (800) 848-2837, (805) 484-8138. Cost: $39.95

This video features occupational therapist Nancy Sebring who gears the program to wheelchair users—children and adults. The 45-minute routine starts with a warm-up, moves to a vigorous cardiovascular workout, and ends with a cool-down.

Keep Fit While You Sit. Available from: Avenues Unlimited, Inc. (Contact information above.) Cost: $29.95 ($2 of each sale is donated to the American Paralysis Association).

This video is for more advanced workouts. It has been designed to increase circulation, respiratory capacity, flexibility, muscle tone, and strength. This video is endorsed by the American Paralysis Association.

Anybody Can Sit and Be Fit. Available from: Accent on Living. Cost: $19.95 (plus $2.50 shipping & handling).

Martha Rounds has had 30 years in the field of health and fitness. She designed a 20-minute routine for people who need to sit while exercising. The program involves the arms and upper body and some leg lifts to help burn calories, increase circulation, and relieve muscle tension.

Sex and Reproduction Resources

Sexual Adjustment: A Guide for the Spinal Cord Injured. Available from: Accent on Living. Cost: $4.95 (plus $1.25 shipping & handling).

This guide contains information about sexual adjustment for males with paraplegia.

Mother to Be: A Guide to Pregnancy and Birth for Women with Disabilities. Available from: Accent on Living. Cost: $24.95 (plus $2.50 shipping & handling).

This handbook gives the reader a sense of what to expect based on the experiences of women with a variety of disabilities. The book discusses finding the right medical care, nutritional requirements, labor, delivery, and more.

Love-Where to Find It, How to Keep It, by Elle Becker, MA. Available from: Accent on Living. Cost: $6.95 (plus $1.25 shipping & handling).

This self-help book includes information about how to meet other single people, communication skills, dating.

Sexuality Reborn. Available from: Kessler Institute for Rehabilitation, 1199 Pleasant Valley Way, West Orange, NJ 07052. Attn: Education Department. (800) 435-8866. Cost: $39.95 (plus $8 shipping & handling).

Sexuality Reborn, (1991), a videotape about sexuality after spinal cord injury, features four couples who talk about and demonstrate techniques they have found helpful for sexual expression. Due to the nature of the material, audiences should be prepared for sexually explicit scenes and frank discussions of sensitive topics. It was produced with grant funds from PVA's Education and Training Foundation at the Kessler Institute for Rehabilitation and features Ben Vereen as the special guest narrator.

Enabling Romance: An Illustrated Guide to Romantic and Sexual Relationships. Available from: Accent on Living. Cost: $22.50 (plus $2.50 shipping).

This guide was written by a man with a disability for his nondisabled wife.

Skin Care Resources

Pressure Sores. Developed by the RTC on Independent Living at the University of Kansas with grant funds from the Paralyzed Veterans of America Education and Training Foundation. Available from: the RTC on Independent Living. (Contact information above.) Cost: $2.50.

Practical information about how to recognize problem spots, how to prevent them, and how to treat them.

Spasticity Resources

Managing Spasticity, by Carol L. Goodman, MSN, CRRN, and Kelly Hill, RN. *Paraplegia News*, February 1992, pp 24-27. Available from: PVA Publications. 2111 East Highland Avenue, Suite 180, Phoenix, AZ 85016-4702. (602) 224-0500. Current price is available from the publisher.

Statistics Resources

Statistical Findings of the Regional Spinal Cord Injury System. Available from: NARIC. *Rehab BRIEFS*, 6(3), 1983.

Resources on Wheelchairs and Other Assistive Devices

How to Select and Use Manual Wheelchairs. (1993). Available from: Rehabilitation Press, P.O. Box 380, Topping, VA 23169. Cost: $12.50.

Selection of the most appropriate wheelchair and seating system can be simplified if one has information about factors to consider and products on the market. This guide helps new wheelchair users select a wheelchair with the right dimensions and seating system depending upon the degree of disability, goals of the user, and the environment in which the chair will be used. The book also provides information about proper use and maintenance of wheelchairs.

ABLEDATA Resource Guide for Wheelchair Information. Available from: ABLEDATA, 8455 Colesville Road, Suite 935, Silver Spring, MD 20910-3319, (800) 227-0216 (V/TT), (301) 588-9284 (V/TT), (301) 587-1967 fax (V/TT). Cost: $5.

Funding Assistive Technology Fact Sheet, Informed Consumer Guide to Wheelchair Selection, Manual Wheelchairs Fact Sheet, Powered Wheelchair Fact Sheet, Wheelchairs for Children Fact Sheet.

Choosing a Wheelchair System. (1990). Available from: Department of Veterans Affairs, Veterans Health Services and Research Administration, Washington, DC 20420. Clinical Supplement #2, *Journal of Rehabilitation Research and Development*, March 1990. Cost: free.

Several years ago the U.S. Department of Veterans Affairs Rehabilitation Research and Development Service (Rehab R&D) issued Clinical Supplement #2 entitled "Choosing a Wheelchair System." This resource was written by people with disabilities who have selected wheelchairs for many years, health care providers who prescribe wheelchairs, and researchers and engineers who participate in the development of new wheelchair designs.

Sports 'n Spokes. Available from: PVA Publications. Price and availability can be checked by phone call. (Contact information above.)

Sports 'n Spokes, a bimonthly publication for active wheelchair users, publishes an Annual Survey of Lightweight Wheelchairs in their March/April issue each year. The most recent survey (March/April 1994) includes a description of how wheelchairs are tested in order to comply with recently-issued American National Standards Institute (ANSI) standards. Also included are photos of a variety of everyday, sports, and junior-sized lightweight wheelchairs from different manufacturers; comparative sizing information; warranty information; delivery time; and retail price. Back issues of the magazine sometimes are available; so are reprints of specific articles.

Homecare Magazine and TeamRehab Reports also publish an annual *Wheelchair Focus* that provides comparative information. It is published once a year (in the spring). Available from: Miramar Publishing. (Contact information above.) Price and availability can be checked by phone call.

Wheelchair Standards

The American National Standards Institute (ANSI) recently approved a complete set of standards for wheelchairs. These standards consist of standard methods of disclosing information (example: How do you measure the width of a seat? Inside to inside of each tube, or width of a cushion, or through some other measurement?); and standard test methods to test a chair's strength, "tip-ability," turning radius, and so forth.

These standards are of interest to manufacturers, therapists, consumers, and others who are going to conduct testing themselves, as they are very technical documents. However, some good summary documents are available that describe the standards for therapists and laypeople.

To date, very few manufacturers have used the standards routinely to test and disclose information about their products. However, once this kind of information becomes more readily available, it can be used by consumers to make intelligent purchasing decisions.

Available from: RESNA, 1700 N. Moore Street, Suite 1540, Arlington, VA 22209. (703) 524-6686. Cost: $180 for the complete set.

Funding Sources for Assistive Technology

Funding for wheelchairs or other assistive devices is dependent upon an individual's eligibility for medical, social services, income support, or vocational assistance from any of a number of different resources. An ABLEDATA funding fact sheet (*Funding Assistive Technology*) is available to answer questions about funding resources.

Available from: ABLEDATA. Cost: free.

How to Get More Information on Assistive Devices

ABLEDATA is a database of information on more than 20,000 products for people with disabilities. Included in the ABLEDATA database are descriptions of wheelchairs currently available in the United States, as well as information about wheelchair manufacturers and local distributors. Cost: Some services are free; nominal charges for specialized searches is dependent upon extent of information required (Minimum charge: $5).

Research to Find a Cure for Spinal Cord Injury

The Quest for Cure. Available from: Paralyzed Veterans of America (PVA) Research and Education. Cost: $22.45 (including shipping & handling).

This book explains what happens after spinal cord injury from a biological point of view and then explores various scientific theories directed toward repairing damaged spinal cords. The book also includes interviews with key scientists in the field of spinal cord regeneration research.

Database Searching

Because new literature is being added continuously especially to the regeneration field, someone interested in keeping abreast of the latest developments in this research may wish to search the medical literature database (MEDLARS or MEDLINE) through local libraries.

NARIC can search its REHABDATA database for specific topics related to spinal cord injury research, treatment, and life after injury. The database contains more than 1,000 citations with abstracts on spinal cord injury.

Available from: NARIC. (800) 346-2742. Cost: Varies, depending upon length of search. Some services are free. (Minimum charge: $5).

National Database of Resources on Spinal Cord Injury. A database developed under the sponsorship of the American Spinal Injury Association (ASIA), at The Institute for Rehabilitation and Research (TIRR), with support from the Education and Training Foundation of Paralyzed Veterans of America (PVA). The database is currently funded through a grant to Baylor College of Medicine and TIRR from the National Institute on Disability and Rehabilitation Research (NIDRR). It contains more than 500 specialized educational materials relating to spinal cord injury, including both audiovisual and written manuals.

To request a search, call or write, and specify the subject area you want investigated. A printed report will be mailed directly to you. All requests, up to two subject areas, are free of charge. A compendium of the holdings in the database is available for $50. Make checks payable to Baylor College of Medicine, TIRR, 1333 Moursund, Houston, TX 77030.

National Audiovisual Database of Educational Materials on Spinal Cord Injury. Available from: Linda Herson, Division of Education, The Institute for Rehabilitation and Research, 1333 Moursund, Houston, TX 77030. (713) 797-5945. Cost: free.

A national database of more than 200 items on SCI, including films, videos, and audiotapes, on coping with SCI, recreation and leisure activities, sexuality issues, safe driving, water safety, and home modifications.

Sports and Recreation Organizations

American Sledge Hockey Association. 10933 Johnson Avenue South, Bloomington, MN 55437. (612) 750-3973.

American Wheelchair Archers. 5318 Northport Drive, Brooklyn Center, MN 55429. (612) 520-0476.

American Wheelchair Bowling Association. 3620 Tamarock Drive, Redding, CA 96003. (916) 243-2695.

American Wheelchair Table Tennis Association (AWTTA). 23 Parker Street, Port Chester, NY 10573. (914) 937-3932.

Canadian Wheelchair Sports Association. 1600 James Naismith Drive, Gloucester, Ontario, K1B 5N4. Canada. (613) 748-5685.

Challenge Air. 12728 Sunlight Drive, Dallas, TX 75230. (214) 701-0456.

Freedom's Wings International. 1832 Lake Avenue, Scotch Plains, NJ 07076. (908) 232-6354.

Handicapped Scuba Association. 1104 El Prado, San Clemente, CA 92672. (714) 498-6128.

International Wheelchair Aviators. 1117 Rising Hill, Escondido, CA 92029. (619) 746-5018.

International Wheelchair Tennis Federation. Palliser Road, Barons Court, London, W14 9EN England. (011) 44-71-610-1464.

National Association of Handicapped Outdoor Sportsmen. R.R.6, Box 33, Centralia, IL 62801 (618) 532-4565.

National Foundation of Wheelchair Tennis. 940 Calle Amanecer, Suite B, San Clemente, CA 92673. (714) 361-6811.

National Handicapped Sports. 451 Hungerford Drive, Suite 100, Rockville, MD 20850. (800) 966-4NHS; (301) 217-0960.

National Wheelchair Athletic Association. 3595 E. Fountain Boulevard, Colorado Springs, CO 80910. (719) 574-1150.

National Wheelchair Basketball Association. 110 Seaton Center, University of Kentucky, Lexington, KY 40506. (606) 257-1623.

National Wheelchair Billiards Association. 325 Hickory Drive, Cleveland, OH 44017. (216) 779-6966.

National Wheelchair Racquetball Association (NWRA). 2830 McGinley Road, Monroeville, PA 15146. (412) 856-2468.

National Wheelchair Shooting Federation. 102 Park Avenue, Rockledge, PA 19046. (215) 379-2359.

National Wheelchair Softball Association. 1616 Todd Court, Hastings, MN 55033. (612) 437-1792.

Paralyzed Veterans of America. Sports and Recreation Department. 801 - 18th Street NW, Washington, DC 20006. (800) 424-8200, (202) 872-1300.

Paraplegics On Independent Nature Trips (POINT). 4144 North Central Expressway, Suite 515, Dallas, TX 75204. (214) 827-7404.

U.S. Quad Rugby Association. 1605 Mathews Street, Fort Collins, CO 80525. (303) 484-7395.

U.S. Wheelchair Swimming. 229 Miller Street, Middleboro, MA 02346. (508) 946-1964.

U.S. Wheelchair Weightlifting Federation. 39 Michael Place, Levittown, PA 19057. (215) 945-1964.

Wheelchair Motorcycle Association (WMA). 101 Torrey Street, Brockton, MA 02401. (508) 583-8614.

Wheelchair Sports, U.S.A. 3595 E. Fountain Boulevard, Suite L-1, Colorado Springs, CO 80910. (719) 574-1150.

Wilderness on Wheels. 7125 West Jefferson Avenue, Suite 155, Lakewood, CO 80235. (303) 988-2212.

Spinal Cord Injury Organizations

American Paralysis Association (APA). 500 Morris Avenue, Springfield, NJ 07081. (800) 225-0292, (201) 379-2690.

APA's mission is to support research to find a cure for spinal cord injury paralysis. Twice yearly, the newsletter *Progress in Research* reports on research efforts funded by the organization as well as other science news that has bearing on cure research. APA's *Walking Tomorrow* (also published twice a year) details association and chapter activities.

American Spinal Injury Association (ASIA). 345 East Superior Street, Room 1436, Chicago, IL 60611. (312) 908-6207.

The American Spinal Injury Association (ASIA) is a corporation organized for the following purposes: to augment and encourage knowledge and investigation of the causes, cure, and prevention of spinal injury; promote and exchange ideas between professionals in the field of spinal injury management; to support, coordinate, and encourage basic research in the field of management of spinal injury and related trauma; to develop teaching and educational material; and to support and develop education of the profession and the laity in the prevention and proper management of spinal injury.

The association sponsors an annual scientific/clinical meeting for physicians and other health care professionals involved in spinal cord injury and its management. Membership available to health care professionals.

Miami Project to Cure Paralysis (MPCP). 1600 NW 10th Avenue, #R-48, Miami, FL 33136. (800) 782-6387, (305) 547-6001.

The Miami Project to Cure Paralysis is a multidisciplinary basic science and clinical research effort dedicated to finding more effective treatments and, ultimately, a cure for the paralysis resulting from spinal cord injury. Founded in 1985 through the efforts of Dr. Barth Green, an internationally renowned neurosurgeon in the field of SCI, and the family of Nick Buoniconti, a former professional football player, the project is located on the campus of the University of Miami School of Medicine/Jackson Memorial Medical Center.

The basic science research group is comprised of an international team of basic research scientists studying the repair and regeneration of the injured spinal cord. These scientists, trained in the disciplines of cellular and molecular biology, neuroanatomy, and electrophysiology, believe that the time is right to apply the recent technological advances in each of these fields to experimental models of spinal cord injury. The project is forming collaborations with scientists at institutions around the world working on SCI.

The clinical research group is characterizing and defining what happens to the human spinal cord following a traumatic injury. As part of this study, clinical researchers employ magnetic resonance imaging (MRI) to better visualize the damaged spinal cord and the technique of focal stimulation to map remaining functional spinal cord pathways.

The rehabilitative research group evaluates therapies designed to maximize the physical condition of the person with spinal cord injury. Research topics investigate functional electrical stimulation modalities, exercise physiology, and male fertility.

The project raises funds from individuals, corporations, foundations, civic organizations, and federal agencies in the form of donations, grants, bequests, and sponorship of special events.

National Spinal Cord Injury Association (NSCIA). 545 Concord Ave., Suite 29, Cambridge, MA 02138. (800) 962-9629, (617) 441-8500.

The NSCIA, formerly the National Paraplegia Foundation, is the oldest nonveteran spinal cord injury organization in the United States. NSCIA has 32 chapters and 20 developing chapters across the country. They also have an extensive information dissemination program through their National SCI Resource Center and SCI hotline.

Paralyzed Veterans of America (PVA). 801 - 18th Street NW, Washington, DC 20006. (800) 424-8200; (202) 872-1300.

PVA is a federally chartered national veterans' service organization. In addition to a strong national presence in the areas of legislation, advocacy, research, and education, they have chapter offices and service offices located throughout the United States. PVA has many excellent publications available in virtually all areas of interest to people with spinal cord injury. PVA also publishes two nationally distributed magazines, *Paraplegia News* and *Sports 'n Spokes*.

Spinal Cord Injury Network International (SCINI). 3911 Princeton Drive, Santa Rosa, California 95405-7013. (800) 548-2673, (707) 577-8796, (707) 577-0605 (fax).

SCINI offers information and referral services to individuals with spinal cord injuries and to their families. SCINI sponsors Spinal Cord

Injury Video Access, a lending program of educational audiovisuals, which was established in 1993 under a grant from the Paralyzed Veterans of America Education and Training Foundation.

Spinal Cord Society (SCS). Wendell Road, Fergus Falls, MN 56537. (218) 739-5252, (218) 739-5261.

The Spinal Cord Society's motto is "Cure, Not Care." Their only emphasis is one of supporting cure-oriented research. SCS has more than 200 chapters throughout the world, and it publishes a monthly newsletter about research advances and SCS chapter activities.

Toll-Free Information Numbers

National Spinal Cord Injury Hotline: (800) 562-3456.

Paralyzed Veterans of America: (800) 424-8200.

Other Organizations

FES Information Center: 11000 Cedar Avenue, Suite 322, Cleveland, OH 44106. (800) 666-2353, (216) 231-3257.

The center has developed resources for people interested in functional electrical stimulation and makes them available at no cost or low cost.

Professional Organizations

The following organizations are professional societies whose members work directly in the field of spinal cord injury, or in a closely-related field. While these organizations do not produce consumer-oriented literature, they may be able to provide information about practitioners in the requestor's geographic area.

American Association of Spinal Cord Injury Nurses and AASCI Psychologists-Social Workers. c/o Eastern Paralyzed Veterans Association, 75-20 Astoria Boulevard, Jackson Heights, NY 11370. (718) 803-3782.

American Paraplegia Society. c/o Eastern Paralyzed Veterans Association. 75-20 Astoria Boulevard, Jackson Heights, NY 11370. (718) 803-3782.

American Spinal Injury Association (ASIA). 250 East Superior Street, Room 619, Chicago, IL 60611. (312) 908-3425.

International Medical Society of Paraplegia. Rehabilitation Services, The Institute for Rehabilitation and Research, 1333 Moursund Avenue, P.O. Box 20095, Houston, TX 77225. Contact: Dr. Edward Carter, Corresponding Secretary.

National Spinal Cord Injury Statistical Center. Spain Rehabilitation Center, Room 544, 1717 6th Avenue South, Birmingham, AL 35233-7330, (205) 934-5359.

Supervises and directs the collection, management, and analysis of data from the Model Regional SCI Care Systems resulting in the world's largest SCI database.

RESNA. 1700 N. Moore Street, Suite 1540, Arlington, VA 22209. (703) 524-6686.

Periodicals of Interest

Accent on Living. Accent on Living, P.O. Box 700, Bloomington, IL 61702. (800) 787-8444. Cost: $10/year (4 issues).

Careers and the Disabled. Equal Opportunity Publications, Inc., 44 Broadway, Greenlawn, NY 11740. (516) 261-8899. Cost: $10/year (3 issues).

Journal of Neurotrauma. Wise Young, MD, Department of Neurosurgery, New York University Medical Center, 550 - 1st Avenue, New York, NY 10016. Cost: $115/ first class, $38/third class (4 issues).

Mainstream. Mainstream, Inc., 3 Bethesda Metro Center, Suite 830, Bethesda, MD 20814. (301) 654-2400 (V/TT). Cost: $60/year (6 issues).
New Mobility. c/o Miramar, 23815 Stuart Ranch Road, Malibu, CA 90265. (800) 543-4116. Cost: $18/year (6 issues).

Paraplegia. Scientific and Medical Division, MacMillan Press Ltd., Houndmils, Basingstoke, Hampshire, RG21 2XS England. Cost: $350/ year (12 issues).

Paraplegia News. PVA Publications, 2111 East Highland Avenue, Suite 180, Phoenix, AZ 85016-4702. (602) 224-0500. Cost: $15/year (12 issues).

Progress in Research. American Paralysis Association (APA), 500 Morris Avenue, Springfield, NJ 07081. Cost: Free (2 issues).

Progression. Northwestern University/Rehabilitation Institute of Chicago, 345 East Superior Street, Chicago, IL 60611. Cost: Free (4 issues).

The Project. The Miami Project to Cure Paralysis, 1600 NW 10th Avenue, #R-48, Miami, FL 33136. (800) 782-6387, (305) 547-6001. Cost: Free (3 issues).

Rehabilitation: Spinal Cord Injury Update. University of Washington, Rehabilitation Medicine RJ-30, Seattle, WA 98195. Cost: Free (4 issues).

Research Update. University of Birmingham (UAB), Spain Rehabilitation Center, RRTC Training Office, Room 506, 1717 - 6th Avenue South, Birmingham, AL 35233-7330. (205) 934-2088. Cost: Free (1 issue).

SCI Life. National Spinal Cord Injury Association, 545 Concord Avenue, Suite 29, Cambridge, MA 02138. (800)962-9629, (617) 935-2722. Cost: free to members; $30/year to nonmembers (4 issues).

SCI Nursing. Available from: American Association of Spinal Cord Injury Nurses (AASCIN), Eastern Paralyzed Veterans Association, 75-20 Astoria Boulevard, Jackson Heights, NY 11370-1177. Cost: $50 (4 issues).

Sports 'n Spokes. PVA Publications. Cost: $12/ year (6 issues).

Government-Sponsored Research Related to Spinal Cord Injury

National Institute on Disability and Rehabilitation Research (NIDRR)

The National Institute on Disability and Rehabilitation Research (NIDRR) provides funding to a number of research and treatment centers that are related either directly or indirectly to spinal cord injury. Information about the specific responsibilities of each NIDRR-funded project can be obtained from NARIC.

Model Spinal Cord Injury Systems. NIDRR provides financial assistance to 13 Model Spinal Cord Injury Systems throughout the country for the delivery, demonstration, and evaluation of comprehensive medical, vocational, and other rehabilitation services to meet the wide range of needs of individuals with spinal cord injury. Model Spinal Cord Injury Systems are located at the following facilities:

Thomas Jefferson University, Jefferson Medical College, 11th and Walnut Streets, Philadelphia, PA 19107. (215) 955-6579.

University of Alabama/Birmingham, Spain Rehabilitation Center, Room 529, 1717 - 6th Avenue South, Birmingham, AL 35233-7330. (205) 934-2088.

Rancho Los Amigos Medical Center, HB117, 7601 East Imperial Highway, Downey, CA 90242. (310) 940-7161.

Shepherd Spinal Center, Inc., 2020 Peachtree Road NW, Atlanta, GA 30309. (404) 355-9772.

Northwestern University Medical Center, Northwestern Memorial Hospital, 250 East Chicago Avenue, Suite 619, Chicago, IL 60611. (312) 908-3425.

University of Michigan, Department of Physical Medicine and Rehabilitation, N12A09-0491, 300 North Ingalls, Ann Arbor, MI 48109-0491. (313) 763-0971.

The Institute for Rehabilitation Research, 1333 Moursund Avenue, Houston, TX 77030. (713) 797-5910.

Santa Clara Valley Medical Center, 950 South Bascom Avenue, Box A421, Suite 2011, San Jose, CA 95128. (408) 295-9896.

University of Washington School of Medicine, Department of Rehabilitation Medicine, RJ-30, BB919 Health Science Building, Seattle, WA 98195. (206) 543-8171.

Kessler Institute for Rehabilitation, University of Medicine and Dentistry of New Jersey, 1199 Pleasant Valley Way, West Orange, NJ 07052. (201) 243-6805.

Mount Sinai Medical Center, Department of Rehabilitation Medicine, One Gustave L. Levy Place, Box 1240, New York, NY 10029. (212) 241-9657.

Rehabilitation Institute of Michigan, 261 Mack Boulevard, Detroit, MI 48201. (313) 745-9770.

Craig Hospital, Rocky Mountain Spinal Injury Center, 3425 Clarkson Street, Englewood, CO 80110. (303) 789-8220.

Rehabilitation Research & Training Centers (RTCs). NIDRR funds 49 Research and Training Centers (RTCs), which conduct research and training in a variety of areas related to all aspects of disability. Of particular interest to people with spinal cord injuries are the RTCs on the prevention and treatment of secondary complications of spinal cord injury, aging with spinal cord injury, and community integration:

Aging: Craig Hospital, Research Department, 3425 South Clarkson, Englewood, CO 80110. (303) 789-8202.

Los Amigos Research and Education Institute, Inc. (LAREI), Rancho Los Amigos Medical Center, 12481 Dahlia Street, Building 306, Downey, CA 90242. (310) 940-7402.

Secondary Complications: University of Alabama/Birmingham, Department of Rehabilitation Medicine, 1717 - 6th Avenue South, Birmingham, AL 35233-7330. (205) 934-3283.

Community Integration: Baylor College of Medicine, Department of Physical Medicine and Rehabilitation, One Baylor Plaza, Houston, TX 77030. (713) 797-5910.

Rehabilitation Engineering Research Centers (RERCs). One of NIDRR's major missions is to fund research related to the development and use of assistive devices for people with disabilities. To address this mission, NIDRR funds several Rehabilitation Engineering Research Centers (RERCs) that conduct research on specific areas of assistive technology. Of particular interest to people with spinal cord injuries are the RERCs on wheelchair technology, transportation, and children with orthopedic disabilities:

Wheelchairs: University of Pittsburgh, Rehabilitation Technology Program (RTP), 915 William Pitt Way, Pittsburgh, PA 15238. (412) 826-3138.

Transportation: University of Virginia, Transportation RERC, 1011 Linden Avenue, Charlottesville, VA 22902. (804) 296-4216.

Children: Rancho Los Amigos Medical Center, Los Amigos Research and Education Institute, Inc. (LAREI),7503 Bonita Street, Bonita Hall, Downey, CA 90242. (310) 940-7994.

Field-Initiated Research (FIRs). NIDRR funds projects to encourage eligible applicants to originate valuable ideas in areas which represent their own interests, yet are directly related to the rehabilitation of people with disabilities. One project currently funded studies aging and adjustment after SCI:

Sheperd Center for Spinal Injuries, Inc., 2020 Peachtree Road NW, Atlanta, GA 30309. (404) 352-2020.

National Institutes of Health

The National Institutes of Health (NIH) provides funding for research related to the care, treatment, and prevention of many diseases and conditions. NIH is comprised of 13 separate institutes that address specific disease categories or parts of the body. Of direct relevance to people with spinal cord injuries are the National Institute of Neurological Disorders and Stroke (NINDS) at NIH, Building 31, Room 8A-06, Bethesda, MD 20892; (800) 352-9424 and the National Institute of Maternal and Child Health's National Center for Medical Rehabilitation Research (NCMRR) at 6100 Executive Boulevard, Room 2A-03, Rockville, MD 20852; (301) 402-2242.

U.S. Department of Veterans Affairs

The U.S. Department of Veterans Affairs (VA) provides funding to researchers in VA hospitals throughout the country to conduct research on all aspects of spinal cord injury, from the development of new assistive devices to improved treatment for spinal cord injury-related health problems and research toward a cure for SCI. The agency also sponsors a biannual regeneration research symposium that is attended by scientists from all over the world.

Private Organizations that Fund Spinal Cord Injury Research

American Paralysis Association. 500 Morris Avenue, Springfield, NJ 07081. (800) 225-0292, (201) 376-8884.

Miami Project to Cure Paralysis. 1600 NW 10th Avenue, #R-48, Miami, FL 33136. (800) 782-6387, (305) 547-6001.

PVA Spinal Cord Research Foundation. c/o Paralyzed Veterans of America, 801 - 18th Street NW, Washington, DC 20006. (800) 424-8200, (202) 872-1300.

Spinal Cord Society. Wendell Road, Fergus Falls, MN 56537. (218) 739-5252, (218) 739-5261.

National Spinal Cord Injury Association. 545 Concord Avenue, Suite 29, Cambridge, MA 02138. (800) 962-9629.

Appendix

Other Sources for Further Help and Information

Chapter 45

Public Education Books and Videos on Low Back Pain

The following list of books and video recordings provides information to patients and the general public about the prevention and treatment of low back pain. This is not a comprehensive list nor does it constitute an endorsement of the materials by the National Institute of Arthritis and Musculoskeletal and Skin Diseases. Many of these materials are available through book stores and libraries; all may be obtained from the publisher of the item.

Books

Back Care: Supporting Good Health, Spence, W.R., Available from Health Edco, Waco, TX. 1991. 15 pages.

Back Pain: How to Help Yourself and When to Use Professional Care, Great Performance, Beaverton, OR. 1990. 16 pages.

Care of the Low Back: A Patient Guide, Russell, G.S. and Highland, T.R., Spine Publications, Columbia, MO. 196 pages. (Distributed by F.A. Davis Company, Publishers, Philadelphia, PA.)

Goodbye Back Pain, Faye, Leonard, Berkley Books, New York, NY. 1990. (reprint 1992).

National Institute of Arthritis and Musculoskeletal and Skin Diseases, nd.

Good News for Bad Backs, Swezey, R.L., Swezey, A.M., Knightsbridge Publishing Company, New York, NY. 1990. 303 pages.

Low Back Pain, Baxter Healthcare Corporation, McGaw Park, IL. 1990. 8 pages.

On the Job Exercises, Krames Communications, Daly City, CA. 1989. 16 pages.

Relief from Chronic Backache: Diagnosis, Therapy, Exercises, Blair, Edward, Dell Medical Library, New York, NY. 1990. 132 pages.

Remember Your Back, Krames Communications, Daly City, CA. 1989. 16 pages.

Taking Care of Your Back, American Physical Therapy Association, Alexandria, VA. 1990. 12 pages.

Your Lower Back, Potash, W.J., Gratch, M.J., et. al., Paragon Communications, Inc., Jenkintown, PA. 1993. 203 pages.

When You Need an Operation: About Low-Back Pain, American College of Surgeons, Chicago, IL. 1989. 10 pages.

Video Recordings

Your Aching Back, Renmar Productions, Ltd., Wantagh, NY 1990.

Bum Back, Acupressure Institute of America, Berkeley, CA. 1989.

Daily Living Back School, Cronin, K.M., Health Sciences Consortium, Chapel Hill, NC. 1989.

Chapter 46

Directory of
National Information Sources
and Related Services for
Back Patients

Arthritis Foundation
1314 Spring Street NW
Atlanta, GA 30309
(404) 872-7100

Disabilities served: Arthritis, rheumatic diseases.

Users served: People with arthritis and rheumatic diseases and their families, health care professionals.

Description: The Arthritis Foundation is a national, voluntary health association committed to supporting research to find the cure for and prevention of arthritis and improve the quality of life for those affected by arthritis. Programs include support for scientific research, specialist training, public information and education, and help within the community for people who have rheumatic diseases. The 71 local chapters and divisions of the foundation provide basic information as well as assistance in locating treatment specialists, clinics, and other agencies to help with physical, financial, and emotional problems caused by arthritis. The chapters support a variety of local services, including information and education programs, support groups, exercise classes, arthritis clinics, home care programs, and rehabilitation services.

Excerpted from Directory of National Information Sources on Disabilities, U.S. Department of Education, Office of Special Education and Rehabilitative Services, National Institute on Disability and Rehabilitation Research, 1994-95 ed.

Information services: The foundation disseminates information about arthritis care to its chapters and to professionals in the arthritis treatment field. A variety of pamphlets are available from the foundation's local chapters, including information on specific forms of arthritis, various treatments, and solutions to physical and emotional problems associated with arthritis. Some materials are available in Spanish. Chapters maintain lists of medical and community services and make referrals upon request. The foundation holds national and regional scientific meetings and continuing community education programs to advise local physicians of the latest clinical advances.

Combined Health Information Database (CHID)

National Institutes of Health
Box CHID
9000 Rockville Pike
Bethesda, MD 20892
(301) 468-6555
(301) 770-5164 (fax)

Description: CHID contains more than 104,000 citations and abstracts which provide information relevant to health professionals, health educators, people with disabilities, and the general public. Topics include: AIDS information and education programs, Alzheimer's disease, arthritis, asthma, blood resource information, cardiovascular disease, cholesterol education, deafness and other communication disorders, diabetes, digestive disease, eye health, kidney disease, cancer, cancer information and education materials, comprehensive school health, disease prevention, health promotion, heart attack, smoking, high blood pressure, maternal and child health, oral and dental health, post-traumatic stress disorder, and veterans' health.

Vendors: BRS Online, A Division of CD-Plus Technologies.

HEALTHSOUTH Corporation

Two Perimeter Park South
Birmingham, AL 35243
(800) 768-0018
(205) 967-7116
(205) 969-4741 (fax)

Disabilities served: Spinal cord and head injuries, musculoskeletal trauma and orthopaedic conditions, sports and work-related injuries, stroke, arthritis, neurological and neuromuscular disabilities.

Users served: Patients with the above listed disabilities, including support services for their family members.

Description: HEALTHSOUTH Corporation was established in 1984 to build a national rehabilitation network of inpatient and out-patient rehabilitation facilities that are capable of providing the full spectrum of medical rehabilitation services. All HEALTHSOUTH facilities offer comprehensive medical rehabilitation services; a coordinated, interdisciplinary team approach; physician direction and supervision; top quality, highly-motivated rehabilitation professionals; state-of-the-art technology and techniques; and barrier-free physical environments.

HEALTHSOUTH operates 52 locations in 21 States, with a network of 1,400 beds and an employee base of 3,500. Since the company's founding, the comprehensive rehabilitation network has provided services to more than 100,000 patients and experienced more than a million outpatient visits.

Information services: HEALTHSOUTH publishes newsletters for medical professionals and is expanding its national, regional and local speakers' bureaus, to address medical/rehabilitation topics, current treatments, and technical innovations.

Missouri Arthritis Rehabilitation Research and Training Center (MARRTC)
University of Missouri—Columbia
Department of Medicine, Division of Immunology and Rheumatology
MA427 Health Sciences Center
One Hospital Drive
Columbia, MO 65212
(314) 882-8097
(314) 882-8096

Disabilities served: Arthritis and musculoskeletal diseases.

Users served: People with arthritis, families, faculty for education of rehab personnel, physicians.

Description: The Missouri Arthritis Rehabilitation Research and Training Center is a project funded by the National Institute on Disability and Rehabilitation Research (NIDRR) to evaluate techniques for assessing performance; evaluate new techniques; demonstrate rehabilitation models; and provide training to professionals, persons with arthritis, and their families.

Information services: MARRTC publishes curricula and training materials, journal articles, monographs, and a newsletter.

National Arthritis and Musculoskeletal and Skin Diseases Information Clearinghouse
Box AMS
9000 Rockville Pike
Bethesda, MD 20892
(301) 495-4484

Disabilities served: Rheumatoid arthritis, osteoarthritis, gout, systemic lupus erythematosus, scoliosis, scleroderma, sports injuries, and approximately 600 other rheumatic, musculoskeletal, and skin diseases.

Users served: Physicians, nurses, occupational and physical therapists, librarians, researchers, educators, members of the media, patients, and their families.

Description: The National Arthritis and Musculoskeletal and Skin Diseases Information Clearinghouse is a service of the National Institute of Arthritis and Musculoskeletal and Skin Diseases, a division of the National Institutes of Health.

Established in 1978, the clearinghouse is a national resource center for information about professional, patient, and public education materials; and federal programs related to rheumatic, musculoskeletal, and skin diseases.

Information services: The clearinghouse maintains a file on the Combined Health Information Database (CHID), an online computerized database available to the public via BRS Information Technologies. Bibliographies, fact sheets, and brochures are compiled and distributed.

The National Scoliosis Foundation
72 Mount Auburn Street
Watertown, MA 02172
(617) 926-0397

Disabilities served: Scoliosis, kyphosis, lordosis.

Users served: General public, school personnel, health care professionals (anyone seeking information on scoliosis).

Description: The National Scoliosis Foundation is a nonprofit organization focusing on educating the public, promoting school screening, and maintaining a resource center of information.

Information services: The foundation offers packets of information to parents and young people, adults with scoliosis, and health care professionals. It publishes a biannual newsletter, *The Spinal Connection*, which includes an overview of the foundation's activities and services and a Medical Update Information column.

Policy Barriers that Impede Utilization of Technology to Maintain the Independence and Employment of Individuals Aging with a Disability Project (PAD)
Andrus Gerontology Center
3715 McClintock Avenue
Los Angeles, CA 90089
(213) 740-1750
(213) 740-8241 (fax)

Disabilities served: Rheumatoid arthritis, cerebral palsy, postpolio, stroke, and spinal cord injury.

Users served: Professionals in rehabilitation and related fields, people with disabilities, and researchers.

Description: PAD is a research project examining the responsiveness of current public policy to the dynamic needs of people "aging in" with lifelong disabilities. PAD research investigates policies affecting the availability, affordability, and accessibility of assistive technologies aimed at maintaining community-based living and the employment of middle-aged and elderly individuals with longstanding disabilities. In addition, PAD develops and critically evaluates recommendations for improving the responsiveness of current disability/aging programs.

Information services: PAD can provide general policy information to inquirers by phone or by letter. Technical publications on project research can be obtained by contacting the PAD office.

Resources for Rehabilitation
33 Bedford Street, Suite 19A
Lexington, MA 02173
(617) 862-6455
(617) 861-7517 (fax)

Disabilities served: Hearing and speech impairments, arthritis, stroke, diabetes, osteoporosis, epilepsy, multiple sclerosis, mobility impairments, low back pain, spinal cord injuries, vision impairment and blindness, and Parkinson's disease.

Users served: Professionals who provide services to individuals with disabilities and chronic conditions and individuals with these disabilities.

Description: Resources for Rehabilitation is a nonprofit organization dedicated to providing training and information to health and rehabilitation professionals, employers, and the public.

Information services: The organization provides directories, desk references, anthologies, and special large print publications designed for distribution by professionals to individuals with disabilities and chronic conditions. It also conducts custom-designed training programs, workshops, and seminars. Program evaluations are also performed.

One publication is *Resources for People with Disabilities and Chronic Conditions*, 2nd Edition, 1993. This directory contains chapters on spinal cord injuries, low back pain, diabetes, multiple sclerosis, hearing and speech impairments, vision impairments, blindness, and epilepsy. Information on organizations, publications, environmental adaptations, and assistive equipment is provided as well as special information for children and youth.

Resources for Rehabilitation has available *Meeting Needs of Employees with Disabilities* 2nd Edition, 1993. The publication provides employers and counselors with the information they need to help people with disabilities retain or obtain employment. It contains information on government programs and laws, supported employment, training programs, environmental adaptations, and transition from school to work. Chapters on mobility, vision, hearing, and speech impairments include information on products and services that enable employers to accommodate the needs of people with disabilities.

Spina Bifida Association of America (SBAA)

4590 MacArthur Boulevard NW, Suite 250
Washington, DC 20007-4226
(800) 621-3141
(202) 944-3285
(202) 944-3295 (fax)

Disabilities served: Spina bifida with related hydrocephalus

Users served: Parents, teachers, professionals, and anyone interested in spina bifida

Description: Organized in 1974, the Spina Bifida Association of America (SBAA) emphasizes local parent and patient support groups. Activities also include public education, research, advocacy, and sponsorship of an annual conference for professionals and lay people on medical, social, educational, and legal issues relating to this disability. A Medical Advisory Board identifies national medical needs and evaluates current medical advances, reporting on these to the membership. The Professional Advisory Board for Education studies current educational programs for children with spina bifida. SBAA continues to work closely with the National Easter Seal Society and the March of Dimes Birth Defects Foundation, and the American Academy of Pediatrics.

Information services: Publications and public education materials are available through the national office in Washington, DC, or 100 local chapters in the United States and Canada; chapters also sponsor parent, teenage, and young adult support groups. Publications include: *Introduction to Spina Bifida*; *You are Special — You're the One*; *A Guide to Hydrocephalus*; the bimonthly newsletter *Insights*; and manuals for parents and teachers. Material on organizing SBAA chapters, copy for radio spots, publicity and media presentations, and a directory of chapters can be requested.

There is a nominal charge for publications; price lists are mailed. SBAA makes referrals to local chapters and/or treatment centers as necessary. Video and audiotapes are also available for purchase.

Spinal Network
23815 Stuart Ranch Road
Malibu, CA 90265
(800) 543-4116

Disabilities served: Paralysis due to spinal cord injury, multiple sclerosis, spina bifida, postpolio.

Users served: People who use wheelchairs, physical rehabilitation professionals.

Description: Spinal Network was formed in 1985 to provide a central database for people who use wheelchairs to find answers, connections, and resources. As a result of this organization, Spinal Network published the second edition of *Spinal Network: The Total Resource for the Wheelchair Community*, a resource guide with chapters on medical information, sports and recreation, travel, computers, sex and romance, civil rights, a description of disability organizations in North America, and a state-by-state listing of resources.

Information services: Spinal Network sells and distributes a wide variety of books on all aspects of disability, and the journal *New Mobility*, a lifestyle magazine for people who use wheelchairs.

United States Wheelchair Swimming
229 Miller Street
Middleboro, MA 02346
(508) 946-1964
(719) 574-1150 (Membership)

Disabilities served: Spinal cord injuries, amputation, spina bifida, and multiple sclerosis.

Users served: People with spinal cord injuries, amputations, cerebral palsy, spina bifida, and multiple sclerosis.

Description: United States Wheelchair Swimming is a nonprofit organization that promotes recreational and competitive swimming to enhance the health and quality of life of persons who have disabilities. As a part of Wheelchair Sports U.S.A., the organization is a member of Section E of the U.S. Olympic Committee. Members will participate in the Paralymic Games in Atlanta in 1996.

Competitions use a functional classification system based on effective function of muscle groups in swimming, body position, and locomotor ability. They are conducted for youth, adults, and older persons. An Elite Training Camp is held each spring.

Information services: A quarterly newsletter is published.

Vermont Rehabilitation Engineering Research Center in Low Back Pain
University of Vermont
Department of Orthopedics and Rehabilitation
One South Prospect Street
Burlington, VT 05401
(800) 527-7320 (Nationwide, except in Vermont)
(802) 656-4582
(802) 660-9243 (fax)

Disabilities served: Low back pain, back disorders, and related disabilities.

Users served: Manufacturers, employers, legislators, policy makers, social planners, researchers, vocational rehabilitation personnel, allied health personnel, physicians, and people with disabilities

Description: With support from the National Institute on Disabilities and Rehabilitation Research (NIDRR), this center works to improve the employability of people with low back disorders and disability by developing and testing assistive technology and by modifying jobs and workplaces. Engineering projects include studies of lifting, posture, seating, vibration, and materials handling in connection with back pain and disability. Applied research projects include the testing of rehabilitation engineering products, evaluation of exercise programs, and the development of a statewide model program to hasten return to work of back-injured workers. The center's Information Services Division provides toll-free assistance in locating research and rehabilitation programs, as well as bibliographic searching and factfinding.

521

Information services: The center produces journal articles, brochures, fact sheets, and annual reports; develops technology; conducts conferences; and develops curricula/training materials.

Wheelchair Motorcycle Association, Inc. (WMA)
101 Torrey Street
Brockton, MA 02401
(508) 583-8614

Disabilities served: Spinal cord injuries, spina bifida, amputation, cerebral palsy, multiple sclerosis, and other physical disabilities.

Users served: People with spinal cord injury, spina bifida, cerebral palsy, multiple sclerosis, and amputation, and recreational therapists.

Description: Founded in 1975, the Wheelchair Motorcycle Association, Inc., is a private, nonprofit, all-volunteer organization. The purpose of the organization is to offer mobility options and choices for outdoor transportation and recreation. WMA offers information on off-road vehicles, which members test. The organization also researches three-wheel motorcycles for highway use. WMA has also adapted an ordinary wheelchair into an all-terrain wheelchair called The Turtle.

Information services: WMA publishes a newsletter and sends out a kit on various vehicles such as sit-down lawn mowers, tractors that hold wheelchairs, all-terrain wheelchairs, and three-wheel mopeds.

Index

Index

Page numbers in *italics* refer to graphics and tables; the letter n following a page number refers to a note.

A

abdominal muscles 8, 26, 46, 313
  exercise 52, 78
  support 67
  tightening 56
ABLEDATA 473n, 474, 477, 479, 485, 494, 496
ACA *see* American Chiropractic Association
acetaminophen 206
AcroMed Corporation 254-59
acromiohumeral region, defined 29
activities of daily living (ADL) 29, 224
activity alteration, acute low back pain 207-8
acupressure 69, 150, 183, 512
acupuncture 69, 150, 183, 206, 222, 248, 394
Acute Low Back Problems in Adults 195n
acute stage, defined 29

ADA *see* Americans with Disabilities Act
Adams, M. 66
Adams, M. A. 23, 28
adaptive equipment 29
  see also assistive devices
adjustment
  defined 305
  spinal cord injury 345
ADL *see* activities of daily living
adolescents, low back pain 22
adults, posture 15-16
advocate, defined 29
age factor
  ankylosing spondylitis 136
  back pain 47-48
  disabilities 517
  low back pain 22, 216
  osteoporosis 10, 103, 114, 115-16
  posture 16-17, 18
  spinal cord injuries 335
  spinal disks 57-58
  spinal injuries 316-17
  spinal stenosis 78, 100
  syringomyelia 125
  tumors 157
Agency for Health Care Policy and Research (AHCPR) 244, 267n, 287, 289, 299

AHCPR *see* Agency for Health Care Policy and Research
Air Carrier Access Act (1986) 451-52, 459, 464, 466
air travel, spinal cord injury 451-71
airway management, defined 29
alcohol 156, 333-34
  cirrhosis of the liver 31
  osteoporosis 48, 105, 119
alendronate (Fosamax) 118, 120
Alexander, G. 72
AMA *see* American Medical Association
Amador, Marie, RN 435
American Academy of Orthopaedic Surgeons 90, 94, 259
American Academy of Pediatrics 90
American Association of Spinal Cord Injury Nurses (AASCIN) 504
American Brain Tumor Association 178
American Cancer Society 178
American Chiropractic Association (ACA) 290, 297n
ACA Journal of Chiropractic 303
American Chronic Pain Association 130
American Family Physician 45
American Journal of Physical Medicine 28
American Medical Association (AMA) 286
American Paralysis Association (APA) 131, 411, 413n, 419, 434, 500, 504, 508
  Consortium on Spinal Cord Injury 414, 417
American Physical Therapy Association 231n, 232, 237
American Spinal Injury Association (ASIA) 497, 500, 503
Americans with Disabilities Act (ADA) 315, 366-69, 457
American Syringomyelia Alliance Project, Inc. 130
amitriptyline 70, 297-98, 392
analgesics 70, 192, 205
Anaprox DS 192
anatomical relationships, physical fitness 22-23, *24*

anatomic defects 210, 213
anemia 30, 139
aneurysm 77
angiography 162
ankle dorsiflexion 75
ankylosing spondylitis 40, 48, 133-53
ankylosis, defined 133
annular cysts 57, 58, *58*
annulus fibrosus 8, 10, 213, 239
anorexia nervosa 114
anticonvulsants 392
antidepressants 243, 297, 392
anti-inflammatory medication 47, 48, 73, 408
anxiety 71
APLD *see* aspiration percutaneous lumbar diskectomy
appearance, posture 17, 140
appliance, defined 30
arachnoiditis 126, 391, 398
Arachnoiditis Information and Support Network 132
arches 7-8, 50
argon 240
arm pain 291, 294-96
Arnoczky, S. P. 268, 274
arthritis 48, 96, 136, 182, 236, 246-47, 305
  degenerative 95
  facet 65
  rheumatoid 105, 517
  systemic 64
  wear and tear 13, 102
  see also ankylosing spondylitis; spinal stenosis
Arthritis and Rheumatism 102
The Arthritis Foundation 149, 513-14
Arthritis Today 99n
artificial limbs 37
Ascher, P. W. 241
Asher, Marc 259
aspiration percutaneous lumbar diskectomy (APLD) 52
aspirin 205, 395
assertiveness training 341, 348-49
assistive devices 29, 454, 462-65
  spinal cord injury 473-85
Assistive Technology Funding & Systems Change Project 484

astrocytomas 174-75
ataxia 160, 311
atherosclerosis, defined 30
atlas 181, 191
atrophy
  acute low back pain 198
  defined 30
  muscles 47, 332, 397
  vertebrae 55-56
attendant, defined 30
automobiles
  accidents 313, 317, 409, 488
  adaptive equipment 30, 477-78
  posture 12, 17, 142-43
  whiplash 294
automobile seats 49, 52
avocational, defined 41
avulsion 398
Axelson, Peter 475
axis 181
axons 404, 417-18, 422-23, 425, 426-27
Ayuayo, Albert 416

B

backaches 52-53, 96, 136
back bones *see* vertebrae
back curvature 123
back extensor muscles 26, 27
back muscles 8, *9,* 19
  exercise 52
  quantity 8
  see also *individual muscles*
back pain
  causes 8-10, *9,* 46, 99
  chronic 15, 219
  location 3, 6-7
  surgical relief 50-51, 243-51
  see also low back pain
back schools 220, 224, 512
back strain 136
Baer, Jean 370
Bailin, P. 239
balance problems 159, 161
Balazy, Thomas E., MD 393, 400
bamboo spine *135*
Barbach, Lonnie 387

barbiturates 169
Barnicle, K. 478
Battié, M. C. 25, 27, 84
BCNU drugs 167
Becker, Elle 493
bed rest 49, 69, 78, 97, 121, 244
  ankylosing spondylitis 143
bedridden, defined 30
bed sores *see* pressure sores
behavioral symptoms, tumors 159
Belknap, Katherine 473n
Bell, G. R. 83
benign, defined 155
benign tumors 165
Beninger, Paul R., MD 406
Bennett, G. 400
Ben Said, R. 28
Bernini, P. 72
Biering-Sorensen, F. 27
Bigos, S. J. 25, 27, 289
Bigos, Stanley 250
biofeedback 183, 206, 248
biomedical engineering 431
biopsy 163-64
  see also surgery
Bird, Edward D., MD 173
birth defects, syringomyelia 129
bladder 30, 31, 34, 40
  residual urine 38
  see also catheterization; Credé;
    Foley catheter; intermittent
    catheterization program
bladder function 246, 313, 314, 328
  degenerative back disease 96
  ejaculations 378-79
  resources 491
  sciatica 74, 76, 79
  sexual function 378-79, 381
  spina bifida 86-87
  spinal cord injuries 403-4
  spinal stenosis 100
  syringomyelia 127
blood-brain barrier 168-69
blood circulation
  spinal degeneration 95, 160
  whiplash 293
Bloom, B. A. 87
blue pads *see* chux
Blumenthal, S. 84

BMD *see* bone mineral density
body composition, bone mass 112
body mass index (WT/HT²) 26
body weight, disk pressure 57
Boeing Corporation 25
Bogos, S. 195n
Boline, Patrick D., MD 297
bone alignment 11
bone density 103, 104, 106
bone grafts 33, 129, 263, 268, 273
bone mass 111-14
bone mineral density (BMD) 111-14
bone remodeling 104, 114
bone scans 65, 210
bone scintigraphy 268
bone spurs 9, 95
bone strength 103, 111
botulinum toxin (Botox) 186-87
bowel function 313
  cauda equina 47
  degenerative back disease 96
  posture 17
  resources 491
  sciatica 74, 79
  sexual functions 381
  spina bifida 86
  spinal stenosis 100
  syringomyelia 127
bowstring test 76
Bowyer, O. 195n, 289
braces 37, 222
  ankylosing spondylitis 143, 151-52
  defined 30
  osteoporosis 123
  scoliosis 91-92
brachytherapy 168
Bracken, M. 434
Bradbard, Linda 89-90, 92
Bradley, Laurence A. 401
Braen, G. 195n, 289
Bragg, C. 273
brain, described 305
Brain Tumor Information Service 178
brain tumors 155-79
The Brain Tumor Society 178
breathing exercises 144, 148
Bregman, Barbara S., Ph.D. 418
Bridges, A. 267, 271, 273
British Medical Journal 303

Brodsky, A. E. 269, 274
Brophy, Brian P. 400
Brown, C. W. 274
Brown, M. D. 82
Bubis, J. J. 269, 274
bulging disks 58, 246
Bunge, M. B. 435
Bunge, R. P. 434, 435
Buoniconti, Nick 500
bursitis 56, 295

C

Cady, L. D. 25, 27
Cailliet, R. 22, 28, 66
Calcimar 117
calcitonin 104, 108, 117, 120
calcitriol 104
calcium 104
  deposits 97
  osteoporosis 48, 105, 119
  sources 106, *109*
calcium supplements 106-7, 110
Calvo, Mona, Ph.D. 104-5, 106
Cameron, H. U. 267, 271, 273
Campbell, J. N. 400
cancers 48, 105
  endometrial 108
  see also brain tumors; spinal cord
    tumors
carbamazepine 392
carbohydrates, defined 30
carbon dioxide 240
cardiopulmonary conditions 236
cardiovascular disease 48, 101
cardiovascular fitness 227, 228-29
  low back pain 25
caregiver, defined 30
carmustine drugs 167
Carragee, Eugene J., MD 84
Cartesegna, M. 79, 83
cartilage 7, 8, 9
Casavant, D. A. 26, 28
Cassidy, J. D. 83
Cassidy, J. David, DC 303
cath *see* catheters; intermittent
  catheterization program
catheterization, defined 30

catheters 383, 384
  spina bifida 86-87
CAT scans *see* computerized axial
  tomography
cauda equina 7, 10, 47, 78, 325, 332
  syndrome 30-31, 71, 79, 196, 246
CBC *see* complete blood count
CCNU drugs 167
central nervous system (CNS) 156-57,
  162, 166, 167, 305, 312, 406, 413,
  422, 423
central stenosis 9, 10
cerebral palsy 235, 517
cerebrospinal fluid 126, 129, 158, 391
cervical, defined 31, 305
cervical dystonia 185-87
cervical spine disorders 181-84
cervical vertebrae 3, *5*, 133, 160, 294,
  312, 324
  flexibility 6
Chalker, Rebecca 491
Chanaud, Cheryl, MD 435
Cheever, Raymond C. 491
chemonucleolysis 31, 247
chemotherapy 166-67, 168-69, 177
  see also drug therapy
Cherkin, D. C., Ph.D. 302
Chesney, Denise 475
Chiari I malformation 126, 127, 131
children
  adoption 386
  disability benefits 439-40
  low back pain 22
  posture 15-16
  resources 491-92
  scoliosis 96
  spina bifida 85-87
  spinal cord injuries 338, 362-63
  tumors 174, 176-77
  wheelchairs 494, 507
The Children's Brain Tumor Foundation 179
Chilgren, R. 387
chiropractic facts 283-86
chiropractic terms 305-8
chiropractors 49, 69, 288, 293, 296,
  301, 305-6
  patient emotional state 250
  see also manipulation

cholesterol, defined 31
chondroitin sulfate 240
chordomas 174
Choy, D. S. 241
Christodoulides, A. N. 82
chronic pain
  defined 31
  management 389-401
Chronic Pain Letter 130
chux, defined 31
chymopapain 31, 51-52, 81, 247
circulation examinations 234
circulatory conditions 236
circumferential measurements 199
cirrhosis of the liver, defined 31
claudication 60-61, 78, 216
cleft spine *see* spina bifida
Clinical Practice Guideline 195, 299
clothing allowance, defined 31
CNS *see* central nervous system
Coale, John 256
COBRA 152
coccyx 3, 7
cognitive symptoms, tumors 159
Cohen, J. M. 82
Cole, T. 387
colitis 48, 139-40
collagen fibers 8
collagenous disorders 235
comfort, acute low back pain 203
communicable diseases 453, 461-62
communicating syringomyelia 126
communication skills 358-59
community resources, spinal injuries
  369
Complaints Resolution Officials 453,
  470
complete blood count (CBC) 211
compression fractures 64
computer imaging 35, 50, 80
computerized axial tomography (CAT
  scans) 50, 65, 106, 268
  sciatica 76-77
computerized tomography (CT scan)
  96, 127, 129, 162-63, 211
  defined 32
  neck pain 280
computer terminals, posture 12, 17
congenital disorders 88

congenital tumors, defined 155
connective tissue conditions 235
Connolly, J. F. 274
constipation *see* bowel function
Consumers Reports 275n
contact placing 418
contractures 31, 397
contraindicated, defined 31
convulsions 159
cord cysts 398
cordotomy 399
cortical bone 105
corticosteroids 105, 408
cosmetic restorations 37
costs
  back pain 45, 65
  back surgery 244, 254
  low back pain 22, 219
  osteoporosis 105-6, 118
  spinal injuries 318, *319*
Cotrel-Dubousset surgery 93
Cousins, Norman 346
craniopharyngiomas 174
Credé, defined 31
Crenshaw, R. L. 26, 28
Cronin, K. M. 512
crossover pain 202
crutches 476
CT-myelography, defined 31
CT scan *see* computerized axial
  tomography
Cuckler, J. M. 72
Cummings, John 256
curls 20
Currier, B. 84
curvature of spine *see* scoliosis
Cutrow, Michelle 248-49
cyclobenzaprin HCl (Flexeril) 70
cystic myelopathy 391, 399
cysts 57, *58,* 125, 398

D

Dabezies, E. J. 84
Daffenr, R. H. 66
Danish Medical Bulletin 27
Davidoff, G. 400
Davis, Alexander A., MD 84

Davis, G. W. 241
Davis, Martha 352, 369
deafferentation 399
Decade of the Brain 414, 416
decompression 32, 101-2, 249
decubitus ulcer, defined 32
degeneration, defined 306
degenerative back problems 95-97, 249
degenerative changes of spine 8, 9,
  47, 57-62
  see also age factor
degenerative diseases 56, 58, 71, 137
DeLisa, Joel A. 308
DeLuca, C. J. 26, 28
Demos Publications 335
demyelination 425, 427
dendrites 422
denervation pain 399
densitometry 118, 119
DePalma, A. F. 268, 273
Department of Education 513n
Department of Health and Human
  Services 244, 299
Department of Transportation (DOT)
  451, 463, 465, 469, 471
Department of Veterans Affairs (VA)
  41, 475, 507
Department of Veterans Benefits
  (DVB) 32
depression 71, 346-47
  ankylosing spondylitis 137
dermatome 80, 328
DeVries, H. A. 26, 28
DEXA *see* dual energy x-ray
  absorptiometry
dexamathasone 167
Deyo, R. A. 78, 83
Deyo, Richard, MD 248, 249
diabetes 59
diagnosis
  ankylosing spondylitis 139
  cervical spine disorders 182
  low back pain 62-65, 233-34, 244-45
  osteoporosis 105-6, 117-19, 120
  sciatica 74-76
  spinal stenosis 100
  syringomyelia 127
  tumors 155, 161-64, 167, 199
  whiplash 292-93

diagnostic tests 49-50
diathermy 67, 78, 206
Didronel 117
diet *see* nutrition
dietitian, registered 151
diffuse idiopathic skeletal
  hyperostosis (DISH) 59
disability, defined 438
Disability Determination Services
  442-43
Disabled Sports USA 480
DISH *see* diffuse idiopathic skeletal
  hyperostosis
diskectomy 241, 247
  defined 32
  sciatica 79, 80-81
disk excision 71
diskography 32, 96, 268
disk prolapse 56-57, 58
disks 56-58, 294
  defined 306, 323
  degeneration 95
  see also spinal disks
distal nerve entrapment 78
distended, defined 32
dizziness 191, 292, 392
doctor of medicine (MD) 283
  described 35
  see also physicians
Dolan, P. 66
dorsal horn 399
dorsal root entry zone surgery
  (DREZ) 395-96
dosage, defined 32
dowager's hump 105
  see also osteoporosis
DREZ *see* dorsal root entry zone surgery
drugs, defined 32
drug therapy 166-67, 168-69, 190, 297
  acute low back pain 205-6
  ankylosing spondylitis 141
  chronic pain 392-93
  spinal cord injury 408-9, 422, 428-30
  see also chemotherapy; nonsteroidal
    anti-inflammatory drugs
    (NSAID)
dual energy x-ray absorptiometry
  (DEXA) 118-19

Dunn, Michael 369
dura mater 129, 161
duritis 59, 69
Dutta, Chhanda, Ph.D. 104, 105, 106
Duvauferrier, R. 82
DVB *see* Department of Veterans
  Benefits
Dwyer, A. F. 269, 274
dyesthesia 77, 399
dystonias 185-87

E

edema, defined 32
education
  accommodations 368-69
  acute low back pain 203
  books and videos 511-12
  physical therapy 235
  sexuality 373
  spinal injuries 333-39
Edwards, C. C. 269, 274
EEG *see* electroencephalogram
Eglow, Todd 305n
Eismont, F. J. 84
ejaculations 378-79, 407, 432
Elavil 70, 298
electrical bone growth stimulation
  267-73
electrical nerve stimulation 396-97
electric muscle stimulation 92, 222
electroencephalogram (EEG) 163
electromyogram (EMG) 50, 63, 77,
  127, 210
  analysis 26
  defined 33
eligibility, defined 32-33
Ellis, Albert 347
Elmer, Charles D. 491
embolus, defined 33
EMG *see* electromyogram
Emley, M. S. 26, 28
emotions
  chronic pain 397-98
  posture 12
  spinal cord injury 344-49
  stress 53
emotive imagery 398

Endep 70
endocrinologists 118
endometriosis 77
endorphins 68, 69
endurance examinations 234
enkephalin 70
enthesopathies (trouble spots) 138
environmental factors 157, 158
ependymoblastomas 177
ependymomas 175
epidural scars 77
epidural steroids 69-70, 78
epilepsy 173
erections 377-78, 382, 410
ergonomic issues 190
  see also work space design
erythrocyte sedimentation rate (ESR)
  test 139, 211
Eshelman, Elizabeth R. 352, 369
Essei, M. 66
estrogen 117
  bone mass 112
  osteoporosis 104, 105, 108, 114, 119,
    122
etidronate 110, 117
evaluation, defined 33
evoked potentials 165
Exercise and Sports Sciences Review
  28
exercises 14, 97
  ankylosing spondylitis 145-48
  assistive devices 480
  back pain 46, 68, 207-8, 216-18,
    227, 244
  disabilities 337
  muscles 19, *21,* 47
  neck 275, 277-79
  osteoporosis 115
  sciatica 78
  videos 481, 492
extension 33, 68, 220
extensor muscles 19, 68
extradural tumors 161
extramedullary tumors 161
extremity, defined 33
eyeglasses 37
eye problems 12, 14, 138
  tumors 159

F

FABER test 63
fabricate, defined 33
facet arthritis 65
facet joints 7, 9, 62
  degeneration 95
  sciatica 74
  steroid injections 70
  stretched 56
Fager, C. A. 84
fall prevention 116-17, 124, 233
family members
  back pain 220
  physical therapy 235
  spinal injuries 333, 360362
Farley, Dixie 94
fascia 22, 26
Fast, A. 83
fatigue 12, 335
Faye, Leonard 511
FCER see Foundation for
  Chiropractic Education and Research
FDA Consumer 3n, 45n, 89n, 103n,
  403n
femoral nerve stretch test 76
femoral stretch test 63
Fensterheim, Herbert 370
Ferguson, Gregory M. 387
FES see functional electrical stimulation
fibrocartilage 57
Fine, P. R. 400
Fisher, L. D. 25, 27
fitness components 26
fitness levels, exercises 20, *21*
fitness videos 481, 492
flaccid, defined 33
Flexeril 70
flexibility 369
  exercises 20
  low back pain 26
flexion 57, 75, 220
  defined 33
  spinal 78
Florida Workers' Compensation
  Study 301

flouride therapy 120
flourine intake 59
Foley catheter 33
  see also catheterization
folk remedies 145
foot problems 12, 73, 74
foramenotomy 80, 216
foramina 7, 60, 78, 183
Forristall, R. M. 82
Fosamax 118
Foundation for Chiropractic Education and Research (FCER) 297-98
4-aminopyridine 416-17
fractured vertebrae 45, 265
Freedox 429, 433
Friedreich's disease 311
Frocrain, L. 82
Frymoyer, J. W. 66, 72
functional electrical stimulation (FES) 336, 406-8, 431, 433, 502
furniture design
  back pain 243
  posture 14, 17-18
fusion 33
  see also spinal fusion

G

Gage, Fred 417
gait 33, 233, 293
gallbladder disease 48
Gallinaro, P. 79, 83
Gallup Poll (1991) 303
gamma knife 169
ganglioneuromas 175
Garfin, Steven, MD 258, 259
Gehweiler, J. A. 66
Geisler, F. H. 435
Geisler, Fred H., MD 409
gender factor
  ankylosing spondylitis 149
  low back pain 22
  spinal cord injury 410
  spinal injuries 317
  spinal stenosis treatment 101-2
gene therapy 169-70
genetic engineering 425-26
  see also heredity

genital function 374-77, 379-80, 385
  see also sexual function
Gill, K. 84
glioblastoma multiforme tumors 175
gliomas 174-76
glucose injections 162
GM-1 ganglioside 409, 430
Golden, Linda, MD 106, 108
Goodman, Carol L. 494
grafts 33, 129, 263, 268, 273, 409
Gratch, M. J. 512
Grecovetsky, S. 28
Green, Barth, MD 500
Greenwald, Harold 352, 370
Grieve, Gregory P. 306, 308
growth factors 172, 416, 424, 425, 427
Guarracina, M. 400
Guenard, V. 435
Guttmann, Ludwig 416

H

Haldeman, S. 83
Hall Bartelson, J. 66
halo, defined 34
Halverson, Lynn 473n
Hambrecht, F. Terry, MD 407-8
Hamburger, Viktor 416
hamstrings 19, 20, 26, 27, 227
Hanley, Edward 245
Hannon, K. M. 273
Hansson, T. H. 25, 27
Harper, Robert 347
Harrington, I. 72
Harrington Rod surgery 93
HBHC *see* hospital based home care
headaches 125
  chiropractic relief 297-98
  posture 16
  tumors 158
  whiplash 292
head retraction exercise 277
health care professions 283
health insurance 152
  chiropractic 304
  see also insurance reimbursements; Social Security disability insurance

health maintenance organizations (HMO) 302
health promotion, defined 34
health risks, defined 34
HEALTHSOUTH Corporation 514-15
Healthy People 2000 19, 20, 22, 28
hearing aids 37
hearing problems
 air travel 454, 460
 diagnosis 161
 tumors 159
heat therapy 67, 97, 144, 206, 220, 223, 295
Helie, J. 28
hemangioblastoma 177
Hendler, N. H. 400
Hendrix, M. 66
heparin 105
heredity
 ankylosing spondylitis 149
 bone mass 112
 osteoporosis 104-5, 119
Herkowitz, H. N. 267, 273
Herman, Robin 243n
herniated disks 9, 10, 31, 49, 51, 56, 95, 182, 213-14, 247
 defined 34
 laser therapy 239-41
 sciatica 73, 75
 tests 63
 young people 57
 see also ruptured disks
herniation, defined 306
herpes zoster 77
Herson, Linda 497
Highland, T. R. 511
Hill, Kelly, RN 494
Hingley, Audrey T. 411
hip flexors 19, 313
hip fractures 105-6, 108
hip joints 7, 22, *135*
hip muscles 112
hobbies 481
Holets, V. R. 435
hormone replacement therapy 108, 117
Horner's Syndrome 391
hospital based home care (HBHC), defined 34

hot baths 48, 150
 see also heat therapy
hotlines
 American Paralysis Association 411
 National Spinal Cord Injury 502
 National Spinal Cord Injury Association 411, 487, 489
 Paralyzed Veterans of America 502
hot packs 78, 150
Hotta, S. Steven, MD 274
Howley, Susan 418
hubbard tank, defined 34
Hueftle, M. G. 82
humerus 29
hurdler's stretches 20
Husson, J. L. 82
Hutton, W. C. 23, 28, 66
hyaluronic acid 240
hydrocephalus 86-87, 126, 165, 519-20
hydrocollator moist pads 150
hygiene, defined 34
hyperextension injury *see* whiplash
hyperextension posturing 68
hyperflexion injury *see* whiplash
hyperinfraction 166
hyperkyphosis 90
hyperlordosis (sway back) 56, 90
hyperreflexia 391
hyperthermia 170
hyperthyroidism 105
Hypokinetic Disease 28
hypokinetic disease 22

I

ibuprofen 243
ice packs 150, 206, 293
ICP *see* intermittent catheterization program
idiopathic, defined 89
ILU *see* independent living unit
immunotherapy 170-71
impaction, defined 34
incentive spirometer, described 34
incontinence 31, 34, 100
 see also bladder function

independent living 356-57, 474
independent living unit (ILU) 34
infections 196, 248
injection therapy 70, 78, 162, 192, 206, 247
The Institute for Rehabilitation and Research (TIRR) 334, 497
insurance reimbursements 65
ankylosing spondylitis 152-53
chiropractic 289
intermittent catheterization program (ICP) 34
International Chiropractors Association 11n, 283n, 286, 291n
International Spinal Research Trust 434
internet addresses
ABLEDATA 485
American Chiropractic Association 287n, 297n
American Paralysis Association 419
Chiropractic OnLine Today 305n
internists 49
interstitial chemotherapy 169
intervertebral disks 5, 8, 306
intervertebral foramena 35, 39
intradural tumors 161
intramedullary tumors 161
intrinsic muscle atrophy 56
inversion therapy 68
iritis 138
iron supplements 151
ischemia 59
ischemic vertebrae 55
ischiatica 73
ischium 138
isometric exercises 280
isotretinoin (Accutane) 59

J

Jackson, Tom 359
Jarvis, Kelly B., DC 302
jaw pain 16
Jayson, M. 72
The Johns Hopkins Medical Letter After 50 103n

joint dysfunction, defined 306
joints 7, 11, 306
pain 335
and soft tissue injuries 235
spinal disease 58, 95, *135,* 137, 138
stiffness and posture 13
Journal of American Health Policy 304
Journal of Bone and Joint Surgery 259
Journal of Family Practice 302
Journal of Health, Physical Education, Recreation and Dance 28
Journal of Manipulative and Physiological Therapeutics 302
Journal of Occupational Medicine 27, 302

K

Kahanovitz, N. 268, 274
Kahanovitz, Neil, MD 244, 245, 250, 256
Kane, W. J. 269-72, 274
Kapandji, I. A. 241
Karwasky, R. J. 25, 27
Kary, M. 28
Katz, Jeffrey, MD 100-102
Katznelson, A. 274
Kegel exercises 382-83
keratin sulphate 240
Kessler Institute for Rehabilitation 336, 493
ketorolac tromethamine (Toradol) 192
Khalil, M. A. 269, 274
kidney disease 105
kidneys 40
King, A. 66
Kirkaldy-Willis, W., MD 303
Kleitman, Naomi, MD 435
knee pain 293
Kostuik, J. 72
Kraus, H. 22, 28
KTP *see* potassium titanyl phosphate
Kuo, P. P. 83
Kushner, Harold S. 344
kyphosis 123, 265

L

Lakein, Alan 352, 370
laminaplasty, defined 35
laminectomy 50-51, 67, 71, 97, 239, 247, 248
  alternatives 52
  defined 35
  spinal stenosis 100-101
Langford, K. 84
laser surgery 165, 206, 239-41
  KTP laser 240
Laslett, M. 72
lateral stenosis 10
Laws, Edward R., Jr., MD 50-51
LBP *see* low back pain
legal rights 363-69
leg length 63, 207
leg pain 73, 74, 201, 293
lesions 63, 77, 294
lethargy 293
leukemia 105
Levi-Montalcini, Rita 416
Levin, John 256
Levy, S. 28
licensed practical nurse (LPN) 35
Liehman, W. P. 27, 28
life expectancy, spinal injuries 314-15, 319, 404, 421-22
life style changes 224-27
  see also activities of daily living; sedentary life styles
lifting 224, 244
  acute low back pain 208
  posture 18
ligaments 8, *9*, 22, 239, 292, 323
  anchors 7
  posterior longitudinal 74
  posture 11
  sprains 46
  stretched 56
  vertebrae 7, 59
ligamentum flavum 60
Lindahl, Olov 395, 400
Lipson, S. 72
Loh, Z. C. 83
lomustine drugs 167
Long, D. M. 400

lordotic curve 22
  see also lumbar lordosis
Love, Anthony 401
Low Back Pain 3n
low back pain 244, 521
  acute 55-72, 74, 195-218
  chronic 55-72
  motion and progress 219-29
  physical fitness 19-27
  posture 16
  spinal stenosis 100
  surgery 47, 50, 51, 71, 73
  whiplash 293
  see also back pain
Low Back Pain Syndrome 28
lower extremity, defined 33
lower motor neurons (LMN) 326-27, 328-32, 423
LPN *see* licensed practical nurse
lumbar, defined 35, 306
lumbar lordosis 55, 56, 63, 66, 75
lumbar muscles 19, 20, 56, 160
  flexibility 27
lumbar nerves 78
lumbar roll 276
lumbarsacral region 22
lumbar spondylosis 58
lumbar vertebrae 3, *5*, 6-7, 7, 133, 239, 312, 324
lumbosacral strain 46, 49
lumbosacral supports 67
lung capacity 16, 35, 38
Lyons, J. P. 26, 28

M

MacCornack, Frederick A., Ph.D. 301
Maddox, S. 483, 489
Maddox, Sam 433
magnetic resonance imaging (MRI) 50, 65, 96, 162-63, 211, 246, 268, 501
  defined 35
  dynamic 129
  neck pain 280
  sciatica 76-77
  syringomyelia 126, 127
mainstreaming 87

male fertility 432, 501
male genitalia 374-75, 377, 386-87
malignant, defined 155
malignant tumors 155-56, 176-77
Manga Report 300
manipulation 190, 191, 287-90, 298, 301
  defined 306-7
  low back pain 68-69, 206
  sciatica 79
  see also chiropractors
manual therapy, described 307
March of Dimes Birth Defects Foundation 88, 132
Marsh, H. O. 82
Martin, D. C. 78, 83
massage therapy 69, 150, 206, 287, 307
mattresses 53, 123-24
maximal oxygen consumption (VO$_2$max) 25
Mayo Clinic Health Letter 185n
McCay, M. 352, 369
McKenzie, R. 68, 72
McKenzie, Robin 276
McKenzie extension exercise 227
McKinley, William O., MD 407, 410
McLone, D. 87
MD *see* doctor of medicine; physicians
Meade, T. W., MD 303
medical history
  acute low back pain 197-98
  defined 35
Medicare 446, 450
medication, defined 35
Medicine and Science in Sports and Exercise 28
Medletter Associates, Inc. 3n
medullablastomas 177
medullar vessels, defined 35
medulloepitheliomas 177
Melkerson, Mark N. 92-93, 264
meningiomas 176
meningitis 126
meningocele 85, 86
Meredith, R. L. 400
metastatic tumors 157, 158, 174
methadone 393

methylprednisolone 167, 313, 408, 428-29
metronidazole 169
Miacalcin 117
Miami Project to Cure Paralysis (MPCP) 433, 434, 435, 500, 504, 508
microsurgery 165
migraine 191
military posture 15
Miller, Marc 403-4
Minkel, Jean 475
misonidazole 169
Missouri Arthritis Rehabilitation Research and Training Center (MARRTC) 515-16
Mitchell, W. 359
mobility
  air travel 456, 462-63
  osteoporosis 121
  spina bifida 87
  spinal cord injury 311
  see also wheelchairs
mobilization therapy 287
Model Regional Spinal Cord Injury Care System 320-22, 505-6
Modern Medicine 55n, 239n, 240
Modic, M. T. 82
monoclonal antibodies 171
Mooney, T. 387
Morris, Elliot K. 302
Morris, J. 84
motorcycle accidents 25
motor function examinations 233
motor neurons 325-32, 377, 423
motor problems 159, 160, 313
Mrganit, B. 269, 274
MRI *see* magnetic resonance imaging
multiple sclerosis 77, 235, 420
Munzner, Robert F., Ph.D. 407
muscle contractions 185-87
muscle performance examinations 233
muscle relaxants 47, 70, 220
muscles 22
  anchors 7
  bone mass 112
  posture 11, 12
  see also *individual muscles*

muscle stimulators 336, 406
muscle strength 52, 112, 116, 199
  exercises 20
  low back pain 26
muscle tightness 27
muscular endurance 20, 26, 207-8
myelin sheath 422
myelography 50, 65, 127, 163, 211
  defined 36
  sciatica 76-77
myelomeningocele 85, 86, 87
myelopathy 36, 182, 391
myths and sexuality 372-74

N

NA *see* nursing assistant
Nachemson, A. L. 25, 27, 66, 72
Nachemson, Alf, MD 49
naproxen sodium (Anaprox DS) 192
narcotics
  low back pain 70, 71
  sciatica 80
NARIC *see* National Rehabilitation
  Information Center
Nashold, B. S., Jr. 400
National Academy of Sciences 106
National Arthritis and Musculoskel-
  etal and Skin Diseases Information
  Clearinghouse 516
National Board of Chiropractic Ex-
  aminers 299n
National Brain Tumor Foundation 179
National Center for Education in Ma-
  ternal and Child Health 88
National Chronic Pain Outreach As-
  sociation, Inc. 130
National Easter Seal Society 88
National Handicapped Sports 480
National Information Center for Chil-
  dren and Youth with Disabilities 85n
National Institute for Occupational
  Safety and Health 225
National Institute of Arthritis and
  Musculoskeletal and Skin Diseases
  29n, 95n, 181n, 511n
National Institute of Mental Health
  173

National Institute of Neurological
  Disorders and Stroke (NINDS) 128,
  129, 171, 173, 177, 407, 408, 434
National Institute on Disability and
  Rehabilitation Research (NIDRR)
  473n, 484, 504-5, 513n, 521
National Institutes of Health (NIH)
  49, 51, 173, 507
  Combined Health Information Da-
    tabase (CHID) 514, 516
  Consensus Development Confer-
    ence on Osteoporosis 106-7
National Organization for Rare Disorders (NORD) 132
National Osteoporosis Foundation
  103n
National Rehabilitation Information
  Center (NARIC) 88, 479, 487n, 489,
  494, 497, 505
National Scoliosis Foundation, Inc.
  92, 94, 517
National Spasmodic Torticollis Association 187
National Spinal Cord Injury Association (NSCIA) 131, 311n, 316, 411,
  421n, 434, 436, 484, 490, 501, 504,
  508
nausea 159, 191, 392
neck exercises 275, 277-79
neck pain 181-84, 275-80
neodymium:yttrium aluminum garnet 240
neoplasms, defined 155
Nepomuceno, C. 400
Nerubay, J. 269, 274
nerve blocks 394-95, 396
nerve cell replacement 426
nerve compression 74-76, 100
nerve growth factor 416, 424, 425, 427
nerve impairment 211, 295
nerve injury 235
nerve interference 16
nerve root compromise 57, 59, 196,
  198, *200,* 214
nerves
  defined 307
  inflamed 73
  regeneration 406, 426-27
  see also spinal nerves

nervous system, described 307, 312
Neuman, B. P. 269, 274
neural foramina 60
neural grafts 409, 434
neuritis 59, 295
neuroblastomas 177
neurofibromatosis 156, 173
neurogenic, defined 36
neurogenic claudication 60-61, 78, 216
neuroglial cells 426, 427
neurologic conditions 235, 317-18
neurologic examinations 63-64, 75, 183, 190, 199, 210
neurologists 49
neuromotor development examinations 234
neuromuscular exercise 20, 27
neurons 325-32, 377, 422
neurosurgeons 49, 50, 52, 129, 245
New Zealand Commission report 300-301
noncommunicating syringomyelia 126
nonsteroidal anti-inflammatory drugs (NSAID) 69, 97, 100, 151, 183, 192, 220
Novation, Inc. 334
nucleus pulposus 8, 10, 56, 57, 58, 80, 213, 239, 240
nurses 504
   see also licensed practical nurse; registered nurse
nursing assistant (NA) 36
nutrition
   ankylosing spondylitis 151
   bones 104
   chronic pain 395
   defined 36
   degenerative back disease 97
   osteoporosis 106-8, 119
   pregnancy 129
Nyiendo, Joanne, Ph.D. 302

O

obesity 46, 224
   see also weight factor
occipital cephalgia 189, 190-92
occupational therapy, defined 36

occupations
   acute low back pain 208
   back strain 46
   neck pain 182
   spinal injuries 318, 359-60
   stiff neck 189-92
O'Connor, S. M. 83
Office of Cancer Communications 178
Office of Scientific and Health Reports 130
ogliodendrocytes 427
O'Hara, Jim 260
oligodendrogliomas 175
omentum transposition 431, 433
oncogenes 171
Onifer, S. M. 435
Onik, G. 241
Onofrio, B. 66
oral, defined 36
Oregon Workers' Compensation Study 302
organizations
   spinal cord injury 500-503
   sports activities 498-99
Orlock, Carol 102
Orme, T. J. 274
orthopedic conditions 235
orthopedic shoes 37
orthopedists 49, 52, 90, 245
orthosis, defined 36
osseous protrusion, defined 36
ossification 59
osteoarthritis 13, 39, 48, 307
osteoblasts 104, 105
osteoclasts 120
osteogenesis 273
osteoid matrix 104
Osteomark urine test 120
osteopaths 49, 283
osteophytes 9, 59, 60, 216
   defined 36
osteoporosis 10, 48, 49, 50, 96, 103-24
   ankylosing spondylitis 151
Osteoporosis and Related Bone Diseases - National Resource Center 103n
OT see occupational therapy
Ouellette, E. A. 84
Overmyer, Robert H. 241

P

Paget's bone disease 110, 117
pain
  ankylosing spondylitis 137, 141
  arthritis 64
  crossover 202
  mechanical 64
  peripheral 395, 399
  poor posture 12-13
  radicular 58, 59, *61*, 73, 247
  referred 48-49, 58-59, 64, 73, 295
  sciatica 82
  sclerotomal distribution *60*
  surgery 97
  syringomyelia 127
  tumors 160
  see also back pain; low back pain
pain behaviors 202
pain management 335
Palmer, Richard 400
Papazian, Ruth 110
para *see* paraplegic
paralysis 38, 246, *405*, 488
  defined 37
  genital function 373, 410
  see also functional electrical stimulation
Paralyzed Veterans of America 29n, 37, 131, 323n, 337, 339, 341n, 371n, 401, 434, 484, 487n, 490, 492, 496, 497, 501, 508
paraparesis, defined 37
paraplegia 312-13, 318, 391, 396
paraplegic, defined 37, 312
parasympathetic nervous system 312
parathyroid hormones 104
paresthesia 74
Parkinson's disease 235
pars interarticularis 61
Patient Care 189n, 190, 219n
Patient Disability Comparison 302
Pay, N. T. 82
Pearce, J. M. 82
Pearson, Jeffrey K., DO 192
Peck, Connie 401
pedicle screws 253-66
Pedinoff, Seymour, DO 229

pelvic abscess 77
pelvic bones 7
pelvic tilt 63
pelvis 22, 26, 56, 133
peptic ulcers 48
Perdue, Gloria 253
periosteum 74
peripheral nervous system 312, 413, 423
Perr, A. 478
personal care 482, 492
personality, defined 37
PET *see* positron emission tomography
phenylbutazone 205
Philips, L. 483, 490
Phillips, Reed B., DC 302
photodynamic therapy 172
photon absorptiometry 106
photosensitivity 191
physical activity 111-14
Physical Activity and Fitness Research Digest 19n, 103n
physical appearance 17
physical examinations 141, 196, 198
physical fitness 19-27
physical therapists 236-37
physical therapy (PT) 190, 192
  ankylosing spondylitis 140, 144-45
  defined 38
  general information 231-37
  neck pain 183
  osteoporosis 123
  sciatica 78
physical working capacity 25
The Physician and Sportsmedicine 73n
physicians 49
  chronic pain 392
  patient emotional state 250
  sciatica 74-75, 78
  tumors 167-68
physiological mapping 172, 210
physiotherapy, defined 37
Pinals, Robert S., MD 229
pineal tumors 176
pineoblastomas 177
Pitchen, I. 28
pituitary tumors 176

Plowman, Sharon Ann 19n, 22-23, 25-27, 28

PNET *see* primitive neuroectodermal tumors

polar spongioblastomas 177

polio 311, 517, 520

poor posture
 back pain 46
 proper alignment 15
 reasons 12
 spinal stenosis 100

Porter, Kent 400

Porter, R. W. 23, 28

positron emission tomography (PET) 162, 171-72

postural evaluation 18

posture
 ankylosing spondylitis 139-40, 141, 142-43, 145
 back pain 46
 exercises 48
 guide 11-18
 importance 52
 neck pain 275-76, 296
 neck problems 184
 scoliosis 90
 self-tests 13

Potash, W. J. 512

potassium titanyl phosphate (KTP) 240

prednisone 167

pregnancy
 ankylosing spondylitis 149-50
 hyperlordosis 56
 nutrition 129
 spinal cord injury 373, 379

President's Council on Physical Fitness and Sports 19n

pressure reliefs, defined 37

pressure sores 335, 476, 494

primary care, defined 37

primary tumors 156, 157

primitive neuroectodermal tumors (PNET) 176-77

progestin 108

Progress in Research 413n

Prokop, Charles K. 401

prone, defined 37

prostaglandins 104

prostate problems 48

prosthesis, defined 37

prosthetic appliances 37, 387

pseudoarthritis 267, *268,* 270

pseudoclaudication 216

psoas abscess 77

psoriasis 139

psychoactive analgesics 70

psychogenic erections 377

psychological, defined 38

psychological pain 49, 245

psychosocial, defined 399

psychosocial factors
 low back pain 70-71
 sciatica 76, 80
 spinal cord injury 341-69, 397-98

PT *see* physical therapy

Public Health Service 20, 22, 28

pulmonary, defined 38

pulmonary disease 101

PVA *see* Paralyzed Veterans of America

PWC *see* physical working capacity

Q

quad *see* quadriplegic

quadriparesis, defined 38

quadriplegia 312, 392, 406, 488

quadriplegic, defined 38, 312

quantitative computed tomography 118-19

The Quest for Cure 339

Quon, J. A. 83

R

Raab, W. 22, 28

Rabin, Barry J. 387

race factor
 osteoporosis 119
 spinal injuries 317

radiation therapy 166, 169, 174, 177

radiculopathy 63, 64, 69, 71, 78, 182, 191, 206
 defined 38

radiology 64-65, 106, 270-72

radiosensitizers 169

Radwanski, Maria 401
Raisman, Geoffrey 416
Ramón y Cajal, Santiago 415
RAND study 300
range of motion (ROM)
  acute low back pain 199
  defined 38, 307
  exercises 31, 227, 397
Rapoff, Michael 400
Recommended Dietary Allowances
  (RDA)
  calcium 106-7
reflexes 161, 332
  tests 198, 199-200
reflexogenic erections 377-78
regeneration, spinal cord 421, 423-28
registered nurse (RN) 38
rehab *see* rehabilitation
rehabilitation
  chronic pain 392
  defined 38
  low back pain 219
  sexuality 372
  spinal injuries 315, 332, 350
  see also therapies; treatment
Rehabilitation Act (1973) 87
Rehabilitation Research & Training
  Centers (RTC) 337, 506-7
Reigel, D. H. 87
relaxation training 341, 350-51
remodeling of bones 104, 114
reproduction 373, 432
The Research and Training Center on
  Independent Living 389n, 401
residual, defined 38
RESNA 496, 503
Resources for Rehabilitation 518-19
respiratory, defined 38
respiratory examinations 234
respiratory problems 96
respiratory therapy (RT), defined 38
retroverted uterus 48
rheumatologists 49, 100, 513
Richards, J. S. 400
Richardson, H. D. 274
RN *see* registered nurse
roentgenograms 268
ROM *see* range of motion
Ross, J. S. 82

rotary torque 57
Roth, E. 400
Rothman, R. H. 83, 268, 273
Rounds, Martha 492
Rowley-Kelly, F. L. 87
Roy, S. H. 26, 28
RT *see* respiratory therapy
ruptured disks 47, 50, 52, 247
  defined 34
  see also herniated disks
Russell, G. S. 511

S

Saal, J. A. 79, 83
Saal, J. S. 79, 83
Sack, Burton, MD 72
sacral, defined 38, 325
sacroiliac joints 3, 48, 133, *135,* 137
sacrum 3, 7, 133, *135*
Sadao, K. 66
saddle anesthesia 31
Samuels, Todd L., MD 47
Saskatchewan Clinical Research 303
Saskatchewan University Study
  (1985) 304
scapula 29
scars 424
Schifrin, L. G., Ph.D. 303
schools
  scoliosis 90
  spina bifida 87
Schroeder, Marie A. 407
Schwab, Martin E., Ph.D. 415, 416,
  417, 418
Schwann, Theodor 415
Schwann cells 426-27
schwannomas 177
Schwartz, John 260
Schwartz, S. Andrew, MD 229
SCI *see* spinal cord injury
sciatica *9,* 47, 71, 73-82, 96, 196, 210,
  214, 244
  defined 39
sciatic nerve 77, 198, 247
sciatic notch 78
sciatic pain 51
  see also back pain; low back pain

sciatic tension tests 201-2
sclerotomes 73
scoliosis 48, 89-94, 96, 262, 265, 271-72
  causes 62
The Scoliosis Association, Inc. 94
Scoliosis Research Society 90, 92, 94
Seater, Stephen R. 298
seating systems 476
sedentary lifestyles 46, 105, 119
seizures 158-59
Selby, David 246, 247, 249
self image 12
Seljeskog, E. S. 87
sensation 39, 161
sensory evoked potentials (SEP) 211
sensory examinations 200, 234
sensory messages to brain 7, 10
sensory problems 160
SEP *see* sensory evoked potentials
serotonin 70
service animals 468
sexual functioning
  after spinal cord injuries 315, 335-36, 363, 371-87, 393, 493
  in spondylitis 149
Sharpe, G. L. 27, 28
Shiu, S. 66
shoe lifts 207
shoulder pain 291, 294-96
shunts 165, 391
sidebend exercise 278
side effects
  amitriptyline 298
  carbamazepine 392
  defined 39
  drug therapy 167
  isotretinoin 59
Silvers, H. R. 84
single photon absorptiometry 118
Siris, Ethel S., MD 118
sitting knee extension test *202*
sit-ups 20
sleeping habits
  back pain 46
  neck pain 276
slipped disks 10, 46-47, 50, 136
  see also herniated disk
Sliwa, J. 400

slumped posture 15
Smith, Manual J. 370
smoker's robot, defined 39
smoking *see* tobacco
Snodgrass, L. B. 27, 28
Snyder-Mackler, L. 26, 28
social rights 363-69
Social Security disability insurance 437-50
social survival tactics 357-63
sodium flouride 110
somatization 71
spasmodic torticollis 185-87, 294-95
spasms 46, 67, 150, 181
  defined 39
  sciatica 75
spasticity 332, 335, 384, 391, 396, 432, 494
  defined 39
Spence, W. R. 511
Spengler, D. M. 25, 27, 83, 84
Spengler, Dan M., MD 229
spina bifida 85-87, 311, 519-20
Spina Bifida Association of America 88, 131, 519-20
spina bifida occulta 85, 86
spinal canal 8, 60, 95
spinal column 156, 181, 307, 324, 404
  diseases 85
spinal cord *6, 7,* 181, 307, 311-12, 422
  cysts 125
  described 323, 325-27, 404
  nerves *9*
  tumors 155-79, 265
Spinal Cord Injury Network International (SCINI) 501
spinal cord injury (SCI) 93, 128, 295, 403-11
  air travel 451-71
  causes 311-20
  chronic pain management 389-401
  defined 39
  general information 323-39, 413-19, 421-36, 489-508
  psychosocial adjustments 341-69
  technology 473-85
Spinal Cord Society 131, 502, 508
spinal cord tethering 391

spinal degeneration 95-97
spinal diseases 69, 311
spinal disks 7-8
  degeneration 9, 47-48, 58
  see also disks
spinal flexion 78
spinal fractures 49-50, 196, 262
  see also spinal cord injury
spinal fusion 51, 71, 249, 265, 267-73
  scoliosis 92
spinal infections 48-49, 100
spinal joints 48
spinal nerves 6, 7, 8, 10, 39, 47, 96,
  325-28, 404, 422
  quantity 8
  see also nerves
Spinal Network 520
spinal osteophytosis 59
spinal shock 332
spinal stenosis 8, 9-10, 51, 52, 60-61,
  78, 95, 99-102, 214-16, 246-47
  diagnosis 62
Spine 27, 28
spine 38, 134
  architecture 5-7, 323-24, 325
  curvature 55, 89
  described 3-8, 99-100, 133
  low back pain 25-26
  movement 8
  parts 4
  posture 16, 17
  stresses within 22, 46
  three-joint complex 55
spine immobilizers, defined 39
spine stabilization 39, 261
spinous (thorn-like) processes 8
splint, defined 39
spondylitis 95, 133
  see also ankylosing spondylitis
Spondylitis Association of America
  133n, 153
spondylolisthesis 39, 61-62, 77, 243,
  247, 262, 265, 307
spondylosis 39, 58, 77
Sportelli, Louis 250
sports activities
  ankylosing spondylitis 144
  assistive devices 480
  bone mass 111-13

sports activities, continued
  resources 498-99
  spinal cord injury 410
  warming up 52
sports injuries 25, 236, 317
  back pain 46
  posture 15-16
  whiplash 291
sports medicine 226
Sports 'n Spokes 480-81, 495, 501, 504
sprains 46
SSI see Supplemental Security Income
standing aids 481
Stano, Miron, Ph.D. 302
Stano Cost Comparison Study 302-3
statistics
  back pain 45
  chiropractic 283
  low back pain 55, 195, 219
  malpractice 285, 290
  physical therapy 231
  spina bifida 86
  spinal cord injury (SCI) 311-20
  tumors 157-58
Steffee, Arthur, MD 254, 257
Steinkopff, Glen 253
Steinmann, J. C. 267, 273
stenosis 39-40, 95
  see also spinal stenosis
stereotactic procedures 165
steroids 69-70, 313, 408
stiff neck 189-92
stiffness 48
stones, defined 40
straight leg raising (SLR) test 63, 64,
  75, 80, 201, 202, 227
  contralateral 76
strain injuries 292
stress 46, 71, 223-24
stress fractures 77
stress management 341
stretching exercises 97
stroke 235, 517
studies
  aging 507
  back pain psychology 250
  chiropractic 284-85, 288, 299-304
  chronic pain 389
  exercise intervention 113-14

studies, continued
  low back pain 23-27, 210-13
  manipulation 287-88
  osteoporosis 107, 108, 110, 115
  sciatica 78, 79
  scoliosis 271-72
  spinal cord injury 409, 429
  spinal fusion 268
  spinal stenosis 101-2
stump socks 37
sublaxation 40, 192, 284, 292, 306
suctioning, defined 40
Summers, Jay 400
Supplemental Security Income (SSI)
  437, 448-49
support system, defined 40
surgery 97
  ankylosing spondylitis 145, 153
  back 243-51
  brain tumors 156
  cervical spine disorders 183-84
  low back pain 71, 213-14
  sciatica 73, 79-81
  scoliosis 92-93
  shunting 86
  slipped disks 47
  spasmodic torticollis 186
  spinal cord injury 430-31
  spinal fusion 51, 71
  spinal nerves 50
  spinal stenosis 100-101, 216
  syringomyelia 127-28
  tumors 164-66
sway back *see* hyperlordosis
Sweeney, Beverly 243
swelling, defined 32
Swezey, A. M. 512
Swezey, R. 72
Swezey, R. L. 512
Sygen 313, 433
sympathetic nervous system 312
symptoms
  acute low back pain 196, 198, *205*
  ankylosing spondylitis 137-38
  cervical spine disorders 182
  defined 308
  degenerative back problems 96
  occipital cephalgia 190-91
  sciatica 74, 80

symptoms, continued
  syringomyelia 125, 126
  tension neck syndrome 189-90
  tumors 158-61
synapses 422-23, 424
synovitis 69-70
Synthes (U.S.A.) 256
syringomyelia 125-29
syrinx 125, 126, 127
  see also cysts
systemic arthritis 64
systemic diseases 236

T

tailbone 3, 38
  see also coccyx
Taylor, Frances 179
technology
  spinal cord injury 473-85
  tumors 157
television
  assistive devices 479
  back pain 46
  neck pain 190
  posture 12
temporomandibular joint disease
  (TMJ) 16
tendons 8, *9,* 59, 292
tenodesis, defined 40
TENS *see* transcutaneous electric
  nerve stimulation
tension neck syndrome 189
testosterone 115
tetraplegia 317-18, 391
tetraplegic, defined 38, 399
therapeutic recreation specialist
  (TRS), defined 40
therapies
  defined 40
  hormone replacement 108
  humor 346
  low back pain 66-70
  spinal cord injury 413-19
  tumors 166-67
  see also treatment
thermal therapy 67
Thermophores 150

Thiel, Haymo, DC 303
thigh joints 22
thigh muscles 52
thigh pain 73
Third International Symposium on
  Osteoporosis 106, 108
Thomas, P. C. 25, 27
thoracic, defined 40, 308
thoracic vertebrae 3, *5*, 133, 160, 312,
  324
  size 6
thrombus, defined 40
thyroid hormones 104
time management 341, 351-56
tipped uterus 48
tirilizade mesylate (Freedox) 429
TMJ *see* temporomandibular joint
  disease
TNS *see* transcutaneous electric
  nerve stimulation
tobacco 52, 156, 224
  osteoporosis 48, 105, 119
tomography *see* computerized axial
  tomography; positron emission
  tomography
Toradol 192
torticollis *see* spasmodic torticollis
Tourtellotte, Wallace W., MD 173
Toyoi, O. 66
trabecular bone 105, 268
traction 68, 78, 192, 206, 222
training principles *114*
transcutaneous electric nerve stimulation (TENS) 67, 78, 150, 206, 222,
  393-94, 399
trauma 126, 146, 216, 265, 293, 311
traumatic brain injury 235
Travis, John 435
treadmill tests 25
treatment
  acute low back pain 195-218, *209*
  ankylosing spondylitis 140-45
  cervical spine disorders 183-84
  chronic pain 390, 391-98
  degenerative back problems 97
  lumbosacral strain 49
  occipital cephalgia 190-92
  osteoporosis 117-18, 120, 122-24
  sciatica 78-79

treatment, continued
  scoliosis 90-993
  spasmodic torticollis 186-87
  spinal cord injury 403-11, 408-11,
    421-36
  spinal stenosis 100-101
  syringomyelia 127-28
  tension neck syndrome 190-92
  tumors 164-68
  whiplash 293
  see also therapies
Treat Your Own Neck (McKenzie)
  276
tricyclics 70, 297
trigger point injections 70, 78, 192
trochanters 56
TRS *see* therapeutic recreation specialist
trunk exercises 20, 79, 228
trunk extensor endurance 26
trunk muscles 52, 313
tuberous sclerosis 156, 173
tumors 196, 199

U

Ullian, Arthur D. 414
Uloka, G. 66
ultrasonic aspirators 165
ultrasound therapy 78, 171, 206
underwater weighting studies 26
United Cerebral Palsy Associations,
  Inc. 484
upper extremity, defined 33
upper motor neurons (UMN) 325-27,
  328-32, 377
urinalysis 40, 211
urinary system, described 40
urinary tract
  infections 335
  spinal injuries 319-20, 383-84
  stones 40
  see also bladder
Utah Workers' Compensation Study
  302

V

VA *see* Department of Veterans Affairs
Varghese, George 400
vasa nervorum 59
vascular claudication 60-61, 216
vascular tumors 177
venous obstruction 59, 60
ventilation examinations 234
ventilators 41, 312, 313, 462
Vermont Rehabilitation Engineering Research Center in Low Back Pain 521
vertebrae 49-50, 292, 308, 311-12
  cervical 181
  diseases 85, 137
  number codes 3
  periosteum 74
  quantity 3, 8, 22, 133, 324
vertebrae alignment 26, 39
vertebral compression 8-9, 10
vertebral fractures 121, 181
vertebral laminae 97
  see also laminectomy
veterans 37, 323n
  benefits, described 32-33
vibration 225
videos 481, 492, 512
Virginia Comparative Study 303-4
vision problems 138, 159, 392, 456
  posture 12, 14
vitamin C 151
vitamin D 104, 107, 122
vocational, defined 41
vocational rehabilitation, defined 41
vocational rehabilitation specialist (VRS), defined 41
voc rehab *see* vocational rehabilitation
void, defined 41
Volvo automobile seat 49
VO$_2$max 25
Von Hippel-Lindau disease 177
VRS *see* vocational rehabilitation specialist

W

Wagner, Edward 254-55, 256, 257, 258
walkers 476
Walsh, N. E. 78, 83
Walter, O. P. 83
Washington HMO Study 301-2
Washington Post 29n, 243n, 253n
Watkins, M. B. 273
Weber, H. 79, 83
Weigel, M. C. 269, 274
weight factors 52
  ankylosing spondylitis 151
  low back pain 26
  posture 12, 13
Weinreb, J. C. 82
Weiser, Benjamin 260
Werder, Richard 259
Wetta, W. J. 273
Wheelchair Motorcycle Association, Inc. 522
wheelchairs 37, 314, 337, 357, 404, 406, 410
  air travel 455, 463-64
  carriers 478
  information 474, 475-76, 494-96, 507
  sexual functions 381
  spina bifida 87
  swimming 520-21
whiplash 181, 291-96
White, Arthur, MD 245-46, 249, 250, 251
White, Mary C. 401
white blood cells 136, 139, 149
Whitmore, Kristene, MD 491
Whittemore, S. R. 435
Wickham, G. G. 269, 274
Wiesel, S. 72
Wiesel, Sam 246
Wight, J. S., DC 303
Wight Study on Recurring Headaches 303
Wilk, Chester A. 286
Williams flexion exercise 227
Wilson, A. Bennett 476
Wise, T. N. 400
Withers, Lyonne 244

Wolbarsht, L. B. 82
Wolk, Steve, Ph.D. 301
women
  ankylosing spondylitis 138, 149
  genitalia 376-77, 379-80
  hyperlordosis 66
  osteoporosis 48, 96, 103, 104-6, 114
  spinal stenosis 101-2
workplace injuries 236
work space design
  posture 12, 14, 17
  spinal injuries 315, 482
  see also ergonomic issues
Wortley, M. D. 25, 27
WT/HT² 26

X

X-rays 31, 49-50, 52, 64-65, 96, 127, 210
  neck pain 280

X-rays, continued
  sciatica 76
  scoliosis 90, 93-94
  tumors 161-63
Xu, X. M. 435

Y

Yahiro, Martin, MD 90-93
Yarkony, G. 400
Yasuma, T. 66
Young, Wise, MD 408, 417, 503
Yuri, H. 241

Z

Zamula, Evelyn 53
Zeh, J. 25, 27
Zunin, Leonard 370
Zunin, Natalie 370